Moritz Meyer, William Alexander Hammond

ELECTRICITY in its RELATIONS to PRACTICAL MEDICINE

Moritz Meyer, William Alexander Hammond

ELECTRICITY in its RELATIONS to PRACTICAL MEDICINE

ISBN/EAN: 9783741122422

Manufactured in Europe, USA, Canada, Australia, Japa

Cover: Foto ©Lupo / pixelio.de

Manufactured and distributed by brebook publishing software (www.brebook.com)

Moritz Meyer, William Alexander Hammond

ELECTRICITY in its RELATIONS to PRACTICAL MEDICINE

ELECTRICITY

IN ITS

RELATIONS TO PRACTICAL MEDICINE.

BY
DR. MORITZ MEYER,
ROYAL COUNSELLOR OF HEALTH, ETC.

*SECOND REVISED AND CORRECTED AMERICAN EDITION.
TRANSLATED FROM THE THIRD GERMAN EDITION,
WITH NOTES AND ADDITIONS,*

BY
WILLIAM A. HAMMOND, M. D.,
PROFESSOR OF DISEASES OF THE MIND AND NERVOUS SYSTEM, AND OF CLINICAL MEDICINE,
IN THE BELLEVUE HOSPITAL MEDICAL COLLEGE; PHYSICIAN-IN-CHIEF TO THE NEW
YORK STATE HOSPITAL FOR DISEASES OF THE NERVOUS SYSTEM, ETC.

NEW YORK:
D. APPLETON AND COMPANY,
549 & 551 BROADWAY.
1872.

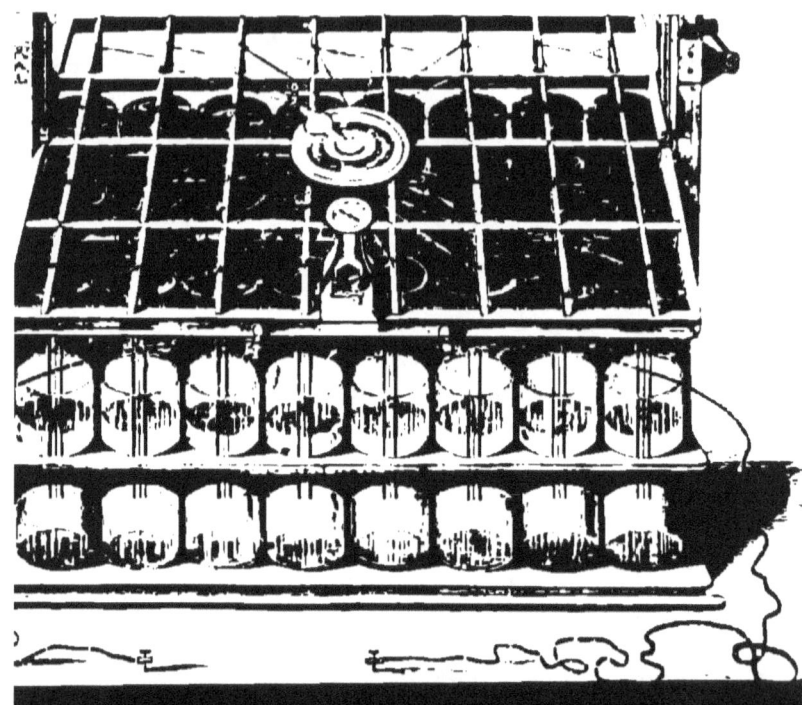

Electricity in its relations to practical medicine

Moritz Meyer, William Alexander Hammond

TO

THE PRIVY COUNSELLOR AND PROFESSOR,

DR. MORITZ HEINRICH ROMBERG,

KNIGHT, ETC., ETC.,

IN HONOR OF THE

FIFTIETH ANNIVERSARY OF HIS DOCTORATE,

AND AS AN EVIDENCE

OF THE

HIGH REGARD AND GRATITUDE

OF THE

AUTHOR.

PREFACE TO THE SECOND AMERICAN EDITION.

THE demand for a second edition of my translation of Dr. Meyer's excellent treatise, has enabled me to make several corrections in the typography, and to call attention to certain improved forms of electrical apparatus for medical use.

WILLIAM A. HAMMOND.

162 WEST 84TH ST., NEW YORK, *September* 20, 1871.

PREFACE TO THE FIRST AMERICAN EDITION.

The belief that Dr. Moritz Meyer's Treatise on Electricity in its Relations to Practical Medicine was the best which had yet appeared on the subject, must be my excuse for presenting it in an English dress to the Medical Profession of America and Great Britain.

I had intended adding largely to it, but attentive perusal convinced me that, by so doing, I would only enlarge the volume, without giving it a corresponding increase in value. I have, therefore, refrained from the citation of cases from my own practice, except in a few instances; or from adding much other matter, except under the head of Infantile Paralysis, which subject, it appeared to me, had not been sufficiently considered by the author.

PREFACE TO THE THIRD GERMAN EDITION.

FROM the publication of the second edition of this book to the present time, has proved to be another important period in the history of electro-therapeutics. The great event has been the reception of the constant current into medical practice generally. True, the founder of this mode of treatment, Robert Remak, has, during this period, been taken from his place among the living, while valiantly contending for the correctness and the recognition of his theories. But his unexpected death and the involuntary termination of his brilliant labors led, perhaps, to a more candid examination of his assertions, and to an earlier acknowledgment of their correctness, than would have been the case had he lived. This intimation might be so construed as to mean, that either mental apathy, jealousy, or perversity, prompted the partisans of the intermitting current to oppose the constant current; this reproach, however, may be emphatically denied. It was not the constant current as such, but the manner in which Remak—especially at the beginning of his career as practitioner—denied that the interrupted current possessed any therapeutical value whatever, that made of natural allies unwilling opponents.

I hope that the present volume, while it recognizes, on the one hand, the superiority of the constant current in certain directions, on the other it aids the interrupted current to recover its full and well-founded rights, of which it has of late been deprived by a sort of distinguished and unmerited distrust, and that it advances the true object of therapeutics in securing to the greatest possible number of the afflicted either a radical cure, or, at least, some relief. Then, we must not forget that the interrupted current is to-day the common property of the profession, while the constant current will, perhaps, never come into so general use. At all events, it has thus far comparatively few advocates, and these are found only in the larger cities.

A retrospective glance at the progress made in electro-therapeutics, especially during the last few years, is in the highest degree encouraging. The possibility of the constant current acting on the brain or spinal marrow—which has been until late so generally doubted—the electrotonic action of the constant current on the living, the galvanic irritation of the sympathetic nerve, etc., have been stricken from the list of hypotheses, and elevated to places among scientific facts. In surgery, the electro-chemical action begins to attract more attention. It is now being used not only in cases of varices and aneurisms, but also in the treatment of strictures, tumors, etc. In regard to obstetrics, we would repeat the wish expressed on a former occasion—that more extended experiments may be made by our honored colleagues, especially by those who have charge of our public hospitals.

Dr. Moritz Meyer.

Berlin, *March* 29, 1868.

CONTENTS.

FIRST SECTION.

	PAGE
Historical Sketch of the Applications of Electricity in Medicine,	1

SECOND SECTION.

I. Friction Electricity,	9
II. Contact Electricity (Galvanism),	11
III. Induction Electricity (Faradism),	30

THIRD SECTION.

Of the Electro-Motor Properties of the Animal Body,	35

FOURTH SECTION.

The Action of the Electric Currents on the Organs and Tissues of the Animal Body, ... 44
   A. The Action of the Electric Current on the Nerves and Muscles, 44
      I. Action of the Current on Motor Nerves and Muscles, . 44
      II. The Effect of the Electric Current on the Nerves of Sense and the Sensory Nerves, ... 68
   B. The Influence of the Electric Current on the Brain and Spinal Marrow, ... 74
   C. The Influence of the Electric Current on the Sympathetic, 79
   D. The Effect of the Electric Current on the Organs furnished with Organic Muscular Fibres, ... 81
      I. Digestive Organs, ... 82
      II. Urinary and Sexual Organs, ... 84
      III. The Iris, ... 85
      IV. The Heart, ... 86

xii   CONTENTS.

	PAGE
E. The Effect of the Electric Current on the Blood-vessels and Lymphatics,	88
F. The Effect of the Electric Current on the Blood,	89
G. The Effect of the Electric Current on the Skin,	90
H. The Effect of the Electric Current on the Bones,	92
I. Accessory Effects of the Current,	92
Conclusions,	94

FIFTH SECTION.

I. Galvanic Apparatus,	97
II. Induction Apparatus,	113

SIXTH SECTION.

Methods of Using Interrupted and Constant Currents, . . . 139

SEVENTH SECTION.

Electricity in its Application to Anatomy, Physiology, and Pathology,   167

EIGHTH SECTION.

The Importance of Electricity in the Diagnosis and Prognosis of Paralytic Affections,	180
General Application,	180
I. Cerebral Paralysis,	192
Hysterical Paralysis,	203
II. Spinal Paralysis,	209
A. Paralysis arising from Injury to the Independent Motor Power of the Spinal Cord,	209
B. Paralysis caused by Interruption in the Conducting Power of the Spinal Cord,	243
III. Paralysis of the Sympathetic,	247
IV. Nervous Paralysis,	254
V. Muscular Paralysis,	267
A. Paralysis from the Poisonous Action of Lead,	281
B. Progressive Muscular Atrophy,	287

NINTH SECTION.

Electricity as a Curative Agent, ... 305

CHAPTER I.

The Use of Electricity in Medicine,	307
I. Electricity in Nervous Diseases,	307

	PAGE
A. Hyperæsthesia—Neuralgia,	307
B. Anæsthesia,	334
C. Spasms,	343
D. Paralyses,	372
Cerebral Paralysis,	376
Spinal Paralysis,	385
Locomotor Ataxia,	393
Nervous and Muscular Paralysis,	408
Rheumatic Paralysis of the Muscles of the Eye,	420
Traumatic Paralysis,	422
Secondary Paralysis,	424
Lead Paralysis,	427
Asphyxia,	429
Incontinence of Urine,	433
Laryngeal Paralysis,	435
II. Electricity in Diseases depending upon Anomalies of Secretion and Excretion,	439
A. Rheumatic Exudations,	439
B. Arthritic Articular Exudations,	447
C. Suppressed Secretions and Excretions,	449

CHAPTER II.

The Employment of Electricity in Midwifery and Gynecology,	452

CHAPTER III.

The Use of Electricity in Surgery,	460
I. Electricity for the Generation of Thermic Effects,	460
II. Electricity for Causing Chemical Effects,	467
A. Galvano-puncture in Varices and Aneurisms,	468
B. Electrolytical Treatment of Strictures, Exudations, Tumors, Ulcers, etc.,	474
C. The Galvanic Current for the Solution of Vesical Calculi,	487
D. Electricity for the Removal of Poisonous Metals from the Organism,	489
III. Electricity as a Stimulant in Pseudoarthrosis,	491
APPENDIX,	493
INDEX,	503

ELECTRICITY

IN ITS

RELATIONS TO PRACTICAL MEDICINE.

FIRST SECTION.

HISTORICAL SKETCH OF THE APPLICATIONS OF ELECTRICITY IN MEDICINE.

THE history of electro-therapeutics is the history of electricity. Every advance step in the field of the latter has been quickly followed by an endeavor, on the part of the medical profession, to turn the new discovery to practical account.

The history of electro-therapeutics may be divided into three periods. The first dates back some two thousand years into the dim past, beginning with our primitive knowledge of electricity, the electricity of the raja torpedo—for us a long and unfruitful period—and ends with the therapeutical use of the electrical machine and Leyden jar. The second is comprised within the years 1789, the date of the discovery of contact electricity, and 1831, the year in which induction electricity was discovered. The third extends from the latter date to the present day.

Of the first period only a few isolated facts are known. The ancients often ate of the flesh of the raja torpedo on account of its curative properties. A thousand years ago, the native women of West Africa put their sick children into a hole filled with water, in which there were some of these fish. Scribonius Largus, a physician who lived at the time of the Emperor Tiberius, is known to have done something similar for the cure of gout. Pliny also mentions electricity as a remedy, and Dioscorides records an electrical cure of prolapsus ani. So much for the historical, or rather the mythical, data of this period.

It was not until the middle of the eighteenth century—after the discovery of the electric machine and of the Leyden jar—that modern practitioners began to experiment with the new remedy. Among these we have the Germans Kratzenstein, who used friction-electricity with success for a paralyzed finger, and De Haën, under whose direction experiments were made in the Vienna Hospital, and the Frenchmen Jallabert, Sigaud de la Fond, Bertholon, and finally, Mauduyt, who are especially worthy of notice. The last-named, by his masterly report to the Société Royale de Médecine, 1773, made his colleagues enthusiastic partisans of the new method of treatment. Thus manifold uses were made of electricity—as, electric baths, electric streams, electric inhalation, or electric sparks or shocks, in which latter a powerful irritant for impaired nervous sensibility was recognized. Cavallo collected the varied observations in his "Essay on the Theory and Practice of Medical Electricity," London, 1780. He found electricity efficacious in paralysis of the muscles, impaired vision or hearing, chorea, epilepsy, chronic rheumatism, scrofulous enlargement of the glands, tape-worm, and especially as a means of reanimating the apparently dead. Soon, however, after the failure of many a hope, and after the discovery of an incomparably more abundant source of electricity in galvanism, had attracted the attention of the learned world, they turned their backs on the electric machine and Leyden jar, in order to employ the new panacea with still more sanguine expectations.

Let us glance, for a moment, at the therapeutical application of the magnet, which we could not well pass unnoticed. Although its power was not unknown to the ancients, it was not until the middle ages that the attention of the physician was particularly directed to it. Paracelsus, especially, recommended it "as a remedy which possessed such mysterious properties, that one, without it, could accomplish nothing, and, further, it was an agent so excellent in the hands of the medical inquirer, that none could be found, far or near, of which so much could be said." The results, however, were very insignificant so long as the feeble action of the loadstone only was at command; these were rendered more important about the middle of the last century by the preparation and use of artificial magnets, particularly by those of Maximilian Hell, of Vienna.

After Galvani, in 1789, discovered contact electricity, and had found that, by touching an exposed nerve or muscle with two connected metals, convulsive contractions are produced, which, however, immediately disappear, when the connection is broken, he concluded that there must be present in animals an electric fluid upon which all muscular action depends. To this fluid he gave the name Animal Electricity, and so, in appearance, prematurely made an assertion, the correctness of which, after long battling, has recently been recognized. Alexander Volta opposed this theory, and showed that the metals necessary to the production of this phenomenon must be heterogeneous; that it, on the contrary, was not necessary to bring the nerve and muscle into contact with both metals, but that the simultaneous contact of two points of a nerve or muscle was sufficient to produce the phenomenon. Through the construction of the pile that bears his name, he at the same time became the originator of the present system of galvanism and of the discoveries that are the pride of our century. But Volta, as well as Valli, still contended that the nerve-fluid was electric in its nature, and only by contact with different metals could be put in motion; while Reil, Gren, Fontana, and others, denied the existence of animal electricity, and saw in the electricity generated by different metals an irritant for the sensitive muscular fibres.

In 1797 Humboldt published his celebrated work,[1] in which he showed the power of galvanism to effect an immediate change in the secretions, studied the action of galvanism on the nerves and muscles, and demonstrated the dependence of nervous sensibility on external circumstances, such as muscular exertion, diseased conditions, etc., and thus gave to science the results of his experiments with a power which, since then, has played so important a part in physiology. In the mean time Valli proposed electricity as a test in cases of apparent death. Hufeland and Sömmering designated the phrenic nerve as the one best adapted to the use of galvanism as a means of resuscitation. Pfaff, Reil, Humboldt, and others, recommended contact electricity as especially efficacious in cases of paralysis of certain organs. Until now, however, the experiments had been made only with certain chain-connections. But when Volta's pile, constructed in 1800, attracted the more general attention of the profession with its magnificent revelations, Loder, in Jena, assisted by Bischoff and Lichtenstein, Grapengiesser and Hers, in Berlin, and the medical school under the direction of Haller, in Paris, resorted to it in cases of paralysis of the extremities and the nerves of sense. At the same time, Professor Schaub, in Cassel, and Eschke, director of the Institution for the Deaf and Dumb in Berlin, employed it in cases of impaired hearing and of deaf mutes; and Aldini and Bichat were the first to experiment on the bodies of those who had been executed (1802). In general, galvanism had greater difficulties to contend against in Italy and France than in Germany. Nevertheless, in Italy, according to the observations of Gentili and Palazzi, isolated cases of

[1] Versuch über die gereizte Muskel- und Nervenfaser, etc. Band I

melancholy were cured by the new remedy. It, however, frequently failed. This was due, in a great measure, to a want of discrimination on the part of the practitioner, to the incompleteness of the apparatus, and to other causes. In consequence of these failures, the scientifically-educated physicians were slow to recognize galvanism as a therapeutical agent, and as a natural sequence, it fell into the hands of charlatans, who hawked the pile of Volta in the marketplaces as a panacea for every imaginary ailing. With it they pretended to make the blind to see, the deaf to hear, and the lame to walk. Mesmerism also—which made its appearance about this time, and spread rapidly through France and Germany, finding adherents even among physicians, Hufeland, Wolfart, Kluge, and others—contributed to deter the profession from studying electricity with the view of turning it to practical account, and to confuse the people in their conceptions of magnetism and electricity—so that, at last, mineral and animal magnetism, talismans, amulets, charms, and sympathetic cures were all placed in the same category. Thus faith was lost, not only in the miraculous, but also in the healing powers of electricity, and we have in this period only a few names to mention which are of any importance in its history. To these belong G. F. Most,[1] Sarlandière, who, by the adoption of acupuncture, rendered the action of electricity on the deeper organs possible, and Magendie, who, by the authority of his name, sustained the waning confidence in this remedy.

With Faraday's discovery of induction electricity began a new era in its application to medicine. In 1832 Pixii constructed the first magneto-electric rotary machine, to which, later, Saxton, Keil, Ettinghausen, and Stöhrer made important improvements. As the high price of this apparatus prevented its general use, Aldini, Neef, Wagener, Rauch, and others constructed cheaper Volta-electric machines,

[1] Über die grossen Heilwirkungen des in unsern Tagen mit Unrecht vernachlässigten Galvanismus. Lüneburg, 1823.

which Duchenne, Du Bois-Reymond, and Stöhrer considerably improved. Physicians, naturalists, and physiologists now devoted themselves with equal ardor to electricity. Marshall Hall, Golding Bird, Stokes, Phillips, Graves, Donovan, among the English—Poisseuille, Pétrequin, Masson, Duchenne, A. Becquerel, etc., among the French—and Weber, Froriep, Schuh, Heidenreich, Richter, Moritz Meyer, Schulz, Erdman, Baierlacher, Eckhard, Remak, Heidenhayn, A. Fick, Ziemssen, Althaus, Rosenthal, Benedict, Frommhold, etc., among the Germans.

Pravaz was the first to conceive the idea of curing aneurism by galvano-puncture, Liston the first to test the method on the human subject, and Cinisilli the first who succeeded. Bertani and Milani made use of electricity in varices, while Radford, Simpson, Frank, and others used it in obstetrics.

Encouraged by Davy's and Ritter's observations relative to the influence of large plate voltaic cells in producing heat, Crussel, Marshall, Middeldorpf, Alph. Amussat, Zsigmondy, Schuh, etc., made use of the platinum wire loop as a cauterizing apparatus for surgical purposes.

After Nicholson and Carlisle, through the voltaic pile, had decomposed water and Davy the alkalies, here and there was to be found a physician who made use of the chemical action of electricity for physiological and therapeutical purposes. Heidenreich, with the pile, decomposed the blood, Prévost, Dumas, and Bence Jones calcareous deposits in the bladder—Crussel, Colley, Willebrand, and Wells used it in cases of malignant tumors and ulcers—Fabré-Palaprat, Orioli, etc., endeavored to introduce medicines into a part of the human body; and, finally, Verqués, Poey, and Meding to remove metals from the organism.

Besides the advances in therapeutics thus made through electricity in the broad fields of medicine, surgery, and obstetrics, owing chiefly to the researches of Hall, Duchenne, Myer, and Benedict, the new agent was made serviceable in other ways. Thus Duchenne, by perfecting the necessary apparatus, as well as by an improved (localized) application of the inductive current, succeeded in introducing electricity into medicine as an important diagnostic aid. During the last decade, Remak endeavored to become more thoroughly acquainted with the physiological difference in the action of the constant and interrupted electric currents, to assign the diseases of the muscles and nerves almost exclusively to the former, and to extend its efficacy to the treatment of cerebral and spinal affections.

His observations in this field are recorded in his treatise on Galvano-therapeutics, and in a little brochure, as valuable as it is small,[1] which he published a short time before his death, and left as a sacred inheritance to electro-therapeutists. Extravagant as Remak often was in his opinions, unjust as he often was relative to the claims of the interrupted current (which no electro-therapeutist can do without, and to which many owe their greatest successes), and, finally, prone as he was to draw the least favorable conclusions as to the extent of its efficacy from one or a few cures, still those who had an opportunity to closely notice his brilliant services must indorse the words of Graefe,[2] that "Remak, by introducing the constant current into the practice of medicine, enriched it with an invaluable treasure, whose aid, in numerous otherwise incurable cases, is incalculable." It becomes Remak's successors to test his observations without prejudice, to separate the many kernels from the chaff, and to circumscribe within proper limits the immoderately large field over which the application of electricity has extended. At the same time, they should condemn none of his assertions without proper investigation, as he was one of those brilliant geniuses who often instinctively discover the right, and in whose extravagant expressions there is always a healthy germ and more or less truth. Besides, the application of the

[1] Application du Courant constant au Traitement des Nevroses, etc. Paris: Baillière. 1865.
[2] Ber. Klin. Wochenschrift, 1865, p. 479.

constant current, which Remak introduced into practical medicine, at a time when the incompleteness of the galvanic elements rendered a daily cleansing of the battery necessary, is to-day—thanks to the improvements of Meidinger, Smee, Stöhrer, and, above all, of Siemens and Halske in the quality of the elements, for the purposes of telegraphy—attended with far less difficulty, although a convenient, transportable battery still remains a great necessity.

In conclusion, we must also refer to those who have endeavored to establish the laws that govern the electrical currents of the various animal tissues and organs—a Ritter, Pfaff, Nobili, Matteucci, etc.—with the aid of whose researches Du Bois-Reymond was enabled to give to so-called animal electricity a scientific basis, to discover the laws that govern the muscular and nervous currents, and establish the influence, on the latter, of external electrical currents. Adopting as a basis these researches, which Du Bois-Reymond published in his work,[1] his pupils Pflüger, Heidenhayn, J. Rosenthal, V. Betzold and others continue to work on with restless enthusiasm.

[1] Untersuchungen über thierische Electricität.

SECOND SECTION.

OF THE ACTION OF THE ELECTRIC CURRENT IN GENERAL.

ELECTRICITY has thus far been employed in medicine, as obtained from the sources of friction, contact, and induction.

I. FRICTION ELECTRICITY.

If we rub a glass tube lengthwise with a woollen cloth or with a piece of leather, over which an amalgam of quicksilver and zinc or tin has been spread, it will become electric, and, provided the negative electricity generated at the same time is properly conducted away, it will share its electricity with another non-electric body brought in contact with it. In order to produce friction-electricity, we use either an electrophorus, which in a long time produces but little electricity, or an electric machine. With the latter a large quantity of electricity may be communicated to an isolated body by simple contact. The sparks, when they touch the skin, cause an unpleasant twitching and a pricking sensation, and produce small spots not unlike the bites of the gnat, and sometimes little blisters, according to the size and strength of the sparks. The skin, at the same time, is reddened, and the sensibility increased.[1] The action does not extend to the subcutaneous tissues, and is hardly capable of producing any contraction of the superficial muscles. The electricity of the electric machine has been applied in various forms: as electric air-baths, in an uninterrupted electric current, as electric baths, electric inhalation, etc., but all these methods

[1] Sundelin, Anleitung zur medicin. Anwendung der Electricität und des Galvanismus. Berlin, 1822, p. 49.

belong rather to the history of electricity than to its therapeutical application, with which we are here especially occupied.[1]

The Leyden jar produces far more important physiological effects, by transmitting a larger quantity of electricity to a small area of any given portion of the body. If we place one hand on the button and the other in connection with the external rim of the jar, an unpleasant convulsive shock is produced. If the jar be lightly charged, the shock is felt in the fore-arm; if more strongly, it is felt in the upper arm; if still more strongly, the shock causes a penetrating pain in the breast. The action extends to the deeper tissues, and the muscles contract powerfully. If the button of the Leyden jar be brought in contact with a nerve, the sensation of a contusion is produced, and a numbness follows. If the quantity of electricity be still further increased, the limb falls, or perhaps even the body, as though it were struck by lightning. Even a weak battery, that is, a connection of a few small jars, is sufficient to kill small animals, such as birds, rabbits, etc.; more powerful batteries kill even dogs, or as lightning, men. The skin of the part in contact is marked with burnt spots, bruises, and torn wounds. After death no anatomical injuries, sufficient to account for the result, are visible. The blood in the heart and blood-vessels is not coagulated.

In accordance with the above-mentioned phenomena, we may consider the use of the Leyden jar indicated in cases where an irritant is wanted for the superficial tissues. Where deeper action is necessary, on account of the unpleasant and dangerous complication which attends its use, it should not be employed. As, however, the action

---

[1] The English, only make frequent use of the electric machine in cases where a general irritation is intended, as in chorea, rheumatism, and hysterical and lead paralysis, when they generally let the sparks pass over the spinal column. (See, "On the Value of Electricity as a Remedial Agent," by William Gull; Guy's Hospital Reports, Second Series, vol. viii., part i., p. 80, 1852.)

on the superficial tissues may be more perfectly obtained by galvanic and inductive electricity, to which we shall proceed to give our attention, the Leyden jar, for therapeutical purposes, has fallen into disuse.[1]

II. CONTACT ELECTRICITY (GALVANISM).

Galvanic electricity is generated by bringing in contact two dissimilar conductors, whether solids or fluids, or by the contact of metals with gases or fluids. The electricity produced by the contact of two fluids, compared with that generated by the contact of metals, is very weak. But, though all metals are, in general, good electromotors, observation has proved that in this particular a great difference exists between them. Thus zinc, lead, tin, iron, copper, silver, gold, platina, carbon, form a series, the preceding body of which, in contact with any of the following, is electrically positive, the electric antagonism increasing in a direct ratio to the distance of the two metals from each other in the series. Thus a zinc-carbon or a zinc-platina connection, particularly when diluted sulphuric or nitric acid, or a solution of chloride of ammonium or common salt, is used as an intermediate conductor, forms the most powerful battery.

If only one liquid be used as an intermediate conductor, the current is unsteady—at first often powerful, but soon decreasing in strength; while, by using two intermediate conductors, the more perfect, continued, and durable current, the so-called constant current, is produced. This variableness or invariableness of the current depends on a chemical decomposition going on in the conducting fluid, and produces the so-called polarization of the plates. This

[1] Notwithstanding this fact, it is very certain that friction or statical electricity is beneficial in certain diseases, and is sometimes, perhaps, to be preferred to other forms of the agent. Thus, in amenorrhœa it was used with great success, several years ago, by Dr. Golding Bird. In cases of suspended animation, as in that induced by submersion in water, it is more powerful to restore vitality than either galvanism or faradism.—W. A. H.

process causes a decomposition of the fluids in which the metals are immersed, the product of the decomposition collecting on the metal, and generating, in its turn, a current, the so-called polarization-current, which, as it always takes a contrary direction to the one by which it is produced, always more or less weakens the latter, or finally wholly destroys it. If we have, for instance, a zinc and a copper plate, connected by a wire and immersed in a solution of sulphate of zinc, the oxide of zinc is decomposed in such a manner, that the oxygen goes to the zinc plate, forming new oxide of zinc, while metallic zinc collects on the copper plate. When the copper plate has completely covered itself with oxide of zinc, the current ceases, for the reason that two heterogeneous metals are no longer connected, but two homogeneous. If we use, instead of a metal solution, diluted sulphuric acid, the water will be decomposed. On the one side oxide of zinc will be formed, while on the other the copper will be covered with bubbles of hydrogen. Oxygen forms the electro-negative end of the electrolytic series, while hydrogen is certainly more electro-positive than zinc, in consequence of which a current is generated, that passes from the hydrogen deposit to the oxygen deposit, that is, from the copper to the zinc, in the direction contrary to that of the primary current.

On the contrary, if we insert two fluid conductors that are separated by a porous body—an animal membrane or plaster cylinder—the polarization will be prevented. In this case, the metal surfaces will be kept clean by the water-forming process that takes place on the partition-wall. If we have, for instance, a so-called Daniell's element, that is, a zinc cylinder within a closed membrane filled with diluted sulphuric acid, and this within a copper cylinder filled with blue vitriol, the water will be decomposed on the inner side of the membrane; the oxygen goes to the zinc, forming oxide of zinc, which is dissolved in the acid; the hydrogen, on the contrary, goes to the membrane, forming, at the same

time, the positive pole for the current which now goes over
to the other fluid. The oxide of copper, on the contrary,
will be decomposed in such a manner, that the oxygen goes
to the partition-wall to form water by uniting with the hydrogen that is produced on the other side; while metallic
copper is deposited on the copper plate which is thus
always covered with a coating of fresh copper. In order to keep the vitriol solution as highly concentrated as
possible, a surplus quantity of the crystallized salt may be
thrown into it, or, what is better, a gauze bag filled with
pulverized blue vitriol may be suspended in the solution.

The first constant battery was constructed by Becquerel.
It consists of a hollow copper cylinder, that is loosely enveloped in a bladder in such a manner that the intervening
space can be filled with a saturated solution of blue vitriol.
The bladder is surrounded by a hollow zinc cylinder, and
the whole is suspended in a glass or porcelain vessel, containing diluted sulphuric acid, or a solution of sulphate of
zinc, or common salt. The battery of Daniell, already mentioned, is only a modification of Becquerel's. The constant
batteries (elements) now in general use, besides those already
named, are Grove's, or the zinc-platina battery, and Bunsen's,
or the zinc-carbon battery. As for the construction of the
first, it consists of a zinc cylinder, in a vessel filled with
diluted sulphuric acid. Within the cylinder is a cell of porous clay, containing concentrated nitric acid and a thin
plate of platina. The decomposition takes place as follows:
the hydrogen generated by the dissolution of the zinc in the
sulphuric acid is immediately oxidized at the expense of the
nitric acid, whereby nitrous acid is formed, which escapes
in the form of vapor. Owing to the cost of platina, in its
stead, lead, plated with platina, is used. As the lead here
acts only as a conductor, so long as the platina lasts, this
substitute does as well as pure platina.

In the Bunsen battery, instead of platina, carbon is used,
which is still more electro-negative. A Bunsen element con-

sists of a cylinder of prepared carbon, placed in a clay cylinder, closed at the bottom. The latter is surrounded by a zinc cylinder, open at both ends, which stands in a glass vessel. The glass is filled with diluted sulphuric acid, the clay cylinder with concentrated nitric acid. The Bunsen battery is almost as powerful and much cheaper than Grove's, but, like the latter, owing to the production of nitrous-acid fumes, is objectionable. Besides, it has the disadvantage of being less reliable in its action, the consequence of the imperfect composition of the carbon, the causes of which have thus far not been explained. The current, though powerful at first, gradually loses in strength, and often cannot be restored to its original integrity, either by cleansing the elements or by renewed filling. In order to remove the first objection, on Poggendorf's recommendation, instead of sulphuric acid, a mixture, consisting of one pound of bichromate of potash, one pound of sulphuric acid, and a quart of water, is used. Here sulphate of potash and chromic acid are at first formed; the chromic acid is reduced to oxide of chromium, which enters into combination with another part of the sulphuric acid and the above sulphate of potash, forming the double combination, chrome alum (consisting of sulphate of potash and sulphate of the oxide of chromium), which is deposited on the carbon. In order to render the action of the carbon more reliable, of late, instead of the coal cylinder formerly used, artificial plates or cylinders have been employed. These are prepared from the coke that remains in gas retorts. The process consists in mixing together with water a quantity of finely-powdered coke and baked coal-dust, then heating the mixture and saturating the porous mass with a concentrated solution of sugar, and finally drying it and bringing it to a white heat.

As for the zinc cylinder, which, in a large majority of batteries, forms the positive metal, Joh. Wilh. Ritter discovered that, by plunging it into quicksilver after it had been cleaned with sulphuric or hydrochloric acid, it became far more positive, and consequently by this process the element became proportionately more active and durable. This is due, probably, to the fact that the zinc of commerce is always rendered impure by the presence of other metals, and never has a homogeneous surface, so that by contact with the acids little galvanic currents are formed, by which it is rapidly destroyed. By the coating of zinc-amalgam this action is prevented. It is a good plan, in order to make the quicksilver penetrate as deeply as possible into the zinc, to warm the cylinder thoroughly preparatory to the amalgamation. By covering the outer surface with varnish, for instance, amber varnish, the power of the zinc to resist the acids will be still further increased. In general the positive metal is made tolerably large, in order to present to the moist conductor as large a surface as possible; on the contrary, the negative metal should not be so large, since otherwise the coating of hydrogen, formed by the passage of the electric current, will be too considerable to be carried off by the current.

A frequently-used modification of Daniell's battery is that of Meidinger. In the interior of a large glass vessel, a small, conical glass cylinder, with a small opening, is fastened, and is filled with a solution of sulphate of copper, while the larger vessel contains the zinc in a concentrated solution of sulphate of magnesia.

Of the other galvanic elements that have been used for therapeutic purposes, Smee's cell and Hare's calorimeter are worthy of notice. The former consists of a thin plate of platinized silver, which is separated by cushions of guttapercha from the amalgamated zinc plates that are placed on each side of it. The plates are suspended, without any porous diaphragm, in sulphuric acid, twenty-five times diluted. The silver plate of Smee's element must not be too thin, and must possess a certain stiffness, which makes such a battery tolerably expensive. The Engineer Board (Genie-Comité) in Vienna have remedied this objection by constructing the zinc-lead-platina battery, which, besides, possesses the advantage that the lead and platina having a far greater affinity than silver and platina, the platinizing is more rapid, more thorough, and more durable. Hare's calorimeter consists of a large compound zinc and copper plate, the elements of which are separated by strips of cloth, and secured in a spiral form, so that the upper surface presents from fifty to sixty square feet, the whole placed within a wooden cylinder three inches thick and eighteen inches high, in which the dilute sulphuric acid is poured.[1]

When the two metals of a simple battery, or the terminating metals of a series of simple batteries (a compound battery), are connected, the circuit is said to be closed, and the wire connecting the poles is called the connecting arch.

In the closed battery the opposing currents unite through the arch closing the series, and the current—in contrast with the current produced by friction-electricity, which, with all its strength, is of short duration, continuing only so long as is necessary to neutralize the electricity collected on the conductors—continues uninterrupted until the difference in the tension of the two metals, through the complete solution of one metal in the fluid, is adjusted. The direction of the current in the terminal arch is always from the metal standing lowest in the electrolytic series toward the one standing highest; for example, from the copper to the zinc, and therefore the projecting point of the copper is called the positive, the projecting point of the zinc the negative pole. This designation it is all the more necessary to observe, as zinc, by contact with copper, becomes electrically positive, and is consequently the positive, while the copper becomes the

[1] Of late, batteries have also been constructed of one metal only, for instance, of iron. The action of such batteries is due to the fact that certain metals, for example, iron, when subjected to the action of very concentrated sulphuric acid, become passive or electro-negative, being no longer corroded by nitric acid, and taking in a measure the place of platina. Thus, batteries are constructed of common and passive iron, and nitric acid and sulphuric acid can be used as moist conductors.

negative metal. In the conducting fluid the current always
goes in the contrary direction, that is, from the zinc through
the fluid to the copper. In every open battery, no matter
whether simple or compound, each pole has free electricity
of a certain tension, the quantity of which is equal at each
pole. At the positive pole it is represented by +, at the
negative pole by —. The tension increases with the number of the elements in arithmetical progression, so that in
the middle of the pile, at the so-called neutral point, there
is a pair of plates that have no free electricity, and by which
the pile is divided into two equal opposing halves.

If the current is conducted by means of a straight wire,
parallel with and over or under a magnetic needle, the needle
will deviate in proportion to the number of the elements.
The direction of the deviation is variable, depending upon
the current being conducted over or under the magnetic
needle, or whether the direction of the current be changed
or not. In order to determine the direction of the current
from the position of the needle, the following rule of Am-
père is used: Imagine to yourself a human figure, introduced into the current so that it enters at the feet and goes
out at the head. If the figure turns its face toward the
needle, the north pole of the needle will always be turned
toward the left of the figure. By this rule we see that the
several parts of the current which is led in a circle around a
needle all tend in like manner to make the needle deviate,
and also to mutually strengthen one another. In order,
therefore, to produce an observable deviation, it is only necessary to have a greater number of well-isolated coils of the
wire in a parallel direction. Such an instrument, which
serves to recognize weak currents, and to determine their
direction, is called a multiplicator, and may be used as a
galvanometer.

If we turn now to the action of the electrical currents,
we must recognize two distinct series of them, the one going
on in the conducting body itself, the other in the distance—

both always proportionably present. To the first belong:
1. The electro-motor action, which the current produces in the moist conductors in porous vessels, membranes, etc.; 2. The thermal or caustic action, that is, the warming of the conductors; 3. The chemical action, which comprehends the physiological (the phenomena of motion and sensation). To the action in the distance belong: 1. The deviation of the magnetic needle (magnetic action of the electric current); 2. The magnetizing of soft iron (electro-magnetic action); 3. Induction, or the power of an electric current to produce a second current in a distant conductor.

The action of a battery depends, under like circumstances, upon the tension which its poles have when open. This varies with the combination and number of the elements, and is called the electro-motor power. If we imagine a metallic wire, of equal size in its entire length, bent into a circle, and further imagine any point to be the seat of the electro-motor power, then, in any given time, the same quantity of electricity will pass this point. The quantity of electricity, however, which, in any given time, passes the imaginary point of the circuit, is called the current-power, which is measured either by the electro-magnetic power of the stream, as shown by the extent of the deviation of the magnetic needle of the galvanometer, or by the electro-chemical action, as evidenced by its power to decompose chemical combinations. The greater the electro-motor power, the greater will also be the strength of the current; that is, the latter will be in direct proportion to the former. The reverse is true with regard to the opposing power of the conductors. Every substance that possesses the power of conducting electricity lessens the rapidity of the electrical current, and this in direct proportion to its size. This so-called resistance is, consequently, in indirect proportion to the strength of the current. If we let C represent the strength of the current, E the electro-motor power, R the resistance, we have, in accordance with the Ohm law, the formula $C = \dfrac{E}{R}$: the strength of the current equals the electro-motor power divided by the resistance.

This law, the most important for the rational application of electricity in medicine, retains its validity even when several opposing bodies, different in quantity and quality, are found in the circuit. The power of a body to oppose the movement of a current varies, however, very greatly according to form, length, diameter, temperature, peculiarities of composition, etc. Its dependence on form cannot, in most cases, be expressed by a simple formula; on the contrary, however, it can be experimentally demonstrated. On the other hand, it is found to be a general law, that, with the increased length of the wire introduced, the conducting resistance increases, or, what is the same, the strength of the current decreases; and, conversely, with a wire of increased diameter, the resistance decreases, or the current-power increases. So far, therefore, as the resistance depends on the length, L, and the diameter of the conductor, D, it may be expressed by the formula $R = \dfrac{L}{D}$: the resistance equals the length divided by the diameter.

Relative to the influence of temperature, it is found that, with metals, the resistance increases as the temperature is raised; with fluids, however, other conditions remaining the same, the reverse takes place.

An important influence is exercised over the resistance by the quality of the conductor or the substance of which it is made; and here innumerable differences are to be considered—thus, for example, the resistance of copper compared to that of water is as 1 : 4,000 millions, the resistance of copper compared to that of a concentrated solution of sulphate of copper is as 1 : 11 millions, etc. As a general thing, the metals offer the least conducting resistance; but their specific conductive power varies. If, for example, we let the conductive power of pure silver = 100, then that of copper = 50, of gold = 55, of zinc = 27, of iron = 15, of platina = 10, of quicksilver = 2.[1] The resistance of the fluids is far greater; the best conductor, perhaps, among them—sulphuric acid—is about a million times below silver. Sulphuric acid and water, mixed in certain quantities, offers the least resistance of all the fluids thus far tested; while each of these fluids separately is a very bad conductor.

With regard to the conduction resistance of the animal body in general, Cavendish seems to have been the first to represent that the animal tissues are equally as bad conductors as the fluids. Nevertheless, the number of methodical experiments made with the view of ascertaining the conduction resistance of the animal tissues generally, as well as of determining the difference between them, remained very small up to a recent date. It has long been known, that vegetable and animal matter are conductors only by virtue of the water they contain, and, when desiccated, become non-conductors, and that the animal fluids and the parts moistened by them are better conductors than cold water. Ritter had already recognized the formidable resistance offered by the epidermis to the passage of the electric current. For this reason, Humboldt experimented on parts deprived of the outer skin by blistering, and found the resistance of the animal body considerably lessened. Many erroneous opinions were, nevertheless, entertained with regard to the nerves, which were supposed to possess peculiar conductive powers. The researches of Person, Pouillet, Ed. Weber,[2] and Lenz, corrected these errors. Their deductions are founded on a scientific basis. Pouillet estimates the resistance offered by the human body, when the whole hand is immersed in water to which one per cent. of sulphuric acid has been added, to be equal to that which forty-nine thou-

---

[1] According to Heidemann and Franz, the conductive power of the metals for electricity and heat is the same.

[2] Questiones physiologicæ de phænom. galv.-magnet. in corp. hum. observatis. Commentatio pro facultate scholas acad. habendi. 1836.

sand and eighty-two metres of copper wire one millim. in diameter offer to the electric current. According to Lenz and Ptschelnikoff,[1] the resistance of the human body is equal to that of a copper wire 91.762 metres in length and one millim. in diameter. It was further discovered that the human body offers the same resistance as a body impregnated with blood and other salty fluids, namely, a resistance from 10 to 20 times less powerful than distilled water equally warm, and equally as powerful as warm salt water. Finally, it was shown that the epidermis, dry and cold, offered 50 times more resistance than the whole human body, from the right to the left hand, but that this resistance was diminished in proportion as it was warmed and moistened, and in a direct ratio to the conductivity of the moistening fluid.

With regard to the various tissues, Person[2] was the first to express the opinion that the nerves were no better conductors than the muscles or other moist animal tissues. According to Matteucci, the muscles conduct electricity four times as well as the nerves; according to Schlesinger,[3] the conductivity of the muscles to that of the nerves is as 8 : 3; according to Eckhardt,[4] as 1.9 : 1. Eckhardt found, further, that sinews, cartilage, and nerve-tissue offer no perceptible difference as resistants, and that it is difficult to determine which of the three is the best conductor. As for the cartilage, he found the resistance of the compact tissue from 16 to 22 times greater than that of muscle, while the resistance of the porous tissue was considerably less, depending on the quantity of water it contained. The resistance of the skin on the various parts of the body differs in degree.

[1] Über den Leitungswiderstand des Körpers gegen galv. Ströme, in Poggendorf's Annalen, Band lvi., Pag. 429, seq.
[2] Sur l'Hypothèse des Courants électriques dans les Nerfs, Magendie, Journal de Physiologie Expérimentale, 1830, t. x.
[3] Die Electricität als Heilmittel: vom physikalischen und experimental-physiologischen Standpunkt erörtert, Zeitschrift der Wiener Ärzte, 1852, Juli.
[4] Beiträge zur Anatomie und Physiologie. Heft 1.: Über den galvanischen Leitungswiderstand der thierischen Gewebe.

This depends, for the most part, on the structure of the channels through which the moisture of the electrodes or current-bearers comes in contact with the moist parts of the human body—for example, the hair-bulbs and the ducts of the sudorific glands.[1]

The vessels filled with blood conduct better than the muscles, while the aponeuroses and the subcutaneous or intramuscular cellular tissue offer to the electrical current a very considerable resistance. The resistance of the mucous membranes, owing to their thinness, as well as to their moisture, is but slight. The worst conductors in the animal organism are the horny structures, epidermis, hair, and nails. According to Eckhardt (l. c.), the resistance of the animal tissues seems to depend altogether on two factors—the quantity of water and the quantity of soluble salts. Of these two the second differs far less than the first, and consequently the specific conductivity is in a direct ratio with the quantity of water. The death of a muscle is, therefore, as Ranke[2] discovered, accompanied by a decrease of resistance; in a rabbit, one-half, and in a frog, one-third of the original resistance, because the product of the decomposition of the muscle is a far better conductor of electricity than the healthy muscular tissue. The decrease in resistance discovered by Du Bois-Reymond in the muscles by boiling may be explained in the same manner.

In conclusion, the question arises, Is the resistance of the tissues altered by the current itself? The law that Benedict[3] established for the metals, that their resistance is diminished by the constant current, is equally applicable to the animal tissues.

The researches of the above-named observers indicated many other circumstances that influence the increase or de-

---

[1] Remak Galvanotherapie, Pag. 61.
[2] Tetanus, eine physiologische Studie. Leipzig, 1865.
[3] Sitzungs-Bericht der kaiserlichen Academie der Wissenschaften in Wien, Band xxv., S. 590. Juli 1857.

crease of the conditions of resistance. It seems, for example, that the resistance of a part of the body is directly proportioned to the length, and indirectly proportioned to the thickness, just as two wires of the same metal offer an equal resistance, if their respective lengths are in an inverse ratio to their transverse sections.

Lenz, at all events, found that arms and legs, in the six combinations of which they are capable—right arm and left leg, right leg and left leg, right arm and right leg, etc.—offered about an equal resistance. The relation of the surface of the part to its thickness seems, besides, to have its influence; the smaller the surface in comparison to the thickness the less the resistance, which is, perhaps, the consequence of the bad conductivity of the epidermis in comparison with the other animal tissues. Lenz found that the separate fingers of young persons offered a greater resistance to the electric current than those of adults; that, further, the resistance of the separate fingers is comparatively greater than the fingers of the whole hand when closed. For many other phenomena—as, for instance, the one observed by Weber, that the tongue, when the two borders are brought in contact with silver plates, offers as great a resistance as the whole human body from one hand to the other—we have as yet no satisfactory explanation. It may be found in the anatomical formation of the tongue, which consists[1] of two equal halves, separated by a mass of connective tissue, each of which is formed by bundles of muscular fibres, that cross in every direction, and being enclosed in a thick cellular sheath, with numerous fat-cells. The electric current must, therefore, in order to pass from one side of the tongue to the other, go through these various, and, in part, inferior media, which are here found in greater number within the same space than any other part of the human body.

[1] Kölliker's mikroscopische Anatomie, 2. Hälfte der 1. Abtheilung, Pag. 12.

From the law of Ohm, the following important practical conclusions between the intensity of the current, the electromotor power, and resistance may be deduced. If we increase the electro-motor power by a combination of elements, the resistance will also be increased. If 5 represents the power, 100 the resistance, then the intensity of the current $= \frac{5}{100} = \frac{1}{20}$. If a second battery of equal power be added, then the intensity of the current is $\frac{2 \times 5}{2 \times 100} = \frac{1}{20}$, the same figure to represent the same intensity of current. If the object be to increase the intensity of the current, it is necessary to find a combination in which the resistance does not increase in a direct ratio to the number of elements. The resistance, however, is the sum of the two factors—the resistance of the cell, which varies according to its dimensions, and the nature of the active fluids (for example, a Grove's battery has half the resistance of a Daniell's battery of the same size), and which is called the essential resistance, because in a given battery it is invariable, and the resistance of the terminal arch, which is variable, and is called the external, contingent, or variable resistance. If, in a given case, 5 be the intensity, 100 the essential resistance, and 1,000 the variable resistance, then the intensity of the current will be $= \frac{5}{100+1000} = \frac{5}{1100} = \frac{1}{220}$; if a similar battery be added, the intensity of the current will be $\frac{2 \times 5}{2 \times 100 + 1000} = \frac{10}{1200} = \frac{1}{120}$: thus the intensity of the current is notably increased.

Where, therefore, there is a great external or contingent resistance, for example, in electrizing a part of the human body, or in the chemical decomposition of a fluid, it is well to use a battery composed of several elements, in order to overcome the resistance which the animal tissue or the fluid offers to the electric current. If the object be, to bring a short wire to a glowing heat, it will be advisable to increase the quantity of the current by enlarging the transverse section of the elements; while the very considerable resistance of the elements opposed to the short wire will, as we have seen, be lessened; the current-power, therefore, will be increased. Thus we come to the conclusion that, in order to obtain the maximum current-power with a given electro-motor surface, the surface must be so distributed that the resistance of the battery will be as nearly as possible equal to that of the terminal arch. On account of the inconvenience, however, of handling very large cells, a number of small elements may be united to make one large transverse section, so that all their positive and all their negative poles are united, forming a combination, in contradistinction to a connection, when the positive pole of the first is connected with the negative pole of the second, and so on, forming what is called a compound battery.

One more point remains to be explained—the density of the current, and its relation to the current-power. We have already found that the current-power in every transverse section of the circuit must be the same, as it depends upon the collective resistance. Now, if we fix our attention upon a part of the circuit, and reduce the transverse section and longitudinal section one-half, the resistance of the circuit and the current-power will remain unchanged. The quantity of electricity that in a given time passes through the reduced transverse section will consequently be the same, but crowded together on a transverse section of half the size; the current-density is consequently doubled. The smaller, therefore, the transverse section, the denser will be a given current of the electricity passing through it; or, the density is in direct proportion to the current-power, and in indirect proportion to the transverse section. Let D represent the density, T the transverse section, P the current-power, and we have, to represent the relation, the formula, $D = \dfrac{P}{T}$. The density of the current is for the physiological action of the current of the greatest importance, the action being more powerful the smaller the transverse section through which a given quantity of electricity passes.

We will now turn to the chemical action of galvanism. We have already seen that water is resolved into its elements, oxygen and hydrogen, by the galvanic current, and that the oxygen is deposited at the positive, the hydrogen at the negative, pole. The oxides are so decomposed by the current, that the oxygen is deposited at the positive, the base at the negative, pole; and, finally, the salts are so decomposed, that the acids go to the positive, and the bases to the negative, pole. In the decomposition of chlorides, bromides, and iodides, the metals go to the negative, the metalloids to the positive, pole. Faraday has called attention to the fact that we must distinguish the direct and indirect decompositions effected by the acids. The most simple example of direct decomposition is that of water. If, on the contrary, dilute nitric acid be subjected to the action of the current, the water will be decomposed; but the hydrogen, which will be deposited at the negative pole, immediately decomposes the nitric acid, while, on the other hand, water and nitrous acid will be generated. Thus, at the positive pole, oxygen, at the negative, nitrous acid, will be set free. These changes are, however, not effected directly by the decomposing power of the acid, but by intermediate action of the decomposed water. The action is, therefore, secondary. In a similar manner, if a galvanic current be conducted through the white of an egg, serum, or blood, the salts of these fluids will be decomposed, the acids going to the positive pole, where they cause the albumen to coagulate. In bodies that consist of two elements, the proportions of the combination have a marked influence on their susceptibility to decomposition. Faraday has shown that among the dual combinations only those are electrolytes—that is, are decomposed directly by the current—that are composed of one equivalent of one element, and one of the other. This is the reason why sulphuric acid, composed of 1 eq. of sulphur and 3 eq. of oxygen, or nitric acid, composed of 1 eq. of nitrogen and 5 eq. of oxygen, or ammonia, composed of 1 eq. of nitrogen and 3 eq. of hydrogen, cannot be decomposed directly by the galvanic current. It is probable that no galvanic current can pass through a fluid without the passage being accompanied by a chemical decomposition; and, on the other hand, all those fluids that are not decomposed by the galvanic current—as ether, alcohol, etc.—seem to be bad conductors. Distilled and perfectly pure water, which is a tolerably bad conductor of electricity, is also only slowly decomposed. The addition of a drop of acid or a little salt is sufficient to induce a visible increase of conductivity, as well as an active formation of gas.

Thus the galvanic current possesses the power to decompose chemical combinations; it also, however, can cause them to be formed. All metals, gold and platina excepted, oxidize in pure water, and when the air is excluded. The influence that the galvanic current in this manner exerts on the chemical affinities induced Davy to make various experiments. After holding his finger for a length of time in distilled water, he placed it in contact with the positive pole of a Voltaic pile; phosphoric, sulphuric, and muriatic acid immediately escaped from his body to the water. If he placed his finger in contact with the negative pole, alkalies were parted with. The possibility of freeing acid and alkaline compounds from their combinations in the living body suggested to Becquerel, Davy, and Fabré-Palaprat the idea of using the galvanic current in the endermic application of certain substances possessing reactive power. Fabré-Palaprat made the following experiment: After drying both arms of a woman very thoroughly, he bound around one of them a compress saturated with iodide of potassium, covered it with a plate of platina, and brought it in contact with the positive pole of a pile consisting of thirty pairs; the other arm he moistened with a solution of starch, covered it likewise with a platina plate, and brought it in contact with the negative pole. In a few minutes, the starch assumed a bluish color, and thus the iodine—as the perfectly dry skin did not admit of the passage of the current—passed through the body to the negative pole. Davy[1] published the following experiment, made with a pile consisting of one hundred and fifty pairs. He took three vessels, one of which he filled with a solution of sulphate of potash, and placed it in connection with the negative pole; the second vessel he filled with pure water, and placed it in connection with the positive pole; the third he filled with a weak solution of ammonia, and so introduced it as a member of the circuit, that the sulphuric acid could reach the positive pole only by passing through the solution of ammonia. The three glasses were connected by means of pieces of asbestos. In less than five minutes, by means of litmus-paper, the acid was recognized at the positive pole, and in half an hour the experiment was finished. In a similar manner, Orioli succeeded in translating corrosive sublimate; Golding Bird, common salt, etc.

PHYSIOLOGICAL ACTION.—If we bring one pole of a Voltaic pile in contact with one hand, or, rather, with a moistened hand, as the epidermis is a bad conductor, we feel at the moment in which we complete the connection, by bringing the other moistened hand into contact with the other pole, a shock accompanied by a twitching, the so-called connecting shock. The extent of the twitching depends upon the number of the plates—the intensity of the current. So long as the connection remains unbroken, the electric current circulates in the human body without causing a noticeable sensation, or at most, in case the pile be a very powerful one, a

[1] Some Chemical Agencies of Electricity.

burning, trembling sensation at the point where the current enters the body. If we break the connection, we experience a second shock, the so-called disconnecting shock. If we leave one of the fingers of one hand in contact with one pole, while we touch the other pole with one finger of the other hand, withdrawing it from time to time, the shock will follow with proportionable rapidity. The same effect is produced with an apparatus intended to break and reëstablish in quick succession the current that is conducted through the body. Thus continued and intermitting galvanic currents are formed. Nevertheless, the continued current here produced is almost exclusively used for therapeutical purposes, because we possess in induction another source of electricity that yields intermitting currents, and through a small, convenient, and easy-transportable apparatus admirably adapted to the wants of the practitioner.

THERMAL ACTION.—With regard to the thermal action, which has been so variously employed of late in surgery, it is due to the fact that all conductors, irrespective of quality, are warmed by the passing electric current. The greater the quantity of the current, and the greater the resistance of the conductor, the greater the heat produced. Consequently a conducting wire introduced into the closing arch is heated in proportion as it is a bad and the rest of the arch is a good conductor. If we have, therefore, a cell of great electro-motor power and slight resistance—for example, a Bunsen's or Grove's, but not a Daniell's, element of large outer surface—it will be sufficient to bring to a glowing heat and even to melt a platinum wire, which, as we have already seen, belongs to the bad metallic conductors; and, indeed, the shorter and smaller the wire, the easier this effect will be produced. If the wire be long and small and its resistance consequently great, several elements must be connected, the one after the other; while, with a short thick wire, the single-cell combination is the better. In each individual case, therefore, the most efficient combination will depend upon the relation of the resistance between the wire used and the elements.

III. INDUCTION ELECTRICITY (FARADISM).

Faraday discovered, in the year 1831, that a galvanic current, at the moment of closing and opening the circuit, generated in neighboring conductors other electric currents, which he called induction-currents. If we wind a copper wire covered with silk around a wooden cylinder, above or beside this one a second one, also covered with silk, and then connect the ends of the first wire with the poles of a galvanic battery, at the moment the connection is made, an electric current will be established in the second wire, which immediately disappears, in order to return at the moment the connection is broken, and then again to disappear. These second currents are, therefore, of only momentary duration; they arise at each opening and each closing of the connection, and are wanting during the time that the circuit is closed. Duchenne, and after him the other physicians who study the application of electricity, called this the induced or secondary current, in contradistinction to the inducing or primary current.[1]

The induced current is also demonstrable with the galvanometer. The needle, at the moment of the closing of the circuit, diverges toward the primary opposing side, while, at the opening, it diverges in the direction of the primary direct current. During the time that the battery is closed, the galvanometer indicates no divergence; the current does not exist.

Besides these two currents, we observe in the first wire a third current, induced by the several windings of the

[1] We should mention here that physicists call the current, that we, in accordance with Duchenne, call the primary or inducing current, the extra current; while the one we call the secondary current, they call the primary induction current; the one running between the coils of the spirally-wound wire, the secondary, etc. We have thought it advisable to follow the nomenclature of Duchenne, inasmuch as we write for physicians.

primary current. When these windings run near one another, their action is inductive, and they produce what is called the extra current. That this is really so, may be easily seen if we take a simple galvanic battery and close it, at first with a short, and then, for comparison, with a long spirally-wound wire. In the first case we will observe a very weak, in the second a much stronger emission of sparks. From the extra current—which was also known to Faraday, but for a thorough acquaintance with which we are, however, indebted to Dove [1]—originates also an induced current. It arises, as such, at the opening and closing, and takes at the closing a direction opposite to, at the opening a direction corresponding with, the primitive current. That it nevertheless, at the closing, has no effect on a body introduced, that is not so good a conductor, is due to the fact that the current in this case finds in the battery itself a closed metallic conductor, and consequently leaves the secondary connecting body unaffected. At the opening, on the contrary, the action is decided, because here the primary current is interrupted, and consequently the extra current flows through the body that has been introduced in its full intensity. A considerable increase of the extra current will be noticed if we put into the hollow of the wooden cylinder a piece of iron, or better, a split iron cylinder, or better still, a bundle of varnished wire. (Bachhoffner and Sturgeon, in "Annals of Electricity," vol. i., p. 481.) [2]

[1] Poggendorf's Annalen, Band lvi., Pag. 251.
[2] The cause of these phenomena, it was formerly thought, lay in the fact that the metal of which wire is made is softer than a piece of ordinary iron, and consequently susceptible of greater magnetism. Magnus ("Poggendorf's Annalen," vol. xlviii. p. 93) corrected this error. He showed, by the deviation of the magnetic needle, that the bundle of wire was not more strongly magnetized than the piece of iron by the current. He found, moreover, that the physiological action of a bundle of wire was stronger, and was still further strengthened by covering some pieces of the wire with varnish. Magnus's explanation was the following: The current surrounding the iron generates in the iron, at the moment it arises, a counter electric current; during its continuance the iron is maintained in a state of magnetic polarization; when it stops, a current

Here the galvanic current renders the soft iron at first magnetic, and thereby enables it in turn to induce electric currents in the spiral wire. The intensity of the current depends, on the one hand, upon the power of the battery, upon the other on the length of the inductive spiral, the thickness of the wire used, and the size of the bundle of wire. The wire for the inducing current is generally shorter and larger, that for the induced current longer and smaller. The reason will be given in the fifth chapter, where we shall go more into detail with regard to the difference in the action of the two currents. We will now simply observe that the extra current induces currents and causes shocks only when the circuit is opened, while the secondary current does so both when the circuit is opened and closed.

We call a galvanic battery consisting of one or two helices a volta-electric or galvano-electric apparatus. As the induced current produced by such a battery is of only short duration, steps must be taken in order to secure continued generation for medical purposes, to frequently interrupt the primary current. This can be effected either mechanically, by introducing, according to the directions of Sprenger and Aldini, a toothed wheel, the teeth of which, as the wheel is turned, continually open or close the circuit, as in Güterbrock's, Rauch's apparatus, etc., or, much better, by the so-called Neefe's hammer, originally constructed by J. P. Wagner, in Frankfort, a clever contrivance, that secures the opening and closing by using the temporary magnetism of the bundle of

---

corresponding in direction with the primary current is produced. This current, however, retards the disappearance of the magnetism, and thereby weakens the action to be anticipated from the sudden discontinuance of the magnetism. What, therefore, operates to lessen the power of this current in the iron, increases the action of the extra current. But the action of this current will evidently not be so powerful on separate, and especially isolated wires, as on a solid piece of iron. Consequently, in a current induced by a bundle of wire, a given quantity of electricity will be more quickly compensated, and thereby more energetic in its action, than in a current induced by a piece of iron of the same dimensions. A similar result will be obtained with a split cylinder.

wire within the helix. This little hammer, of soft iron, was formerly attached to a steel spring, so that, by drawing it back and letting it strike, the battery could be opened and closed in continued succession. To these self-acting volta-electric batteries belong those of Neef, Wagner, Klöpfer, Romershausen, Hassenstein, Danwerth, Duchenne, Du Bois-Reymond, Ruhmkorff, Erdmann, and others. The more important ones will be discussed in Fifth Section.

Faraday found, further, that, by simply placing a magnet and a closed conductor in close proximity, a stronger current, running counter to the current of the magnet, was induced in the conductor, and that, by removing the magnet to a distance, a weaker current was induced in the conductor, corresponding in direction with the current of the magnet. The continued renewal of the induced current, for medical purposes, is generally secured in the batteries constructed on this principle by winding the ends of an iron, bent in the form of a horse-shoe (or two short bars of iron that rest at right angles on an iron plate), with a copper wire in such manner that the spirals run in opposite directions, and then setting these two pieces of iron with their spirals in motion, by means of a crank, and letting them turn in a circle before the poles of a horse-shoe magnet, lying in a horizontal position. The action of the steel magnet on the spiral is here not direct, but is induced by the magnetism of the soft iron, that appears and disappears with each half revolution. This magnetism in its turn generates a current in the helices. This takes place independently of the fact that the iron is most powerfully magnetized when the helices stand opposite the poles of the magnet, and are always at the moment when the rollers move away from the two poles of the magnet, before which they stood, toward the opposite side, because the inductive action is produced only at the moment of the appearance and disappearance of the current, and not by the magnetism already generated. Saxton was the first to explain the phenomena of the extra current of the so-called magneto-electric apparatus, and consequently the physicists named the apparatus the Saxton battery, which, however, was subsequently changed for the meaningless name of rotary apparatus. It should be stated that the intensity of its current increases with the power of the magnet, the length of the inductive spiral, the proximity of the soft iron, the rapidity of the revolutions, etc. To this class of machines belong those of Pixii, Saxton, Keil, Ettinghausen, Stöhrer, the Bréton brothers, Dugardin, Duchenne, Palmeret, and Hall, etc. (See Chapter V.)

CHEMICAL AND THERMAL ACTION.—The chemical action of induction electricity enables us, by means of the induced current, to decompose water, and a solution of the iodide of potassium, and to effect other electrolytic processes; also, to bring to a glowing heat a short, thin platina wire. But all these phenomena are more slowly and less perfectly accomplished than with the continued galvanic current.

Duchenne called induction electricity Faradism, after its discoverer, Faraday; its action he called Faradic, and its application Faradization, a terminology which has its justification in the nomenclature of contact electricity and its foundation in the difference of the action of contact and induction electricity.

THIRD SECTION.

OF THE ELECTRO-MOTOR PROPERTIES OF THE ANIMAL BODY.

E. Du Bois-Reymond, Untersuchungen über thierische Electricität, vol. I. and II., 1848, 1849. C. Ludwig, Lehrbuch der Physiologie des Menschen, vol. I., 1852, pp. 316, *et seq.* C. Eckhard, Grundzüge der Physiologie des Nervensystems, 1854, pp. 40, *et seq.* A. Fick, die medicinische Physik, 1856, pp. 411, *et seq.* [Morgan, Electro-Physiology and Therapeutics, etc., New York, 1868.]

In order to have a clear understanding of the changes produced by the action of the electric current on the various animal tissues, we shall, in this chapter, speak of the inherent currents that are present in the animal body, as well as of the changes the tissues undergo in their molecular arrangement, during the production and action of the electric current.

Nobili, in 1827, discovered an electric current in the frog, the so-called frog-current, which he—starting on the supposition that nerves, on account of their small mass when compared with the muscles, cool more rapidly through evaporation—mistook for a thermo-electric current. Subsequently Matteucci corrected this mistake, as well as the error that the current is of electro-chemical origin, and proved that the connection of the two points in the long axis of the frog, of which, however, only one must be on the trunk of the animal, shows the presence of an inherent electric current flowing in the same direction. E. Du Bois-Reymond, however, was the first to succeed in demonstrating the presence of specific muscle and nerve currents, by the deflection of the magnetic needle, aided by a very powerful multiplier, to comprehend the laws of the muscle and nerve currents, the changes they both undergo through muscular or nervous action, and to regard the frog-current as being the result of all the several electric currents present in the nerves, muscles, and other tissues.

To this end he distinguished on a long, fresh piece of nerve (sciatic) or muscle (gastrocnemius) of a live frog: 1, the outer surface—the longitudinal section; 2, the transverse section; 3, a line passing around the tissue midway between the apices—the equator. He found that, if, when the muscle was in a state of rest, relaxed, and the nerve in a condition of inaction, two points, lying symmetrically to the equator or the longitudinal axis, were placed in connection with the galvano-multiplier, no deviation of the muscle followed. On the contrary, if the two points lay unsymmetrically to the equator or the long axis, a deflection of the needle took place, which was all the more considerable, the nearer the one and the farther the other point in the longitudinal section was from the equator and in the transverse section from the long axis. The deflection is largely increased when the one point lies on the longitudinal section, and the other on the transverse section.

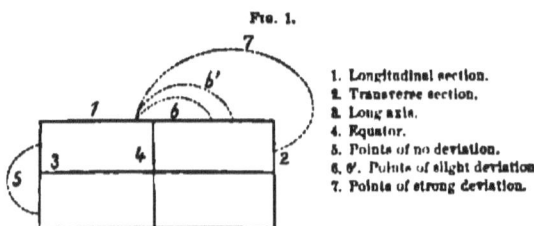

Fig. 1.

1. Longitudinal section.
2. Transverse section.
3. Long axis.
4. Equator.
5. Points of no deviation.
6, 6'. Points of slight deviation.
7. Points of strong deviation.

The direction of the current is always from the longitudinal section to the transverse section, and in such manner that the points of the surface lying near the equator are positive in relation to those near the ends, while these latter are positive in relation to the transverse section.

It further appeared that every artificial transverse section of the brain or spinal marrow is negative in relation to the natural surface of the axis of the brain or spinal marrow. On the contrary, there appears to be no electro-motor difference between the nerves of motion and sensibility, or between the gray and white brain-substance.

Du Bois-Reymond likewise ascertained that if the nerve or muscle be excited by electric currents or by mechanical or chemical irritants, so that the first is rendered physiologically active, and the latter caused to contract, and then placed at two symmetrical points in connection with the galvano-multiplier, a less deflection of the needle is produced than when the nerve or muscle is in a quiescent state. This he called the negative variation of the current. He found, also, that the needle remained in this new position only so long as the nerve or muscle was kept in the state of excitation, and that when the excitation ceased the quiescent nerve-current reappeared. This is the uniform action of the nerves and muscles on the magnetic needle. The piece of nerve or muscle may be thin or thick, short or long; the intensity of the current, as indicated by the deviation of the needle, increasing with an addition to the length or to the size of the transverse section.

From these facts Du Bois-Reymond concluded that nerve and muscle contain innumerable positive and negative electric molecules, which move with great regularity through the tissue. The variation of the negative current seems to be due to the fact that during excitation the electric molecules of the nerves and muscles are kept in motion, and the intensity and direction of the electric current consequently subjected to continual variation. The needle, however, being too slow in its movements to follow, takes a middle position.

In regard to the grouping of the nerve and muscle molecules, if we admit that nerve-tissue consists of an undefined

mass of peripolar molecules, everywhere enclosed by a moist
layer, and that collectively these molecules are composed of
one positive equatorial and two negative polar zones, of
which the last connecting axes collectively run parallel with
the long axis of the nerve, then the peculiarities of the
nerve and muscle currents are explained. In this case we
will imagine to ourselves an illustration similar to the one
we imagined to explain the phenomena of magnetism. Suppose the magnet to be composed of molecules, each one of
which produces precisely the same phenomena as the magnet itself; so here the nerve is composed of molecules, each
one of which produces the same currents as those produced
by the nerve of which it is a component part. We are,
however, justified in this supposition, because we always see
—as Du Bois-Reymond has demonstrated—even in the several small nerves in which we are able to expose a piece of
sufficient size for observation, the currents reappear subject
to the same laws. This arrangement also explains to us
why the needle remains in repose when two points, equidistant from the equator and long axis, are placed in connection. In this case, as well as in all cases of a battery
closed with an arch of like structure in all its parts, what
we said in speaking of the Voltaic pile holds true—namely,
that in the middle there is a neutral point, proceeding from
which on either side the tension increases. It explains
further that, when we connect two points, unsymmetrical in
position to the equator or the long axis, that is, two points
of unequal tension, the needle is deflected in proportion to
the degree of tension; and, finally, it explains the direction
of the currents, since points of less electric tension are to be
considered as positive when opposed to those of stronger
electric tension.

The action of electricity on the non-striated so-called organic muscles of the stomach, intestines, ovaries, urethra,
etc., is analogous, according to Du Bois-Reymond's experiments, to the action on the striated muscles. The only dif

ference which seems to exist between the two forms is, that the current of the non-striated muscles causes a far less deflection of the needle than that of the striated muscles. The lungs, liver, kidneys, spleen, testicles, skin, elastic tissues, etc., also possess electric currents that are demonstrable by the aid of the galvanometer. These currents, however, are not governed by the same laws that govern the muscle and nerve currents. The sinews, fasciæ, sheaths of the muscular fibres, etc., are electrically inactive, and only conduct the currents of the various tissues.

On account of their importance, we must call especial attention to two conclusions resulting from the theory just adduced:

1. Since, according to this theory, every nerve-molecule produces electric currents which are enclosed by the moist membrane that surrounds them and by the entire substance of the nerve, we must always imagine the nerve in the condition of a closed battery.

2. We must not conclude solely from a slight deviation of the needle—which the galvanometer usually shows, despite the powerful multiplicator, when we test the intensity of the muscle or nerve current—that the muscle or nerve current is weak, for every current, in whatever manner taken from an animal, must be sustained as a secondary connection, and considered as a derivative current. Thus the current indicated by the galvanometer shows but a small fraction of the currents that exist, not only in the muscle generally, but even of those currents which pass between the points connected by the wires of the multiplicator.

Du Bois-Reymond has also shown that the phenomena of the negative-current oscillation exist in the human body, and that the multiplicator indicates a weaker current in a muscle when voluntarily contracted than when it is in repose. Joh. Müller[1] describes this experiment in the follow-

[1] Bericht über die neuesten Fortschritte der Physik, Band I., Pag. 843. Braunschweig, 1849–1852.

ing manner: " The copper handle of an induction-apparatus was attached to the ends of the two wires of a multiplicator of 37,000 coils. So soon as we took hold of them with our moist hands, the needle of the multiplicator left the point of equilibrium, made a few oscillations, and then became quiet again, although perhaps not exactly in its original position. If, now, we contracted the muscles of one arm and one hand, while we grasped the handle firmly, the needle immediately turned from 10 to 20 degrees toward one side. Now, if, at the moment the needle began to move in the opposite direction, we relaxed the muscles of one arm and contracted those of the other, we saw the needle go still farther in the contrary direction. If we changed in this wise the contraction of the muscles of the arms at the proper moments, the oscillations ranged from 40 to 45 degrees on each side." The needle, then, remains in repose so long as the circuit continues closed by the relaxed muscles of both arms; the deviation which takes place at the moment of the connection is probably the consequence of the electric dissimilarity arising from the unequal muscular tension of the arms, as well as of momentary difference of time in the touch of the hands. If, for example, we contract the muscles of the right arm, the current passes, in consequence of the lessened electro-motor activity in this arm, from the left arm through the multiplicator to the right arm, causing the needle to deviate in unison with this direction. If we then relax the muscles of the right arm, and contract those of the left, at the moment when the needle begins to return, the current will pass from the right arm through the multiplicator to the left, causing the needle to make another stroke in the opposite direction, that is, in the direction of the current; but this time the deviation will be greater, because the difference in tension between the contracted muscles of the left and right arm is greater than between the contraction of the right side and the relaxation of the left.

We come now to the electrical phenomena exhibited by a nerve when it is brought, at any point in its course, into the circuit of a constant battery—a condition to which Du Bois-Reymond has given the name of *Electrotonus*. This observer[1] found that, when we galvanize a piece of nerve by means of a current of uniform power, the original inherent nerve-current undergoes a change, and, indeed, is increased in power, when the artificial current has the same direction as the inherent current; on the contrary, the inherent current is weakened, or entirely overcome, when the artificial current flows in the contrary direction. These manifestations of the electro-tonic condition are designated in nerve physics by the following expressions: The piece of nerve between the poles of the battery is called the *irritated*, the piece in the circuit of the multiplicator is called the *derivative*. If the nerve-current is increased, it is said to be in the *positive phase*; if it is decreased, it is said to be in the *negative phase*. The increase takes place when the *positive* electrode (the anode) is nearest the transverse section, the decrease when the *negative* electrode (the cathode) is nearest. Since the nerve has a transverse section on both sides of the constant stream, the two conditions appear simultaneously on each nerve. On the side of the positive electrode the nerve-current through the electrotonus is increased (positive phase of the electrotonus, or anelectrotonus); on the side of the negative electrode the current is weakened (negative phase of the electrotonus, or catelectrotonus). The electrotonic condition appears simultaneously with the closing of the generating battery, continues so long as the battery remains closed, and disappears simultaneously with the opening. The degree of the electrotonic increase, as well as of the deflection of the needle caused by the increase, depends on a variety of circumstances. It increases, not only with the length of the galvanized piece of nerve, but also with its proximity to the

[1] *L. c.*, vol. ii., pp. 289-389.

piece of nerve introduced into the circuit of the multiplicator; it is disproportionably greater when the exciting current flows longitudinally than when it crosses the nerve at a right angle. The degree increases further with the density of the exciting current; it, however, soon reaches its maximum, beyond which no increase takes place. It reaches finally, under like conditions, in a fresh and vigorous nerve, a point from which it descends with the decrease of nervous vigor, disappearing when the physiological powers of the nerve cease. If a portion of a muscle be traversed by a constant current, it will also be placed in the electrotonic condition. The electrotonus of the muscles differs, however, from that of the nerves in the following particulars: 1. It continues to increase in strength after the electrotonic current has ceased. 2. It is confined to the portion through which the current flows, while the electrotonus of the nerve extends with diminished strength beyond this limit on both sides.

The illustration we imagined to explain the phenomena of the quiescent current—the current produced by a regular series of peripolar molecules embedded in a moist layer—will serve to illustrate the electrotonus produced by the dipolar-nerve molecules that are arranged in the manner of the Voltaic pile. In this case all the nerve-molecules lying between the electrodes would be so arranged, that they would turn their negative elements toward the positive and their positive elements toward the negative electrode. This is easily imagined if we suppose each peripolar molecule of the quiescent current to be composed of two dipolar molecules with their positive zones touching each other—such molecules as they are resolved into at the closing of the battery. This illustration explains all the phenomena of the electrotonic condition. On the one hand, it shows how opposite phases are exhibited at the ends of a nerve traversed by an electric current; on the other, it explains the degrees of the electrotonic condition incident to the density of the current, the proximity to the electrodes, and finally to the angle at which the electrode is brought into contact with the nerve.

If an uninterrupted electric current be made to pass through a nerve in any part of its course, whether in the same or in various directions, the nerve is said to be *tetanized*—an expression that is justified by the fact that a muscle connected with a nerve treated in the manner just described responds, not only with one simple convulsive jerk, but with a series of twitches which terminate in a contraction of considerable duration, so that the muscle may be said to be in a tetanic state. If the tetanized currents flow in the same direction, the interruptions succeed each other at certain intervals; and, if the intensity of the current is inconsiderable, the action becomes similar to that of the continued current, and the phase of the electrotonic condition appears. If the tetanized currents flow in the same direction, appearing only momentarily, both phases soon follow in their usual form; the positive, however, is generally weaker. In this case the nerve-current quickly decreases, as in the use of Saxton's battery. If, finally, the tetanized currents flow in various directions, the interruptions follow each other in rapid succession, as with the Volta induction-apparatus with a Wagner hammer attached. Thus, under all circumstances, the negative-current oscillation is secured.

Of the action of quiescent electricity on the animal tissues on the parts or the whole of the animal body we know nothing. Furthermore, much as has been said of the effect of the electric tension of the atmosphere on the physical condition, etc., there have thus far been no experiments made which furnish data to justify the assertion that the free constant tension long continued exerts a demonstrable influence on any animal part whatever.

FOURTH SECTION.

THE ACTION OF THE ELECTRIC CURRENTS ON THE ORGANS AND TISSUES OF THE ANIMAL BODY.

A. *The action of the electric current on the nerves and muscles.*

Ludwig's Lehrbuch der Physiologie, vol. I., pp. 102, *seq.* E. Du Bois-Reymond, Untersuchungen über thierische Electricität, vol. I., pp. 303-409—282, *seq.*, etc. Mémoire sur l'emploi de l'Électricité en Méd. par le Dr. H. Valerius. Annales de la Société de Méd. de Gand, vol. xxix., pp. 115-154. A. Fick, Die Medicinische Physik, 1856, pp. 437, *seq.* H. Wundt, Lehrbuch der Physiologie des Menschen. Erlangen, 1865, pp. 430, *seq.* R. Heidenhayn, Physiologische Studien, Berlin, 1856, Art. III., p. 55. Ueber Wiederherstellung der erloschenen Erregbarkeit durch constante galvanische Ströme. C. Eckhardt in Henle's und Pfeuffer's Zeitschrift, 1853, vol. iii., pp. 187, *seq.* Eckhardt, Beiträge zur Anatomie und Physiologie, Heft I. Giessen, 1855, Art. II. Ueber den Einfluss des constanten galvanischen Stromes auf die Erregbarkeit der motorischen Nerven. E. Pflüger in der Medicinischen Central-Zeitung vom 15. März und 16. Juli, 1856. Ueber die durch constante Ströme erzeugte Veränderung der motorischen Nerven. E. Pflüger, Ueber das Hemmungsnervensystem für die peristalischen Bewegungen der Gedärme, Berlin, 1857. R. Remak, Galvanotherapie des Nerven- und Muskelkrankheiten, Berlin, 1858. E. Pflüges, Untersuchungen über die Physiologie des Electrotonus, Berlin, 1859. A. von Bezold, Untersuchungen über die electrische Erregung der Nerven und Muskeln, Leipzig, 1861. H. Ziemssen, die Electricität in der Medicin, III. Auflage, 1866.

I. ACTION OF THE CURRENT ON MOTOR NERVES AND MUSCLES.

If a motor nerve be subjected to the action of only a moderately intense INTERMITTING CURRENT, there will follow, in all the muscles supplied by this nerve, a series of spasmodic contractions, so that, if the several closings and open-

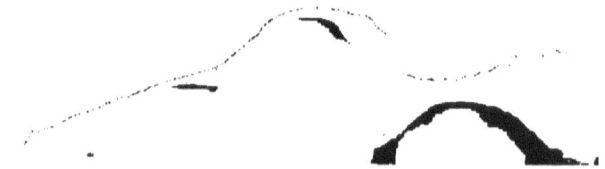

ings of the circuit follow one another slowly, clonic or intermitting spasms ensue, if they follow one another rapidly, in such manner that the new contraction begins before the preceding has ceased, rigid or tonic spasm results. If this condition has continued too long, or if the nerve originally possessed insufficient irritability, intermitting spasms will ensue. In the vigorous muscle of a frog, in the beginning at least, tonic spasms may appear, if even there are not more than two strokes in a second; a less number produce clonic spasms from the first.

The phenomenon, that a muscle contracts only at the closing and opening of the circuit, or only at the moment when the density of the current increases from nought to a certain degree, or descends again from this degree, but not between these two points, when the circuit remains closed and the density remains unchanged, finds its explanation in the fact that the contractions depend on the changing of the density of the current with the greatest possible rapidity. For this reason Du Bois-Reymond gave the following as the first law of the electric-irritation experiments:[1] "It is not the absolute grade of the current density at each moment to which the motor nerve, by a contraction of its muscle, responds, but to the change that takes place in the grade of density from one moment to another. Thus the power of producing the contractions that follow these changes is increased the more rapid the changes are when alike in degree, or the greater they are in a given length of time."

If we have, therefore, a given quantity of electricity, and conduct it in a current of unvarying power through a muscle, the current intensity remains the same from the closing of the circuit to the opening; consequently, during this time, no contractions take place. The same quantity, conducted in an interrupted current, will produce tonic or clonic spasms, according as the interruptions follow one an-

[1] *L. c.*, p. 258.

other more or less rapidly. It is, however, not absolutely necessary, in order to produce the contractions, that the current passing over the nerve should be closed or open, since by this means only the greatest oscillations of the current are produced; more limited variations in the intensity of the current are sufficient for physiological effects: for example, if we suddenly increase or decrease the intensity of the current, or if we suddenly conduct away by a closed circuit a portion of the current that passes over a nerve, or if we conduct, as is the case with Remak's "labile" currents, with the current generators slowly over the surface of the body; in short, if we in any way change the resistance, or if we, by chemical irritation, etc., modify the arrangement of the nerve molecules.

If a muscle be subjected to the action of an interrupted current, only that portion will contract—either exclusively or at least much more energetically—that comes in direct contact with the conductors. As a consequence, in order to irritate a broad muscle by direct action completely and evenly, we must, little by little, bring the conductors into contact with all its fibres. The experiments of A. Fick[1] have also demonstrated that, if an irritant reaches a bundle of muscular fibres only in a limited portion of its length, it contracts only in such portion of its length—the irritated condition, consequently, does not extend over the whole length of the muscle—and that in like manner, by the application of the multiplicator to a portion of the muscle not contracted, the quiescent current continues unchanged, while the contracted portion shows the negative-current oscillation.

Duchenne called the susceptibility of the muscles to contract under the direct action of the current *electro-muscular contractility*, in contradistinction to the indirect action, that is, the irritation of the nerve, called by Flourens motricity.

[1] Ueber theilweise Reizung der Muskelfasern in Moleschott's Untersuchungen zur Naturlehre des Menschen, vol. ii., p. 62, et seq.

The phenomena of the muscular contractions are accompanied by a peculiar sensation. Duchenne calls the power to experience this sensation, *electro-muscular sensibility*. It has not yet been decided whether this sensibility is due to the sensitive nerve-fibres which are found in all nerves, even the motor, or whether it is due to the sensitive nerves of the tissue surrounding the muscle, as Remak[1] is inclined to believe, or finally, whether the muscle-nerves themselves produce the sensation, as Eckhard[2] thinks possible.

The relation of the electro-muscular contractility and sensibility varies in different individuals. Every muscle, in a normal condition, possesses a certain amount of both. Sometimes, however, there is a slight difference between the same muscles of the two sides of the body. In diseased conditions, both, or each separately, may more or less completely disappear; and thus they become an important aid in diagnosis. But this we shall fully consider in Section VIII.

The gradual difference of the electro-muscular contractility and sensibility between the various muscles of the same individual is caused partly by anatomical relations—for example, in the case of the preponderance of the flexors of the hand over the extensors, we require a more powerful current to produce a contraction of the extensor digt. com. than a contraction of the flexor digt. com.—partly by the greater or less abundance of the sensitive fibres that are distributed to the motor nerves, and come in contact with the conductors; and partly by the difference of the resistance offered by the cellular tissue covering the irritated muscle; and, above all, by the thinner or thicker epidermis. Thus the muscles of the face are generally very sensitive, and above all the frontalis, because it lies immediately on the bone, and consequently, in faradizing it, the bone is also electrized, and thus a peculiar pain in the bone will be experienced together with the pain in the muscle. Then fol-

---

[1] Ueber methodische Electrisirung gelähmter Muskeln, Berlin, 1855, p. 19.
[2] Grundzüge der Physiologie des Nervensystems, Giessen, 1854, p. 113.

low the orbicularis palpebr., the levator labii sup. alæque
na-i; then the sphincter oris, the levator ang. oris, the quadratus and triangularis menti; and finally, the zygomatici,
the masseter, buccinator, etc. On the neck, the platysma
myoides possesses an unusual degree of electro-muscular contractility and sensibility, also the sterno-cleido-mastoideus;
on the other hand, the muscles of the back and abdomen
are but slightly sensitive. The anterior muscles of the forearm possess far greater electro-muscular contractility and
sensibility than the posterior muscles. The extensor digt.
com., extensor carpi uln., etc., possess a very low grade.
Finally, the tensor fasciæ latæ and the muscles of the inner
portion of the thigh are much more susceptible than the
muscles of the outer and posterior portions, partly on account of the greater supply of sensitive nerves in the skin
and on account of the large quantity of sensitive fibres distributed to the part by the nervus obturatorius, partly on
account of the thinner epidermis, and partly on account of
the more superficial situation—while the electric current, in
order to reach the muscles of the outer portion of the thigh,
must pass through a thick epidermis, a thin layer, comparatively poor in sensitive nerve-fibres, and a thick layer
of adipose and cellular tissue.

The contractions that arise by direct or indirect galvanic action are accompanied by a notable increase of
temperature. Matteucci[1] found that, by the simple contractions of the muscles in the frog, after the circulation
had entirely ceased, the temperature was increased $\frac{1}{4}°$ C.;
Ziemssen, after a series of careful experiments, concludes that
the muscle-contractions caused by faradic irritation of the motor nerves increase the temperature in the contracting muscles
and in the skin of the part according to the grade and duration of the action. He was able, in a séance of nineteen
minutes (see Experiment IV.), during which he let the cur-

[1] Ueber Muskelcontraction—Referat aus: Proc. of the Royal Society, 1856.
Vol. viii., No. 22, in Virchow's Archiv, 1857. Band xii., Heft I., p. 118.

rent act ten minutes, including interruptions, to cause an increase of temperature of 4.4° C. In the first minute of the muscular contraction, the mercury fell almost invariably from 0.1° to 0.5° C.; it rose, however, in the third minute, if the contraction was prolonged, and then continued unchanged. When the contractions were of moderate duration, after they had ended, the mercury rose in the first minute most rapidly, but reached its maximum height at the first irritation always in from four to six minutes; at the later irritations, it reached its maximum height somewhat sooner. The increase in temperature was accompanied by an increase in volume, which, when the extensors were contracted in the forearm, amounted to from ½ to 1 cm., in the thigh to from 1 to 2 cm. Heidenhain[1] has lately shown that the above-mentioned sinking of the temperature at the beginning of the contractions has its cause in the imperfection of the experiments, and that the temperature immediately rises with the appearance of tetanization, at first slowly, then more rapidly. The tetanus is followed by an increase of warmth caused by oxidation which is produced by the muscular contractions, and seems to promote the circulation in so far, only, as it furnishes material for the oxidizing process.

If a motor nerve be subjected to the action of a CONSTANT CURRENT at the moment when the circuit is closed and at the moment it is opened, the muscle supplied by the nerve will contract: closing contraction—opening contraction. During the time the constant battery is closed, an effect is either not at all or in a much slighter degree noticeable. Remak[2] arrived at the following results: 1. Tonic muscle contractions may also be produced by the constant current,

[1] Mechanische Leistung, Wärmenentwicklung und Stoffumsatz bei der Muskelthätigkeit. Ein Beitrag zur Theorie der Muskelkräfte. Leipzig, 1864.
[2] *L. c.*, p. 56, *et seq.*

but it is necessary to conduct a powerful and painful current over the nerve (from 20 to 50 of Daniell's elements). 2. A current can cause unbearable pain, without producing a tonic contraction, while in another individual, or in the same individual at another time, the same current produces powerful contractions, and very little or no pain. 3. The production of the contractions was generally facilitated by the sudden application of the electrodes to the nerve; cases occurred, however, in which the contractions did not begin in the compass of the nerve until the conductor was slowly withdrawn from the nerve, with which it had been for about a minute in contact. The contractions continued as long as the conductor acted on the nerve by contact with the skin. 4. If the contractions did not appear at the first contact, they often did at the second, after the current had traversed the nerve for a minute or more. Remak called the contraction produced by the constant current in the manner described the galvano-tonic contraction, to distinguish it from the tetanic or clonic contraction, which is produced by frequent induction-shocks, or by the frequently-interrupted constant current. With regard to the explanation of these phenomena, according to Remak, the galvano-tonic contractions, produced in the human organism by the action of the constant current on a nerve, belong to the list of the phenomena resulting from the variations of the current intensity, to which Du Bois's law concerning the current oscillation, already given, is likewise applicable. Remak observed that the tetanus did not appear, however powerful the current, unless the electrodes were connected with the limbs by moist threads, or were in direct contact with the muscles. But if the irritability of the muscular fibres be increased, they undergo a delicate twitching, which prevents the nerve being acted upon in a similar manner. The bearing of the nerve will therefore be the same as when it is alternately brought near to and removed from the most dense current, without ever being entirely withdrawn beyond its influence, that is, the component parts of the nerve will, on account of the variable resistance introduced, be subjected to the action of currents of variable density, and consequently the muscles supplied by these nerves will undergo contractions, which are either really tonic, that is, without any apparent interruptions, or which are concealed from observation by the skin and tissue that cover them.[1] 5. The majority of persons, particularly young, muscular persons, showed, under like circumstances, only tonic contractions in the compass of the galvanized nerve. And further, in the same person a contraction was observed, now within the compass of the galvanized nerve, and now within the compass of its antagonist, on different days, as the result of the same operation. The influence of the will in these cases did not extend beyond preventing the antagonistic contractions; but then there usually followed, on the appearance of the current, tonic contractions in the compass of those muscles and nerves to which the will was directed. This struggle between the antagonistic group of muscles was not unfrequently apparent when it was quite independent of the will; and it happened in some instances that one contraction, for example, the flexion, ceased during the flow of the current, and passed to the antagonistic, that is, into the extension, and *vice versa*. These antagonistic galvano-tonic contractions are said, by the same author, to be reflex contractions, which proceed from the central organs, in consequence of the irritation of the sensitive nerves, which occurs when they are under electric influence.

The opinion also formerly prevailed, with regard to the muscles, that they responded with contractions only to the closing and opening of the circuit. Wundt, Von Bezold, and Fick observed, on the contrary, that the muscles continue contracted so long as the current passes through them. Wundt, especially, found that when he killed animals with curare—which, as is well known, destroys the irritability of

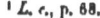
[1] *L. c.*, p. 68.

the nerves, but not of the muscles—the convulsive jerk at the opening and closing disappeared, while the continued contraction remained. The intensity of the current that acts on the nerve and muscle exerts a notable influence on the extent and character of the irritation, as well with regard to the result of each closing and opening as with regard to the result of the continued closing of the circuit. In the first instance, the direction the constant current takes is worthy of notice, according as it is turned from a more central to a more peripheric transverse section (descending current), or from a more peripheric to a more central transverse section (ascending current). When the current is of medium strength, opening and closing contractions follow; on the contrary, when the current is very strong or very weak, only one contraction results, and, indeed, with a weak ascending current, only a closing contraction; with a strong ascending current, only an opening contraction; with a strong descending current, only a closing contraction.

The law observed in muscular contractions accords perfectly with the law that governs nervous contractions, when the part of the muscle directly irritated is separated from the part showing the irritation by its contractions. If, on the contrary, the whole muscle be enclosed in the circuit, the most energetic contractions will generally be the closing, to which, when the current is increased, the opening contractions will be added. But, the worse the nerve in the muscle performs its functions, the more the closing contractions preponderate over the opening contractions. So far as concerns the consequence of the closing, the weakest and strongest currents have no effect on the motor nerves, while currents of medium intensity produce a series of distinct twitches or a tetanic contraction. In the muscle, on the contrary, the contraction that continues during the closing increases with the intensity of the current.

The irritability of the nerve is of notable influence in the production of the contractions. In this regard, Du

LAWS OF THE CONSTANT CURRENT. 53

Bois-Reymond, by experimenting on frogs, arrived at the following results: 1. Contractions of apparently equal power appear with the highest grade of irritability at each closing and opening of the descending current, that is, from the spinal marrow toward the muscle, or with the ascending current, from the muscle toward the spinal marrow. I say apparent, because the energy of the contraction makes a gradual distinction impossible. 2. With a medium grade of irritability, on the contrary, which the frog originally possesses or soon acquires through the weakening of the irritability by the current (see below), at the closing of the descending current, a very powerful contraction appears; at the closing, a very weak contraction, or perhaps none at all. The reverse takes place with the ascending current—that is, at the closing, either a very weak or perhaps no contraction ensues; at the opening, a very powerful contraction. There are many exceptions to the rule established by Ritter[1] and verified by Nobili.[2] For instance, we sometimes see, when under a steady action the irritability has penetrated still deeper, the disconnecting contraction increase in relative strength to the closing contraction, probably because the nerve has, in a measure, lost its susceptibility to this irritation by the preceding energetic closing contractions, while it has retained its susceptibility for the opening of the circuit. According to Longet and Matteucci,[3] this reversion of the usual phenomena takes place normally in the anterior roots of the spinal nerves of the dog, rabbit, frog, etc. For, if we let the current act on these roots instead of on the trunk of the nerve, after it leaves the canal of the spinal marrow, contractions follow at the closing and opening of the ascending and descending cur-

---

[1] Bewels, dass ein beständiger Galvanismus den Lebensprozess im Thierreiche begleitet. See Ritter's phys.-chem. Abhandlungen in chronologischer Folge. Leipzig, 1806.
[2] Annales de Chimie et Physique, Mai, 1833, t. xliv.
[3] Comptes rendus de l'Académie, etc., du 9 Septembre, 1844, t. xix., p. 574.

rent, at first, it is true, later; however, the phenomena arrange themselves invariably so, that a continued contraction follows the closing of the ascending current, and a less durable contraction follows the opening of the descending current, while both are wanting at the opening of the ascending current and closing of the descending current. Since the nerves lose their vitality from the centre toward the circumference, it may be that the excitability in the anterior roots of the spinal nerves decreases rapidly to a degree where a return of the phenomena occurs, until finally, when the irritability is entirely lost, no twitching at all is apparent.[1]

We will now treat of the law in its more specific sense, to which these twitchings are subjected; that is, we will answer the question relative to the *closing and opening of the circuit*, when the current is variously directed, in relation to the motor and sensitive nerves.

The law that applies here is that of Marianini—that the descending current, at the closing, after the closing, and at the opening of the circuit, causes more pain; while the ascending current, at the closing and opening of the circuit, causes greater contraction. Remak[2] succeeded, with a certain intensity of current—between 20 and 30 of Daniell's elements—in producing only pain with the descending current, and only twitching with the ascending current, when he avoided the nerves of the skin running over the biceps muscle. With a greater intensity of current—40 elements, and upward—closing contractions were observed, not only when the current ascended, but also when it descended; they were, however, more powerful when the current flowed in the former direction. By frequently changing the direction of the current, and especially by varying the action of the constant currents, this difference may, it is true, be rendered almost imperceptible. A reversion of the law of con-

---

[1] Gilbert and Ritter's Annalen der Physik, p. 824.
[2] Galvanotherapie, p. 114.

traction often takes place in diseased limbs in such a manner, that the ascending current causes more pain, while the descending current causes more twitching. Remak found further, that, when we let the current act in such manner that one conductor is in contact with a point of the nerve, while the other is in contact with any portion of the body (*unipolar application of the current*), the positive electrode is endowed with nearly all the functions which the descending current discharges, and the negative electrode is endowed with the functions of the ascending current.

If we turn now to the changes in the irritability of the nerve in the electrotonus, which were first studied by Eckhard, and the errors of whose assertions were corrected by Pflüger, we shall find they obey, according to the last-named author, the following law: If a constant current be conducted over a portion of a nerve, during its flow the irritability will be altered, not only in the intrapolar portion, but also in any given extrapolar portion, in either direction, and it is increased within the compass of the negative electrode, the cathode; on the contrary, it is lessened within the compass of the positive electrode, the anode. The law may be thus expressed: Every portion of a nerve in the condition of the catelectrotonus possesses an increased, and every portion of nerve in the condition of the anelectrotonus a diminished, irritability. Between the electrodes there is a point at which the catelectrotonus goes over into the anelectrotonus, and at which the irritability remains unchanged. The position of this point depends upon the constant current; the stronger the current, the nearer the negative electrode. In the extra-polar portions, the irritability decreases with the withdrawal of the electrodes, until at last it entirely ceases.

The changes in the irritability of a muscle when it is in the electrotonic condition differ from the changes that take place in a nerve, therein that they, like the electrotonic condition itself, are confined to the muscle over which the current passes. An irritation produced above or below the portion of muscle over which the constant current passes has, consequently, no influence on the degree of the contractions.

Remak had already [1] endeavored to demonstrate that the changes in the irritability of healthy and diseased nerves and muscles were phenomena resulting from the electrotonic conditions, but he failed to adduce the physical proof of the correctness of his opinion. A. Eulenburg [2] succeeded in placing certain superficial motor nerves (accessorius, medianus, ulnaris, peronaeus) and muscles (deltoideus and opponens pollicis) in the electrotonic condition. For example, by bringing into contact with the N. accessorius, directly at its entrance into the M. trapezius, a small button-shaped negative electrode of the induction apparatus, whose positive electrode, provided with a broader surface, was pressed to the sternum, and then above the negative electrode passing an ascending or descending current—depending on his desire to test the anelectrotonus or the catelectrotonus—over the N. accessorius, in the first case (descending extrapolar anelectrotonus) he was able to prove that there was a negative, and in the second case (descending extrapolar catelectrotonus) a positive increase of the irritability of the portion of nerve lying beyond the current. The experiments demonstrated, further, that the amount of the positive and negative increase, as well as also the duration of the after-effect (especially in the catelectrotonus), generally answered to the strength of the current and the duration of closing.

With regard to the muscles, when the object was to demonstrate the intrapolar anelectrotonus and catelectrotonus, Eulenburg proceeded in such wise that, in examining the ane-

---

[1] *l. c.*, p. 92.
[2] Ueber Electrotonisirende Wirkungen bei percutaner Anwendung des constanten Stromes auf Nerven und Muskeln. Deutsches Archiv. für Klin Medicin, lii. vol., 1867, p. 117, *et seq.*

lectrotonus, he placed the negative electrode of the induction
current, applied to the muscle itself, near the anode, and in examining the catelectrotonus he placed the electrode near the
cathode. Here, also, the positive increase with the catelectrotonus was apparent; the negative increase with the anelectrotonus less so.

Not only, however, is the irritability changed, but the
POWER TO CONDUCT THE IRRITABILITY is also changed, being diminished in the anelectrotonic as well as in the
catelectrotonic portions. Betzold found that this decrease
in the rapidity of transmission reaches its maximum near
the electrodes, and sinks from these points toward the intrapolar as well as toward the extrapolar portions, but the decrease extends farther on the side of the anode than on the
side of the cathode. Another phenomenon, also discovered
by Betzold, is connected with this decreased conductivity
in the electrotonus, that it is longer before the twitching
appears, when the nerve is irritated by the closing of chain
currents (TIME OF THE LATENT IRRITATION), than when by
opening shocks. If it is a descending current, this delay is
noticeable with weak currents only; with stronger currents
the twitchings immediately appear. If, however, it is an
ascending current, so that the stimulus must pass the point
traversed by the current and the anelectrotonic point before
the twitching appears, the moment of the latent irritation
will often be noticeable. These facts can be explained only
by admitting—1. That at every entrance of a constant current into the nerve a moment of preparation transpires
before the irritation appears, which preparatory moment
gradually decreases with the increase in the intensity of the
current; and 2. That at each closing of a constant current,
the irritation takes place only at the cathode, and the portions of nerve and muscle near the anode are only irritated,
if at all, by the transmission of the irritability induced by
the negative pole. A delay in the conductivity takes place
in an electrotonic muscle as well as in a nerve, but the

delay of the conductivity does not extend beyond the electrotonic portion.

THE AFTER-ACTION OF THE ELECTROTONUS is manifold. On the one hand it consists in change of irritability, which remains for a time after the electrotonus ceases, and on the other hand in an irritation that accompanies the transition from the electrotonus to the usual condition. The first of these conditions consists, according to the position of the electrodes, in an increased irritability (positive modification) or in a diminished irritability (negative modification). After its disappearance, the catelectrotonus leaves a negative modification of short duration behind, which soon gives way to a positive modification of greater duration, while the anelectrotonus is immediately transformed into a gradually-increasing positive modification. The second after-action of the constant current—the irritation with the open circuit—is caused by the disappearance of the anelectrotonus, and generally manifests itself by an opening contraction, but sometimes, when the constant current is of a certain duration, by an opening tetanus. Its seat is at the anode. Those transverse sections of nerves or muscles that are near the cathode are placed in an irritated condition, if at all, only by the transmission of the stimulus proceeding from the positive pole.

In the muscle, this after-action, as well as the direct action of the electrotonus, is confined to the portion traversed by the current. The opening of a constant current, that has passed over a muscle for a length of time, is followed by a continued contraction of the muscle, which relaxes very slowly. By closing the antagonistic current, the contraction is increased; by closing the currents flowing in the same direction, it is dissolved. Betzold thinks he is justified, by the results of his experiments, in coming to the conclusion that the irritating action of the galvanic current is due to the chemical effects produced by the current in the conductors over which it flows, and that the electric irritation is nothing else than a certain form of chemical irritation, whose process, like the hydrogen-generating process, during the closing of the current, appears directly only at the negative pole.

We have an additional after-action in the modification of the irritability of the nerves, which is produced by the change in the direction of the current. Ritter, who experimented with weak Voltaic piles, found that, when we let a frog's thigh remain for from thirty minutes to an hour in a closed circuit, its irritability changes. Then, with a descending current, no contraction will follow either the opening or closing of the circuit; with an ascending current, on the contrary, the contractions increase in strength the longer the closing is continued, until at last tetanus follows the opening of the circuit. According to Volta, who experimented with a more powerful apparatus, both directions of the current are depressing in their effects; the nerve, consequently, no matter what the direction of the constant current is, remains motionless. But, if we now change the direction of the current, so that, for example, the nerve is traversed by an ascending instead of a descending current, it will be found to be again irritable (Voltaic change). According to him, therefore, the ascending as well as the descending current would change the irritability of the nerve in such wise, that it renders the nerve insensitive to the stimulus of the direction of its own current, and sensitive to the antagonistic current. J. Rosenthal[1] has given the subject a thorough examination, and has succeeded in bringing all the facts relative to it under the following law: "Every constant current that for a length of time passes over a motor nerve places it in a condition in which the irritability is increased for the opening of the approaching current and the closing of the antagonist; on the contrary, it is diminished for the closing of the former and the opening of the latter."

[1] Monatsbericht der Königl. Preuss. Academie der Wissenschaften zu Berlin, Dec. 1857, p. 640.

A further action of the constant current on the muscles consists in the reëstablishing of their extinct irritability. Heidenhayn was the first to discover[1] that a muscle, that by fatigue or maltreatment of any kind—provided its vitality has not been entirely destroyed—has lost its irritability, will recover it, if the muscle be subjected for thirty seconds or more to the action of a sufficiently powerful (say from twenty-five of Daniell's elements) constant current. The two directions, however, are notably unlike. The descending current is weaker in its action, and loses its powers sooner, than the ascending. If the irritability of a muscle has been reëstablished by a constant current in this manner, the electrical stimulus has a peculiar effect on it. Thus, if a constant current has passed over a non-irritable muscle for a length of time in a certain direction, a contraction can be obtained, under the most favorable circumstances, by opening this current or closing its antagonist. If, also, for example, the ascending current be used to reëstablish the conductivity, contractions will be obtained, under the most favorable circumstances, by opening the ascending or closing the descending current. What Heidenhayn in this manner demonstrated on frogs, Remak observed on the living person. As a result of his experiments, he arrives at the following conclusions: *a.* The constant current increases the irritability in the sensitive as well as in the motor nerves. *b.* It increases the power of a muscle produced by the influence of an induction current. If, for example, we have tested the contractility of a muscle (the biceps, for instance) by means of a weak extra-current conducted over the nerve, and have found it to be feeble, and then conduct a constant current of from 20 to 25 elements, for from 15 to 60 seconds, over the nerve and muscle, the equally-intense induction current will now be able to effect a complete elevation of the upper arm. Fick[2] contends that similar experiments on himself produced negative re-

[1] *L. c.* [2] *L. c.*, p. 461.

sults, and is, therefore, of opinion that the revitalizing of an exhausted muscle on the living subject, by the use of the constant current, as recommended by Heidenhayn, is hardly possible. The result of my own observations inclines me to Remak's opinion. Especially in a case of congenital facial paralysis of the right side in a young man of twenty-four, the reactive power for the intermitting current was always increased, after subjecting the frontalis for 30 or 40 seconds to the action of a constant current of from 12 to 16 elements. The patient also asserted that the feeling of contraction was much stronger than before. In like manner, by means of an intense current, I was enabled, in several cases of lead paralysis, to increase the reaction of the extensors against the induced current. Remak, at the same time, observed[1] that the irritability of the muscles and nerves for induced currents, and for the entrance and exit of constant currents, so far as we can judge, as a rule, is equal; that there are cases, however, in healthy, and, of course, more frequently in diseased, limbs, where the irritability for one or the other current is greater. After Baierlacher, Schulz, Meyer, and Ziemssen had published a series of cases—all of them of facial paralysis—which gave as their result, that in completely paralyzed muscles and nerves the irritability for the constant current is sometimes not only sustained, but even increased, while the irritability for the interrupted current entirely ceases; and after much labor had been expended in vain endeavors to explain these phenomena satisfactorily, Neumann instituted a series of experiments on an appropriate case of facial paralysis,[2] in order to test physically the differential action of the induced and constant currents, which proved that a momentary duration of the constant current produces the irritating effects on paralyzed muscles and nerves, while these effects cannot be obtained by induced currents of momentary duration. Brückner's experiments

[1] *L. c.*, p. 93.   [2] Deutsche Klinik, 1864, No. 4.

on several patients affected with paralysis with fatty degeneration and atrophy,¹ and Ziemssen's observations on paralysis of the nerves of the arm,² prove the correctness of Neumann's views.

In conclusion, we must speak of the so-called paralyzing action of the constant current. Valentine³ was the first to assert that the constant current, so long as it traverses a portion of nerve with a given intensity, renders it incapable of transmitting contraction-producing stimulus. Matteucci attained similar results by a different series of experiments, and consequently recommended the application of the continued current as a remedy for tetanus. He tetanized frogs with strychnia, and then subjected them to the action of a direct continued current. The frogs died without any of the usual convulsions that accompany death caused by strychnia. Later, Eckhard⁴ made some experiments to discover the effect of the electrical stimulus on the nerves of the muscles, when a part of the nerve is subjected to the action of a continued current, and found that in this case contractions followed neither the mechanical nor chemical irritation, nor even the stimulus of the interrupted current. In other words, the nerve is paralyzed so long as any portion of it is subjected to the action of a continued current. The following peculiarities resulted from the application of the interrupted current as an irritant: 1. The relation between the intensity of the interrupted and constant currents is not unimportant. If the latter should neutralize the action of the former, it must not sink below a certain degree. 2. The paralyzing effect of the constant current is more apparent when it is placed between the muscle and the irritating battery than between the irritating battery and free end of the nerve. 3. The ascending direc-

¹ Deutsche Klinik, 1855, No. 30.
² Electricitat in der Medicin, 3d ed., 1856, p. 90, et seq., and pp. 73-95.
³ Lehrbuch der Physiologie des Menschen, vol. ii., sec. ii., p. 655, 1848.
⁴ Henle and Pfeuffer, l. c.

tion of the current in the constant circuit neutralizes more powerful irritating currents than the descending. From these facts Eckhard came to the following conclusions: Every muscular contraction to be expected under the influence of any irritation whatever can be avoided by means of a constant current, and every tetanus already existing may in like manner be removed. An additional series of experiments led Eckhard,[1] in partial contradiction to the above statements, to the following results: 1. If a constant current flows upward in a motor nerve, its irritability is decreased under the influence of every form of irritation, no matter at what point of the nerve it is applied. 2. But, if the current descends, a decrease of irritability will take place in and above the galvanized portion only; on the contrary, the irritability of the portion below the negative electrode will be increased. Pflüger has shown that not only these contradictions, but also the errors in the last two assertions of Eckhard, were due mainly to the fact that he did not consider the great dependency of the phenomena, in these cases, on the intensity of the constant current. In consideration of this fact, the above-named results, according to Pflüger,[2] should be expressed as follows: 1. When we irritate a motor nerve above a constant ascending current whose intensity does not pass a certain grade, the contractions are not weakened, as Eckhard supposed, but the reverse is true of the descending current of like intensity, when the irritation takes place above it. It is only when the intensity of the current passes a certain degree, that results are reversed. 2. The other statement of Eckhard, that with the ascending constant current the irritability of the nerve at every point is decreased, is also in the main incorrect. If, for example, the current does not pass a certain degree, the contractions produced by irritating a portion of the nerve above the portion reached by the constant current are

---

[1] Beiträge zur Anat. Physiol., 1855, l. c.
[2] Ueber das Hemmungs-nervensystem, etc., l. c., p. 8.

by no means weakened—on the contrary, they are singularly strengthened. But if the current passes a certain intensity, then the contrary is true, that is, the contractions are weakened.

Directly connected with the changes that are produced in the nerve and muscle by the electrotonus are those changes of irritability which are occasioned by the irritation itself, as well as by a variety of other influences, temperature, etc.—considerations which, on account of their practical importance, we should not fail to notice in this connection:

1. By the irritation itself sometimes an increase and sometimes a decrease of irritability will be produced. The first is observed when the stimulants follow one another with moderate rapidity, neither too quickly nor too slowly, and do not pass a certain duration and intensity. If the stimulants follow too rapidly, if they are too violent or too durable, a decrease of irritability will be quickly noticeable. The increase of the irritability by the irritation can, according to Wundt's observations, be so considerable, that, for example, an induction shock, that at first only stills a weak twitching, finally produces a forcible and durable tetanus. Wundt found also that, by the use of induction shocks of short duration, a difference existed, depending on the direction of the latter. Descending induction shocks proved much more effective than ascending, probably because in the latter case the irritation at the cathode must pass the anelectrotonic interception before reaching the muscle, while with the descending current the irritation is produced on the side toward the muscle. Hence it is that an increase of irritability produced by a descending induction current is increased by a constant current flowing in the same direction, and, on the contrary, decreased by a constant current flowing in the contrary direction. The decrease in irritability caused by

irritation or fatigue is observed especially when the stimulants follow one another rapidly or are too intense. Thus, frequent interruptions of the current of a powerful battery, as well as the individual shocks of a powerful induction current, have but little influence. So we see, further, not unfrequently, in pathological conditions in which a powerful induction current is necessary to produce muscular contraction, that after a time it fails to produce any contraction whatever. Further, the contraction, when the individual twitchings have become resolved into a continued (tetanic) contraction, decreases, at first rapidly, and later more and more slowly. If a muscle has been contracted for a short time only, its own inherent current—which, by the diminished deviation of the galvanometer needle, has indicated a change in its molecular condition—by the immediate return of the needle to its original position, indicates the undiminished strength of the muscular current; if, however, the muscular contraction has been of longer duration, the needle will take more time to return to its original position. Brown-Séquard's experiments on the enervating effects of the electric current are highly interesting to the student of these phenomena.[1] He subjected the hind-leg of a rabbit to the action of a powerful magneto-electric current, and then killed the animal. Two and a half hours afterward, the electrized limb was found to have stiffened, while the other hind-leg was still limber; two hours later, the rigidity of the faradized limb began to decrease, while it just began in the limb that was not faradized. A week later, the former was in a state of decomposition, while the latter was still rigid. He then took another rabbit, cut off both forelegs, and subjected one of them to the action of an electric current. The muscular irritability decreased slowly, until, at the expiration of ten minutes, it had so far disappeared, that rigidity began to be apparent. The other extremity was still irritable. In half an hour, the rigidity of the fara-

[1] Gaz. Méd. de Paris, 1819, pp. 881 and 999.

dized limb began to decrease, while it was five hours before there was any appearance of rigidity in the other. In a corresponding manner, decomposition had made considerable progress in one extremity, while the other was still rigid.

2. The irritability is preserved by the connection of the nerve with the brain and spinal marrow. In the living animal, a portion of nerve separated from the brain or spinal marrow changes its microscopic character after five or six days, and has then entirely lost its irritability. The muscles retain their irritability longer. In reference to these phenomena, Valli was the first to assert[1] that the vitality of the motor nerves was more in their ramifications than in their origins. In some cases, where the irritation of a portion of nerve situated near the origin failed to produce muscular contractions, they followed the irritation of a portion of the same nerve lying near the periphery. Nysten's law, according to which the rigidity of death proceeds from the portions nearer the brain toward the more distant, in the axis of the brain and spinal marrow from above downward, in every nerve from its origin toward its ramifications in the muscles, is a strong argument in favor of the correctness of Valli's theory. Matteucci and Longet[2] tell us that they have observed directly opposite phenomena in experimenting on the sensitive nerves, which lose their vitality first in their ramifications in the skin, and last at their origin in the brain and spinal marrow, and consequently the portions nearest the nervous centres retain their irritability longer than those near the periphery. These experiments with the sensitive nerves, on account of the difficulties attending them, have not, as yet, been verified. Ritter thought he had also discovered that the irritability of the flexors was much less than that of the extensors; yet the difference between the two consists only in the fact that the flexors sooner cease to react under the influence of the electric stimulus than the

---

[1] See Du Bois-Reymond, l. c., vol. i., pp. 822-326.
[2] Arch. Gén. de Méd., 1847.

extensors, and are the first to undergo decomposition, perhaps because the former are in connection with a higher point of the spinal marrow than the latter.

3. Interruption of the circulation also weakens the irritability. If we separate the lower from the upper portion of a frog in such a manner that they are connected by the nerve only, the irritability nevertheless continues for several days, although the nerves of parts well supplied with blood retain their irritability longer than those of parts poorly supplied. Kilian[1] found that if we open a blood-vessel of one leg of a frog, just killed, and extract the blood, while in the other leg the blood is retained, and then irritate the nerves of both extremities until no more contractions ensue, the nerves of the limb retaining its blood will soon recover so that renewed irritation will reproduce the contractions, while the nerves of the other (bloodless) limb will have entirely lost their susceptibility to electric irritation. Brown-Séquard[2] tied the aorta of a rabbit, above the ateriæ renales, and the muscles of the hind legs a few hours afterward ceased to contract in response to electrical irritation. When he loosened the ligature, however, the muscular irritability returned.

4. Bruises, lacerations, pressure, too high or too low temperature, notable derangement of nervous nutrition, in short, every thing that changes the nerve chemically, decreases the irritability. As for the influence of the temperature, Eckhard found that the nerves of a frog in water of 0° Réaumur became insensible in 45 seconds, and in water from −3° to −5° they become immediately insensible. At +30° R. their susceptibility to irritation continued from 12 to 15 seconds, and at from +55° to +60° R. the susceptibility was only momentary. Rosenthal[3] found that the motor

[1] Versuche ueber Restitution der Nerven—Erregbarkeit nach dem Tode. Giessen, 1857.
[2] Gaz. Méd., 1851, No. 37.
[3] Ueber den Einfluss hoherer Temperaturgrade auf Motersche Nerven. Notiz in der Medc. Central-Zeitung, 1859, No. 96.

nerves lose their sensibility at about +70° C., and that they retain it for a time at a lower temperature, for example, at +60°, about 4 or 5 seconds; at +50°, about 16 seconds; at +40°, more than 10 minutes, etc., that is, much longer than Eckhard states. On the contrary, the higher the temperature, provided it does not pass a certain limit, the greater the irritability. Thus Schelske[1] found, in experimenting with the nerve of a frog, that an irritation that was insufficient to overcome a contraction at 15° C., was quite sufficient at 18° C. An elevation to 36° C. caused a sudden increase, and then a continued decrease of the irritability. Important disturbances of nutrition supervening, the nerve-fibres—the oily matter of which has coagulated—no longer react under electric irritation. A certain decomposition takes place in the muscular fibres of long-paralyzed limbs. They appear paler and softer, lose their contractility, but preserve their transverse fibres. In these cases better nutrition may restore the contractility. If, however, the muscular fibres have degenerated into fat or cellular tissue, the irritability is hopelessly lost.

II. THE EFFECT OF THE ELECTRIC CURRENT ON THE NERVES OF SENSE AND THE SENSORY NERVES.

While on the irritation of the *motory* nerves the resulting phenomena are increased through the fluctuation of the current, it is otherwise with the special nerves of sense and the sensory nerves. It is true that their activity is heightened through the fluctuation of the current's intensity, but this also takes place when there is a gradual lessening of the irritation, even during the closure of the circuit. In other respects the sensory nerves behave as the motory—only,

[1] Ueber die Veränderungen der Erregbarkeit durch Wärme. Heidelberg, 1860.

since, on the other hand, the central nerve-end lies nearer to the organ perceiving the sensation than the peripheral end, the law of the electrical sensations assumes an opposite expression to the law of contraction, i. e., by a descending weak current there is only a sensation on closing the circuit; by a descending strong current there is only a sensation on opening the circuit; while, on the contrary, by an ascending current, the sensation on closing the circuit increases with the strength of the current.

If we allow the interrupted current to work on the skin, the following sensations differ according to the strength of the current, the frequency of the shocks, and the form of the conductors, and vary from a light tickling, pricking, burning sensation to the most severe pain. The increase of the pain with the greater frequency of the shocks, arises from the fact that the nerves of sense and the sensory nerves have the peculiarity of perceiving sensations for some time after the impression is made. A single shock of an induction apparatus causes only a light sensation; if, however, to this there follows quickly a second, the sensation is stronger, for to the effect of the first that of a second is added, and so, according to the quickness of the interruption of the current, the pain is increased in intensity. The form of the conductors we may so modify, by the use of metallic platinum, which easily takes the form of the body, or of cylindrical, globular, or conical tips, or, finally, of metallic threads, bound together in the form of a broom, from the points of which long crackling sparks easily pass to the skin, as to produce a degree of excitement which for the normal skin is insupportable, and which, even to the skin deprived of ordinary sensibility, is exceedingly painful.

If we connect the epidermis with the conducting wires of a Voltaic pile, there arises at the moment of closing the circuit a pricking, stinging, burning sensation which, with currents of certain intensities, may be increased till it becomes unendurable. This sensation, which is strongest at the moment of making the connection, exists with lessened intensity also during the closure of the circuit. The dry skin is much more sensitive than the moist, and, when deprived of its epidermis, a painful, burning point is produced.¹ There is a remarkable difference in the strength of the sensation, both by the use of the Voltaic pile and the induction apparatus, between the positive and negative poles; provided that the electrodes are of equal thickness, the negative pole always produces a more intense effect on the skin. We may easily assure ourselves of this by placing two similar conductors on two corresponding parts of the body; the burning sensation at the point touched by the negative pole will always be the stronger. The negative pole also produces a stronger effect on the motory nerves than the positive. If we expose, for instance, two homologous muscles of the face equally to the working of the current, the contraction of the one affected by the negative pole will be greater than that produced in the other.²

Moreover, all regions of the skin are not equally sensitive —the most sensitive, on account of its richness in nerves, is the face—and in this the most sensitive parts are: the points of issue of the trigeminus nerve, as the N. supraorbitalis from the for. supraorbitale, as the N. subcutaneus malæ from the for. zygomaticum, as the N. alveolaris inf. from

¹ *Vide* Humboldt's Versuche über die gereizte Muskel- und Nervenfaser, 1797. Tom. i., pp. 101, 197, etc.
² The determination of a pole as positive or negative is made most conveniently by the electrolysis of the iodide of potassium. If the conducting wires, tipped with platinum, of a battery, are placed on a piece of blotting-paper, saturated with a solution of starch paste and the iodide of potassium, immediately there appears on the positive pole, from the deposition of iodine, a blue spot. With the induction apparatus we fasten the ends of the secondary coil with the platinum wires (*vide* Section V., Duchenne's apparatus, or the following), secure the spring so that it does not vibrate, and then conduct the induced current, produced by breaking the primary current, through the filter-paper. Of course, if the terms positive and negative are to mean always the same thing, the primary current must always have the same direction, i. e., the positive pole of the battery must always be attached to the same binding screw.

the for. mentale, as well as the line of transition from the skin to the mucous membrane of the nose or of the mouth.

Remak[1] has found that as a law, generally holding good, the excitability of a nerve is the greater the nearer the irritated point is to the brain; and he has further shown that the rule is, not only for each single nerve in its course, but also for the nerves generally of the body, that the nerves of the lower extremities commonly need for their excitation a more intense current than those of the upper. According to this author, the rule appears to be, in regard to the motory nerves, that their excitability is not only greater at their central than at their peripheral end, but that it decreases as we recede from the brain.

As regards the effect of electric currents on the nerves of sense, they are excited both by the constant and interrupted current, yet in a much greater degree by the former. This stronger effect of the constant current is especially remarkable by the irritation of the sense of vision: when we apply one plate of the galvanic element to the forehead, and the other in the region of the trigeminus, a clear perception of light being produced, which even a stronger volta-electrical induction current is hardly able to create. Of the induced currents the magneto-electrical, which, on account of their less frequent interruption, are related to the constant currents, work more powerfully on the sensory nerves than the volta-electrical. If we place a zinc plate on the gums of the upper molar teeth of one side of the mouth, and a silver plate on the corresponding spot of the other side, a sensation of brightness similar to lightning is produced, which is much more perceptible when the current is led directly through the eyes. If we apply an intense constant current, there follows an appearance of fire and flame, and, by careless use of this, even injury to the retina. The light itself, which is perceived when the constant or interrupted current is used,

[1] L. c., p. 87.

is colored, and Purkinje,[1] as well as Ruete,[2] has observed that when we place the positive pole on the closed eyelid, and take the negative in the hand, there appears in the region of the macula lutea a very intense bluish light, which, interrupted by dark-colored circles, fades out toward the periphery. If, on the contrary, we reverse the poles, a reddish-yellow light appears, which, most vivid in the periphery of the field of vision, vanishes toward the centre. When the intensity of the current is considerable, the whole field of vision is lighted up with tolerable uniformity. The interrupted current produces, moreover, when we conduct it in the transverse or vertical direction through the eyeball, a horizontal or perpendicular oval distortion of the pupil, and it increases the tears, but affects the retina, like the continued current, very little.

Brenner[3] has published the following observations in regard to the effect of electricity on the organ of hearing: If the cathode is placed in the auditory passage, filled with water, and the anode is connected with any other part of the body, there arises, when the circuit is closed, a strong sensation of sound, which continues during the flow of the current, but gradually dies away when the circuit is opened. If the anode be placed in the ear, no sound is heard either at the moment of making the connection or during the continuance of the current; yet, when the circuit is broken, a slight sound is perceived. These reactions Schwartze[4] and Lucae have not been able fully to establish; on the contrary, the latter has observed that, when the cathode (zinc pole) is placed in the ear, and the anode on the neck or hand, a painful drawing sensation is perceived in the ear at the closing and during the flow of the current, which immediately

[1] Rust's Magazin für die gesammte Heilkunde, Band xx., pp. 31–50.
[2] Lehrbuch der Ophthalmologie, 1845, p. 73.
[3] Zur Electrophysiologie und Electropathologie des N. acusticus. Petersburger Med. Zeitung, 1863.
[4] Ueber die sogenannte Otiatrik Brenner's. Archiv für Ohrenheilkunde, Band i.

ceases with the opening of the circuit. On the contrary, when the anode (copper pole) is in the ear, a less painful drawing is produced, which also vanishes when the current is interrupted. When the induction current is used, there is, moreover, observed a sensation as of a roaring and rushing wind, which is produced by the presence of water in the auditory passage, besides a tickling, pricking feeling which by means of a very intense current may be made unendurable. At the same time there is perceived, probably in consequence of the irritation of the chorda tympani which descends from the cavity of the drum of the ear against the N. lingualis and in common with it reaches the glandula salivalis int., an unpleasant metallic taste on the middle of the corresponding side of the tongue; and, as Althaus'[1] has remarked, there is an increase in the flow of saliva.

When the conductors are placed in the nose, according to Ritter who made the painful operation with a Voltaic pile of twenty pairs, there arises both at and during the closure of the circuit a peculiar smell, sourish with the ascending and ammoniacal with the descending current. I myself perceived an increase of the mucous secretion, as well as a pricking, stinging sensation in the nose, the latter predominating when the zinc pole was in the nose and the copper pole taken in the hand. If the negative pole were placed in the nose and the positive applied to the neck, I perceived at the same time an alkaline taste on the tongue; by reversing the direction of the current, a sour taste, which spread out from the root of the tongue to its end.

If we place a zinc plate on the back of the tongue and a silver plate under the same, and bring their free ends in contact, we perceive a stinging, sourish taste on the upper surface of this organ, and beneath it a slightly alkaline one, or none at all. If we arm the end of the tongue with zinc, and its back with silver, the sensation of taste is much more intense than by the reverse arrangement of the metals.[2]

[1] Die Electricität in der Medicin, Berlin, 1860, p. 78.   [2] Pfaff.

The sensation of taste lasts during the closure of the circuit with unabated strength.¹

If we touch with the electrodes certain points of the face, and especially of the neck, there arises a decided metallic taste, which appears bitter to some, to others sour or styptic, and which is perceived, not only on the tongue, but also on the gums and on the palate. On the neck, the region of excitation is often limited to the five cervical vertebræ, and frequently, especially in patients suffering from tabes or nervous diseases, it extends even deeper. The zinc pole produces the stronger sensation of taste.

B. *The Influence of the Electric Current on the Brain and the Spinal Marrow.*

For what we know on this subject we are mainly indebted to the investigations of Edward Weber,² whom we follow here in a great measure. If we allow the current of a rotary apparatus to work on the brain of a frog, various phenomena appear, according to the region irritated. If we thus disturb the hemispheres of the cerebrum or of the cerebellum, not only on their surface, but within, there follows either a contraction of the muscles or indications of pain. When the corpora quadrigemina are irritated, there arise contractions of single muscles, which have more the appear-

---

[1] Fehrenbein (Ueber einige mittelbare physiologische Wirkungen der atmosphärischen Electricität, Henle und Pfeufer's Zeitschrift, 1851, Heft iii., p. 365, *et seq.*) supposes that the sour taste produced on the tongue by the galvanic current is not caused by the electricity as such, but by the nitric acid which is formed under the influence of electricity from the nitrogen and oxygen of the air. The smell produced in the nose by the electric current is not directly the result of this, but is more intimately connected with the ozone which is formed by the action of this force on oxygen. Finally, electricity is only the indirect cause of the light and sound phenomena, for these manifestations result from the vibratory movements produced in the particles of the air by the electrical discharges.

[2] Wagner's Handwörterbuch der Physiologie mit Rücksicht auf physiologische Pathologie, Braunschweig, 1846, Theil III., Abth. 2.

ance of clonic than of tonic spasms, and, probably through an appropriate arrangement in the choice of the muscles, resemble the reflex actions.

In regard to the effect of the constant current on the brain of the living animal, Matteucci [1] instituted investigations of which the following are the results: If the poles of a Voltaic pile of sixty pairs of plates are applied to the hemispheres of the cerebrum or the cerebellum, the animal is not disturbed; if, however, the corpora quadrigemina or the crura cerebri are brought in connection with the electrodes, the animal cries out, and at the same time all the muscles of the body contract. These phenomena last several seconds, but disappear with the interruption of the current.

If we allow the current of a rotary apparatus to work on the spinal marrow, by bringing the upper and lower ends of the same in connection with the two poles, there arises a general rigid cramp of all the muscles of the body and extremities, since all their nerves spring from the spinal marrow. In this respect the spinal marrow behaves as a common stem of all the nerves of motion. In two other points, however, it shows itself not to be a common nerve-stem—points which are enough to induce us to yield to it an independent activity:

1. If we place the conducting wires in connection with a deeper-lying portion, or even the lower end of the spinal marrow, all the muscles of the body and extremities are thrown into convulsions, as when their upper end is irritated; if the spinal marrow were only a common nerve-stem, then only those muscles should be seized with rigid cramps, whose nerves pass out from this portion, or lie so near as to be affected by the current. That the convulsion of the muscles of the upper extremities in this case arises directly from the spinal marrow, and not from the effect of the current on the roots of the nerves of these parts, is

[1] Traité des Phenomènes électro-physiologiques des Animaux, Paris, 1844, p. 242.

proved by the fact that, when we make a section through the spinal marrow, and bring the cut surfaces again fully in contact, the upper parts are no longer thrown into convulsions.

2. The electric current working through the nerves produces a rigid spasm which immediately disappears when the current is interrupted; but, when acting on the spinal marrow, it shows its effect even for a considerable time after the breaking of the connection—in frogs, lively and vigorous for one-half or even one minute; and the spasm may be reproduced two or three times, becoming, however, shorter and shorter. When the medulla oblongata is irritated in the same way as the spinal marrow, similar general convulsions ensue.

The constant current behaves differently in regard to the spinal marrow, producing paralysis, at least by long application. If the spinal marrow be exposed to the action of a powerful constant current, convulsions are produced in the extremities at the moment of closing of the circuit; if we allow the current to circulate through the spinal marrow for a long time, applied to whatever points that are convenient, a paralysis is brought about to such an extent, that neither chemical nor mechanical irritants, nor induced currents, are able to move the extremities; if we open the circuit, the spinal marrow responds to their action. As to the direction of the currents, Baierlacher[1] found, when experimenting on frogs, that both directions of the current produce paralysis of the parts affected; that, however, the ascending possesses this peculiarly in a higher degree than the descending. Moreover, as regards the deportment toward irritants of those parts of the spinal marrow whose upper and lower halves are in contact with the electrodes of a constant current, Baierlacher has found that, when the spinal marrow is acted on by a constant galvanic current, the excitability of the same is lessened in all parts, in fact, it is

[1] Die Inductions-Electricität, 1857, p. 102, *et seq.*

paralyzed, which effect is more marked with the ascending direction of the current than with the descending; that, however, this action of the spinal marrow has no influence on the excitability of the motory nerves.

Irritation of the medulla oblongata exercises, according to the investigations of Budge,[1] a decided influence on the motions of the heart, for they become slower, and the heart itself relaxes and spreads out—observations which the brothers Weber have confirmed.

According to Budge and Waller, the pupil of the eye enlarges when that portion of the spinal marrow is acted on by electricity, which lies between the seventh cervical and the sixth dorsal vertebræ—they give to this part the name centrum cilio-spinale, because they consider it the central organ for the cervical portion of the sympathetic, which has the determining of the influence of this nerve on the movements of the iris, and the regulating of the blood-vessels of the head. If, for instance, this part of the spinal marrow is irritated, in consequence of the communication with the cervical portion of the sympathetic, the circular fibres of the M. dilatator contract and prevent the working of the M. constrictor iridis, and there follows an enlargement of the pupil. If, on the contrary, the sympathetic is cut through, the pupil lessens in size, in consequence of the paralysis of the circular fibres and the continuing integrity of the others.

Budge[2] has also found a similar central organ for the sympathetic of the region of the loins, which in rabbits lies in that part of the spinal marrow which corresponds to the fourth lumbar vertebra. If this portion of the spinal marrow is electrically irritated there arise energetic contractions of the ductus deferentes, of the urinary bladder, and of the lower part of the rectum. These movements, however, also follow by the electrical excitation of a little ganglion, which lies in the neighborhood of the fifth lumbar vertebra, and

---

[1] Archiv von Roser und Wunderlich, 1846, Band v.
[2] Virchow's Archiv, 1850, p. 115.

has connection with the third and fourth lumbar nerves. Budge has named this ganglion genito-spinale. If the sympathetic of one side be bisected, the electrical irritation of the centrum genito-spinale produces energetic movements in the ductus deferens of the uninjured side, and slight movements in that of the injured side, in consequence of the connecting branches which exist between the two nerves.

As regards the possibility of galvanizing the brain and spinal marrow through their bony covering, the views of authors differ greatly. For instance, Ziemssen[1] denies the therapeutical effects of available currents. S. Rosenthal[2] believes that the central organs of the nervous system are as accessible through their bony coverings as the other organs lying at similar depths. W. Erb has established the correctness of the latter view by the following experiment: From the top of the skull of a still undissected human body a piece of bone of about 2″ in diameter was sawn out, the skin and periosteum carefully removed, and then the exposed edges of the bone were allowed to dry for several hours. Then a part of the upper surface of the brain was removed, and a well-isolated frog-preparation was brought into contact with the mass of this organ in such a way that its nerve touched it for about 2‴ of its length. Now the electrodes of the constant current were placed on the upper halves of both ears, and a current of considerable strength was conducted through. Ten Bunsen elements gave by reversing the current with the rheotrope,[3] also fourteen elements, with the simple making and breaking of the circuit, lively contractions of the frog-preparation. If the current were conducted from the chin to the back part of the head, it needed to be considerably increased in strength, in order to pro-

---

[1] *l. c.*, p. 58.
[2] Electricitätslehre für Mediciner, 1862.
[3] *Vide* section v., Remak's apparatus.

duce contraction. Induced currents, even of moderate strength, used in the same way, produced evident contractions.

In regard to the spinal marrow, Erb came to similar results. Direct experiments on the dead body, analogous to those made on the brain, gave a positive result, yet this was always less manifest, because Erb could only operate on dissected bodies, and because the isolation of the frog preparation could not be so fully effected as when experimenting on the head. Nevertheless the investigations place it beyond doubt that the conducting of the galvanic current into the spinal marrow is possible.[1]

C. *The Influence of the Electric Current on the Sympathetic.*

Pourfour du Petit, in the year 1727, made the first experiments on the function of the N. sympathetic. He found that after the cutting through of the cervical portion of the sympathetic there followed contraction of the pupil, flattening of the cornea, redness and injection of the conjunctiva of the eye, etc.—after electrical irritation, enlargement of the pupil set in. Claude Bernard[2] observed, besides the above appearances, more or less marked contraction of the nostril and mouth on the corresponding side, increase of the circulation of the blood, and of the temperature and sensibility of the head. When Bernard electrized the cranial portion of the sympathetic, after the bisection of the nerve, or after the destruction of the ganglion cervicale supremum, he found that all these phenomena again disappeared, and that there was even a preponderance in the opposite direction.

---

[1] Dr. Erb has been so kind as to furnish me with a *résumé* of his not yet published work, "On the Possibility of Galvanizing the Brain and Spinal Marrow," which will appear in one of the coming numbers of the Deutschen Archiv's für Klinische Medicin.

[2] Sur l'influence du nerf grand sympathique sur la chaleur animale. Comptes rendus du 29 Mai, 1852.

The pupil then became larger than that of the other side; the eye, which was sunken in its socket, became prominent; the increased temperature ranked below its usual level, and the conjunctiva, nostrils, and ears, which were before reddened and injected, became pale. When the current was interrupted, all the appearances again set in which we have seen were the result of the bisection. These we can two or three times cause to disappear by electrizing the cranial portion of the sympathetic. These experiments were later confirmed by Waller, Budge, Schiff, Brown-Séquard, etc. The phenomena following the cutting through of the sympathetic, in connection with the circulatory system, find their explanation in the yielding of the tension, as Cl. Bernard discovered, depending on the N. sympathetic, of the arterial walls, and in the consequent relaxation of their muscular fibres. Remak was the first to experiment on the effects of the sympathetic on the voluntary muscles.[1] He cut through the neck-portion of the N. sympathetic of a cat, and immediately the *membrana nictitans* of the eye of the same side moved forward and covered one-half of this organ; soon the pupil contracted as well as the cleft of the eye; in short, the upper eyelid descended and the lower lifted itself up a little. These appearances were caused by the relaxing of the levator palpebr. sup. and the convulsive constriction of the orbicularis. If an induced current were then conducted through the peripheric end of the bisected sympathetic, the eye opened, i. e., the third lid moved back, and the cleft of the eye and the pupil enlarged. When the current was interrupted, the eyelids slowly returned to their former position and the pupil again contracted. During the pause a considerable collection of tears took place, which was probably due to the relaxing of the vessel walls in the lachrymal gland.

If we galvanize the ganglion cervicale infimum of the sympathetic, the beating of the heart is accelerated; the

[1] S. Deutsche Klinik, Bd. vii., 1859, p. 294.

same thing is observed when the sympathetic nerve of the heart is electrized. During the electrical irritation of the vagi, as Weber discovered in 1846, the heart's action is lessened.

Pflüger discovered, in 1856, that the Nn. splanchnici have a similar influence on intestinal movements as the Nn. vagi on the action of the heart. He found, namely, that, when the Nn. splanchnici which spring from the six lower dorsal ganglia of the sympathetic were galvanized, the peristaltic motion of the intestine immediately ceased. Hence Pflüger inferred that a certain nerve-group exists, which has the function of causing the peristaltic motions to lessen or entirely to cease, and named this the checking nerve system.

D. *The Effect of the Electric Current on the Organs furnished with Organic Muscular Fibres.*

The most of the experiments belonging here were made by Ed. Weber,[1] not through the action of the electric current on the ganglia and ganglion nerves themselves, but on the organs innerved by these. All the organs supplied from the sympathetic are furnished with organic muscular fibres, and present, under the influence of the electric current, the following phenomena, in which respects they differ from the animal muscles: 1. The movements of the organic muscles set in much more slowly than those of the animal, to such an extent, that the electric irritation may be even withdrawn before the contraction is evident. The degree of slowness with which the movement follows is in the various organs different, so that in this respect there is a gradual approach to the voluntary animal muscles from the ureters and gallbladder, which contract the slowest, to the cæcum, the stomach, the iris, the urinary bladder, the spermatic ducts,

[1] *L. c.*

the pregnant uterus, the small and large intestines, the œsophagus, and the heart. 2. The phenomena excited in these muscles last, in contradistinction to those excited in the voluntary muscles, after the cessation of the irritation for some time, and spread from the muscular fibres in which they begin to others lying at a distance. 3. The movements which the simultaneously or successively attacked fasciculi of the organic muscles execute ensue, in opposition to the animal muscles whose fibres contract mechanically as soon as they are disturbed, in complete appropriateness corresponding to the functions of the respective organs. 4. While the constant electric current causes the animal muscles to contract most at the time of its opening and closing, the contraction of the organic muscles lasts also during the closure of the circuit.

In regard to the individual organs, experiments have furnished the following results:

1. DIGESTIVE ORGANS.

The muscular coat of the entire intestinal canal is markedly affected by the electric current. Aldini observed that, when he placed a zinc plate in the mouth of a recently-killed ox, and a silver plate in its rectum, and connected them with one another by means of a conducting wire, the abdominal muscles convulsively contracted, and the fæces were voided.

In regard to the salivary glands, Ludwig[1] found that, when the N. lingualis and auriculo-temporalis trigemini, the chorda tympani and the rami parotidei postici of the N. facialis were irritated by currents of weakening density, a profuse flow of saliva followed. If, on the contrary, the sympathetic was irritated, the secretion of saliva was brought to a stand-still.

Irritation of the œsophagus of man produced immediately strong contraction of the long and circular fibres; by con-

[1] Lehrbuch der Physiologie des Menschen, 1858, Band ii., p. 289.

tinued action, the irritation remained not confined to the part in contact with the conductors, but spread both upward and downward. The reason of this deportment is, that the œsophagus of man, and of most of the mammalia, is furnished with striped and with organic muscular fibres, so that by long irritation a combined manifestation of both factors takes place; while, by way of comparison, the œsophagus of birds, which consists exclusively of smooth muscular fibres, when electrically irritated, contracts slowly and continuously, and that of rodents, which consists of striped muscular fibres, promptly contracts, and expands immediately again on the opening of the circuit.

If we open the abdominal cavity of a recently-killed mammal—for instance, of a cat, a dog, or a rabbit—and lay the entrails between two metallic plates which are placed in connection with the conductors of a rotary apparatus, there follow peristaltic movements of remarkable activity; the intestines rise and sink, and their movements are transmitted slowly even to the rectum. The movements which are produced by the action of the air on the exposed intestines are much weaker and cease much sooner than those which we here notice. By means of a momentary action of the current on a certain part, especially on the jejunum, there follows a shrinking, which progresses slowly, and increases even to the complete closure of the intestine, and disappears at the same rate of progress. The rectum is the part of the intestine least sensitive to the electrical irritation.

The *stomach* also reacts powerfully under the influence of the electrical irritation; there ensues, in consequence of the muscular fibres which cross it, not only transverse shrinking, but also shortening of its length, if the electrodes are placed in the corresponding direction. The course of the movement is invariably from the cardia to the pylorus.

If we allow the current to work on the *gall-bladder*, it contracts, and throws out a part of the gall into the duodenum. If we place the electrodes very near to one another, there follows a constriction of the gall-bladder, which may become so great that the entire organ is thereby divided into two parts, not communicating with each other.

As regards the *spleen*, Dittrich, Gerlach, and Hey[1] have not observed contractions through electrical irritation, either in the covering or in the body of the organ; while Wagner,[2] Rayer,[3] Harless,[4] state that they have seen them. Moreover, Cl. Bernard[5] has published the following convincing experiment: He exposed the spleen of a dog, measured its dimensions, and placed the conductors of a powerful rotary apparatus in connection with its upper and lower ends. After some minutes the length of the spleen had shortened two or three centimetres. The same experiment, several times tried, gave the same result. When he allowed the current to pass in the transverse direction through the spleen, there was a diminution in the breadth of the organ.[6]

II. URINARY AND SEXUAL ORGANS.

The *ureters* are little sensitive to the electrical irritation, and contract only slightly, while, on the contrary, the urinary

---

[1] *Vide* Prager Vierteljahrsschrift, 1851, Band viii., Heft 3, p. 65; Beobachtungen und physiologische Versuche an den Leichen von zwei Hingerichteten.

[2] Untersuchungen über die Contractilität der Milz mittelst des electro-magnetischen Rotations-Apparates. Jena'sche Annalen, 1849, Heft 1.

[3] Expériences sur la contractilité de la rate. Journal des Connaissances Médicales. Février, 1850.

[4] Electrische Versuche an einem Hingerichteten. Augsburger Allgem. Zeitung, 1850, No. 172.

[5] Gaz. Méd. de Paris, 1849, p. 994.

[6] [In his Astley Cooper Prize Essay on the spleen, Mr. Gray states that he has never been able to produce contractions in the spleen through electrical irritation. In the course of very many experiments made with the object of determining whether the organic muscular fibres of the spleen were contractible by the electric stimulus, I have rarely failed to obtain affirmative results, both with the induced and constant currents. My experiments were performed upon the exposed spleens of living dogs and cats. The organic muscular fibres of the fibrous coat of the fresh spleen, if placed upon a glass slide, excited by the constant or induced current, and viewed with the microscope, can be seen to contract energetically.—W. A. H.]

bladder contracts quickly and energetically, and forces out its contents. The *vas deferens* also reacts powerfully. Weber found that, when experimenting on the uterus of a pregnant bitch, every part of it contracted strongly under the influence of the uninterrupted current, and that the contraction always was limited to the irritated part, and did not extend itself. In this respect the uterus resembles the animal muscles, but it is also like the organic in that the contraction, after the withdrawal of the irritation, lasts for some time. The non-pregnant uterus shows the same phenomena, but in a less degree. Mackenzie[1] found, as he experimented on the exposed uterus of a pregnant animal, the continued current, conducted from the upper end of the spinal marrow through the uterus, more powerful than the local effect, by the direct application of both poles to the parenchyma of the uterus. He found, moreover, that the electric current, when passed through the length of the uterus, that is, from its base to its neck, produced stronger contractions than when directed transversely through this organ, for then it caused only partial contractions in the direction of the current. That also the pregnant uterus in the living human species may be caused to contract powerfully by means of the electrical irritation has been proved by Höniger, Benj. Franck, and others,[2] through the use of the current for bringing on the pains and expelling the contents.

III. THE IRIS.

The *iris* among the mammalia consists chiefly of organic, among the birds of animal muscular fibres—hence the slow dilatation of the pupil in the former, continuing after the withdrawal of the irritation, and the quick contraction of the pupil in the latter, ceasing immediately on the removal of the electrical excitement. Dittrich, Gerlach, and Hey[2] found, by placing the conductors on the inner and

[1] Lancet, March 6, 1858.   [2] *S.*, section ix.

outer angles of the eye, after the subsiding of the contraction of the M. orbicularis palpebrarum which at first sets in, that the pupil assumed a horizontal oval form; and where the poles were brought in contact with the upper and lower borders of the orbit, the pupil took on a vertical oval form. We may produce, moreover, through the irritation of the iris, either a contraction or a dilatation of the pupil, according as we allow the current to work on the M. dilatator or constrictor. In order to produce a contraction, it is sufficient to place one conductor on the cornea, and the other on any part of the face. If we place, on the contrary, the poles of an induction apparatus or of a simple galvanic pair of plates outward from the pupil, the fibres of the M. dilatator pupillæ running in the radial direction become excited, and the pupil consequently enlarged.

IV. THE HEART.

The *heart*, though resembling, in the size and striation of its fibrillæ, the animal muscles, with which it also in common possesses the energy and rapidity of contraction, behaves in other respects as the organic muscles. When Ed. Weber allowed the current of a rotary apparatus to work on the heart of a frog, pulsating vigorously, by placing the ventricle in connection with the conducting wires, the irritated portion little by little contracted, till it took no part in the rhythmical heart-movement; the contraction lasted for some time after the withdrawal of the electrical irritation: when he, on the contrary, allowed the current to play on the *bulbus aortæ*, the pulsations of the entire heart became more active and stronger; finally, when he disturbed the pulsating portion of the *vena cava*, the heart after a few seconds stood completely still, and began again to pulsate some time after the removal of the irritation, and then in a slower rhythm. Dittrich, Gerlach, and Hey[1] placed one pole on the auricle, and the other on the ventricle of the

[1] *L. c.*

right side of the heart of a man hung half an hour previous: rhythmical contractions of the heart set in—by irritating the left side of the heart these were less marked. The reason of this peculiar phenomena of the heart is that it is supplied by the sympathetic and the vagi; through the irritation of the sympathetic the heart's action is increased, while, by the electrizing of both vagi, the pulsations slowly decrease. Cl. Bernard has also made the following experiments on this organ: When he galvanized the upper ends of the Nn. vagi, not the least effect was produced on the heart's action; with a weak current the respiratory movements continued, but with a strong one these ceased, the blood in the carotids was blackened, the mucous membrane of the mouth became injected, the tongue assumed a brownish-black color, and there was the condition of asphyxia, in which, however, the arteries unhindered continued to pulsate. When Bernard interrupted the current the respiratory movements began again, and with a rapidity even greater than before the galvanizing. Moreover, there has been found, after electrizing the *vagi*, sugar in the blood, in the cerebro-spinal fluid, and in the bile: the urinary secretion seems to stand still, and it is observed that the saliva is increased in quantity. Galvanizing, on the contrary, the *lower* ends of the vagi, the respiratory movements continued, while the pulsations of the heart and arteries ceased. In most cases vomiting followed. If we, after the death of an animal, and the heart no longer beats, conduct an induced current unto this organ, rhythmical contractions appear again. The contractions are much more manifest in the right portion of the heart than in the left, as generally after death the left ventricle is firmly contracted, and does not react to the electrical irritation, while the right ventricle in this condition is almost always filled with blood, and contracts powerfully under the influence of the electrical current. In animals which have been killed by chloroform, the left ventricle sometimes continues to pulsate, though faintly, after the action of the right ventricle has ceased, in consequence of excessive expansion, by means of the black blood: if we in such a case electrize the right ventricle, its pulsations begin again and the expansion lessens. Perhaps we might, as a last means, in case of chloroform-poisoning, try to excite the right portion of the heart with a weak induced current.

E. *The Effect of the Electric Current on the Blood-vessels and Lymphatics.*

Weber's experiments[1] gave, by using the interrupted current, the following results: the mesenteric arteries contracted to about one-half or one-third their usual size; by longer working of the interrupted current, even to one-fifth or one-sixth, so that the circulation of the blood was stopped. With a weaker irritation the effect quickly disappeared, with a too strong current the arteries lost their contractile power and expanded into aneurismal sacs. Kölliker[2] placed one pole on the umbilical artery and vein of a fresh human placenta: there followed contractions, as in the case of the vessels of recently-amputated limbs; the veins forced out their blood and changed into bloodless strings, also the arteries and lymph-vessels showed contraction. The irritability of the veins lasted for one hour and fifteen minutes, that of the arteries for one hour and ten minutes, and that of the lymph-vessels for one hour and twelve minutes. In living subjects an enlargement of the vessels immediately follows their contraction when a tolerably strong interrupted current is used. So we often see by electrical irritation of the skin, using moist conductors, first anæmia through spasmodic contraction, then hyperæmia through paralytic

---

[1] Ed. und E. H. Weber, Wirkung des Magnet-electr. Stromes auf die Blutgefässe in Müller's Archiv, 1847, Heft 2 und 3.
[2] Prager Vierteljahrschrift, 1849, Band vi., Heft i.: Zur Lehre von der Contractilität der menschlichen Blut- und Lymphgefässe.

affection of the vessels; while under very intense irritation apparent hyperæmia sets in immediately, and lasts often long after the end of the operation. Remak, experimenting on a living frog, observed the same phenomena. One leg he electrized by means of a current from five or eight Daniell's elements by placing one conductor immovably on a certain part while he moved the other slowly up and down the limb; the other leg he threw into a rigid spasm by means of an interrupted current: after two minutes the vessels of the skin and muscles of the first were swollen with blood, while those of the other leg were pale and contracted.

F. On the Effect of the Electrical Current on the Blood.

W. Brande was the first to institute experiments in regard to the effect of the galvanic current on albumen, and came to the result[1] that it coagulates on the negative pole, and under certain circumstances on the positive. Gmelin, who experimented with a weaker current, saw the albumen always deposited at the positive pole. Golding Bird finally came to the result, that albumen is precipitated from alkaline solutions at the positive pole, from acid at the negative, and consequently belongs to those bodies which sometimes appear as acids and at others as alkalies. Von Wittich[2] confirmed the observations of Golding Bird, and recognized, as did he, that albumen separates from its alkaline solution very quickly, and in the form of a membrane, while from its acid solution it is precipitated much more slowly and as a diffuse cloudiness in the neighborhood of the electrodes. Albumen may be precipitated by means of the galvanic current also from solutions in which its presence cannot be made evident either through boiling or by the addition of nitric acid. The presence at the same time of various salts

---

[1] Proceedings of the Royal Society, 1809. Gilbert's Annals, lxiv., p. 348.
[2] Ueber den Einfluss des galvanischen Stromes auf Eiweisslösungen und Eiweissdiffusion im Journal für praktische Chemie, lxxiii., p. 18, 1857.

modifies the influence of the electric current on the albumen solution. When the sulphate of soda or potassa, nitrate of potassa, phosphate of soda, or chloride of sodium, are present, the precipitation takes place on the positive pole; when the carbonate or bicarbonate of any of the alkalies, or a free alkali is present, the precipitation is prevented, or much delayed. The serum of the blood behaves much in the same way as the albumen solution. Heidenreich has found that,[1] when we expose fresh arterial or venous blood to the action of a continuous current, the coagulation of the same is thereby hastened, decomposition taking place in such a way, that albumen, fibrin, fat, acids, chlorine, etc., separate at the positive pole, while the watery and alcoholic extracts, the alkaline and earthy bases, iron, and coloring matter, appear at the negative pole. If we allow the constant current to act on the blood in the vessels, there is produced a plug which adheres to the walls of the vessel and stops the circulation. The clot becomes firm in from ten to thirty minutes, and is then sufficient to close the vessel. The clot in the veins behaves as in the arteries, though it is less consistent and darker colored.[2]

G. *The Effect of the Electric Current on the Skin.*

A moderately-strong interrupted current working by means of moist conductors on any part of the skin produces generally paleness, which, soon after the removal of the electrodes, is followed by redness and hyperæmia. Through the action of a strong interrupted current, there arise erythema, swelling, vesicles, and even ulcers, according to the degree of sensitiveness of the skin, the duration of the ap-

[1] Heidenreich, phys.-chem. Untersuchungen des Bluts durch die electrische Säule, in der Neuen Medicinischen Zeitung, 1847, No. 31.

[2] Asson, Rapporto della Comissione che a fatto gli sperimenti sull' électropuntura come mezzo congelante la sangue nelle arterie e sull' obliterazione delle vase. Annal. Univers., Jan., 1847, p. 219. Gaz. des Hôpitaux, 1847, No. 48.

plication, the strength of the current, the rapidity of the interruptions, and the peculiarity of the conductors. The contractible fibre-cells of the skin are simultaneously excited, and there is produced thereby the so-called goose-flesh (cutis anserina). That the elevation of the skin-papillæ is not the result of reflex action, but of the direct working of the electrical current, Kölliker[1] has shown by producing the cutis anserina in a piece of skin cut from the leg of a criminal but a short time previously executed. The contractions of the fibre-cells are seen best when we allow the current to work on the tunica dartos and the nipple; the first forms deep and numerous folds, and makes wormlike, undulatory movements, and the nipple rises and remains erect for some time after the action of the current.

Through the continued working for several minutes of the constant current on the outer skin, there is produced, besides the sense of burning at the negative pole, a visible difference between the positive and negative poles. The positive pole enlarges the blood-vessels and reddens the skin, the negative pole has the opposite effect; the first causes a depression of the skin, the last a swelling of the epidermis and cutis. It brings about, moreover, according to its strength, the duration of its application, etc., a chemical process resulting in simple erythema, or even deeply-penetrating destruction of the part. A simple pair of connected plates (zinc and silver), of the size of a dollar, causes on a moist skin, after twenty-four hours, a considerable reddening, and, after a lapse of from two to five days, blisters and pustules. If the skin is deprived of the epidermis, there sets in immediately a powerful burning pain, a profuse secretion of serum, and, after long action, an ulcerated surface covered with a crust. The most striking effect shows itself always at the zinc pole; for, through the action of the current, the salt-holding fluid which exudes from the surface

[1] Ueber die Contraction der Lederhaut des Menschen und der Thiere, Zeitschrift für wissenschaftl. Zoologie, Band II.

of the skin is decomposed, sodium is set free at the silver pole, and chlorine at the zinc pole, and in this way chloride of zinc is formed, which is in the highest degree destructive. The sodium set free at the silver plate is soon converted into soda by oxidation.

The interrupted current produces a disagreeable pricking and piercing sensation on the mucous membrane, when the conductors are held lightly on; when they are applied tightly, there follows an increase of the mucous secretion, probably in consequence of the effect on the contractile fibres; the constant current is able to cause destruction of the mucous membrane by intense action.

II. *The Effect of the Electric Current on the Bones.*

If we allow the interrupted current to work on a bone which lies immediately under the skin previously moistened, there sets in, in consequence of the irritation of the sensory nerves of the periosteum, a rooting, boring pain, resembling osteoscopic pains. Yet all the bones are not equally sensitive to the electrical irritation—a deportment which probably has its foundation in the greater or less abundance of nerves of the periosteum, of the ligaments, etc. The most sensitive are the frontal bone, the collar-bone, and the inner surface of the shin-bone; much less sensitive are the outer and inner condyles of the lower leg, the breast-bone, and the knee-pan.

I. *Accessory Effects of the Current.*

We will not speak of the effects which the application of the electrical stimulus produces on the human mind, which are more of a psychological nature, and manifest themselves sometimes as a sensation of warmth, sometimes as a sensation of pressure, and sometimes result in fainting. There remain still a multitude of effects, which, with a greater or less number of individuals, set in, and must be considered as immediate consequences of the operation. Here belong: the after-effects, which often appear several hours subsequent to the operation in the part affected, and are clearly the results of being electrized. Quite generally there is an inclination to sleep, which comes on sooner or later after the sitting, so that often those who suffer from sleeplessness are freed from this misfortune on the application of electricity. Frequently the menses set in earlier and more fully, probably in consequence of the increase of the flow of blood to the irritated part, or of the general irritation, especially by electrizing the legs; from the same cause, but not so often, hæmorrhoidal bleedings start anew. Finally, we must mention the quieting effect of a weak current directed to a painful part of the body, which is produced often in a short time, and is frequently lasting. We not seldom see neuralgic pains which have withstood the action of various medicines, or pains in consequence of exudation into the joint of the knee, the elbow, the hand, the finger, etc., fully disappear on the application of a weak current directed for a short time through the affected part, while the effect on the exudation itself, judging from the amount of its diminution, is exceedingly slight.[1]

[1] In this connection we should mention the so-called "electrical anæsthesia" resulting from the use of electric currents in connection with certain minor surgical operations. Dr. Rottenstein, of Frankfort-on-the-Main, and Suersen, dentist, of Berlin, were the first to make successful experiments after the directions of Francis, of Philadelphia (Med. Central-Zeitung, Nos. 72-74, 1858), and "to extract teeth without pain by means of a weak induction current." The patient held one electrode, armed with a moist sponge, in the hand, and the other was secured on the tongue which the operator held in his hand covered with a silk glove. The College of Dentistry in London, under the presidency of Mathews, as well as other dentists, have not recognized electricity as an anæsthetic. On the other hand, Fonssagrives (Gaz. des Hôpitaux, 148, 1856), Dr. Emil Friedrich, and Dr. Max Knorr in Munich (Baier. ärztliches Intelligenz-Blatt, 41, 1858), have used electricity with success in other light surgical operations: the first, in cutting into a felon, and in opening syphilitic buboes;

Through the action of the constant current certain other accessory effects are noticeable, which especially relate to the nerves of sense and the brain. Some men perceive a metallic taste when a strong current is conducted through one arm or one leg; also, with some, there follows a sensation of light on electrizing the neck and back. Patients suffering from tabes and atrophy sometimes perceive the metallic taste when we conduct a current through the pelvis; even irritation of the upper thoracic vertebra by a strong current is sufficient in such individuals to produce a flash of light in their eyes. In feeble persons, sometimes constant currents, from twenty to thirty elements, striking the roots of the N. vagus, produce slowness of the pulse lasting for several seconds or minutes, combined with fainting and paleness of the face.[1] Finally, there arise often, when the currents are directed for a long time through the upper portion of the body, dizziness, numbness of the head, illusions of the senses, and other disturbances of the faculties of the brain.

CONCLUSIONS.

1. The interrupted current is applicable in those cases in which we wish—

    a) To excite the muscles, the nerves of sense, the sensory or the motory nerves.

    b) To produce contractions of the blood or lymphatic vessels.

    c) Or to affect certain organs supplied from the sympathetic.

---

the last, in cutting through the skin, and in tenotomy. Finally, Richardson (Med. Times and Gaz., Feb. 12, April 23, 1859) has presented an experiment, under the name "Volta-narcotismus," of the following nature: he held the electrodes, saturated with a narcotic fluid (aconite or chloroform), for a long time on a part in which he wished to produce anæsthesia. Surely, he would have reached the same result by the use of the narcotics alone. In any case, the anæsthetic action has a very slight therapeutic worth.

[1] Remak, *l. c.*, p. 137.

CONCLUSIONS. 95

2. The muscular contraction produced through Faradization increases the temperature of the disturbed muscle, and is accompanied with an increase in the volume of the same.

3. Through the electrical irritation itself there is induced an increase of sensibility, when the irritations follow one another with tolerable quickness, and when they do not exceed a certain duration and intensity; under opposite influences there is soon a marked decrease in sensibility. Hence we should only use currents of such a strength as are sufficient to produce the desired result. To cause contraction in case of muscular paralysis, or sensation where there is lack of sensibility in the skin, we should not allow the currents to work too long without a proper number of pauses.

4. If we wish to relax a tense muscle or to loosen a peripheric contractor, repeated intermissions of a strong battery current, or single shocks from a strong induction current are indicated, and are generally more powerful than the constant current.

5. The use of the *constant* current is indicated in those cases in which we wish—
    a) To excite the nerves of sense or the skin nerves.
    b) To destroy the outer skin or mucous membrane.
    c) To produce an increase of warmth.
    d) Or to induce a chemical process, and also blood-coagulation.

6. While generally the density fluctuation of the interrupted current produces the most powerful exciting means for the motory nerves and muscles, there are certain peripheric paralyses in which the constant current, probably in consequence of its uninterrupted duration, produces effects which cannot be brought about by the induced current.

7. The sensitiveness of a muscle to the interrupted current can in many cases, through the application of a tolerably strong constant current, be increased.

8. In galvanizing a nerve it is advisable often to change

the direction of the current, because the conductivity of a current, flowing long in the same direction, decreases, while with a change in the direction it increases.

9. The extrapolar descending *anelectrotonus* is above all to be used when we wish to bring back to the normal condition a pathologically increased excitability, or abnormal irritation at the periphery of a nerve. The intensity of the desired effect is as the strength of the current, the length of the time of closure of the circuit, the greatness of the interpolar tract, and, finally, the shortness of the distance between the anode and the affected organ.

10. The extrapolar descending *catelectrotonus* is, on the contrary, to be used where we wish again to excite the sunken excitability or lessened sensation at the periphery of the nerve of the respective muscle.

11. From the same points of view the indications for the local production of extrapolar ascending anelectrotonus and catelectrotonus are to be sketched out, and consequently there come into consideration the extrapolar ascending anelectrotonus with increased, and the ascending catelectrotonus with decreased irritability, as applicable respectively to the cerebro-spinal shoots and the central sources of the nerve fibres.

12. There is no doubt that we can, by means of a constant current, even of tolerable strength, affect through their bony coverings the brain and spinal marrow.

FIFTH SECTION.

ON THE VARIOUS KINDS OF APPARATUS CONSTRUCTED ESPE-
CIALLY FOR THERAPEUTICAL PURPOSES.

I. GALVANIC APPARATUS.

AMONG the many apparatuses which have been constructed for the purpose of exciting galvanic electricity for special therapeutic uses, and which have been described and praised according to their different forms, as chain, curved, and binding apparatus, we find some which have no appreciable physical effect—as the Goldberger chain; others whose working is rendered much simpler by means of movable zinc and copper plates combined with one another, which may be laid on any portion of the body—as Romershausen's galvano-electrical curve, Récamier's *cataplasme galvanique*, Kunzeman's apparatus, etc. All these we will pass by in silence, and notice only Pulvermacher's chain, which produces a much more marked physical and chemical effect. This consists of a smaller or greater number of movable members combined with one another, each one of which consists of a small wooden cylinder, around which there are laid, yet without touching each other, a zinc wire and a gilded copper wire having a spiral form. The individual members are connected with one another by means of small metallic rings which take up the zinc wire of one member and the copper wire of the next following. Each time before using it, the series is placed in vinegar, by means of which a tolerably strong electrical current is produced, lasting for about half an hour. To increase the *quantity* of the electrical current, a series composed of larger members must be used; but, to increase the *intensity*, the number of members must be increased. This apparatus deflects quite perceptibly the galvanometer needle, decomposes water, and causes reddening, swelling, and blistering of the skin, and, in short, brings about chemical and physical acts.[1]

[1] [In the NEW YORK MEDICAL JOURNAL for November, 1865, I described a form of galvanic battery similar, in general features, to those referred to in the text, but possessed of many advantages. I referred to it in connec-

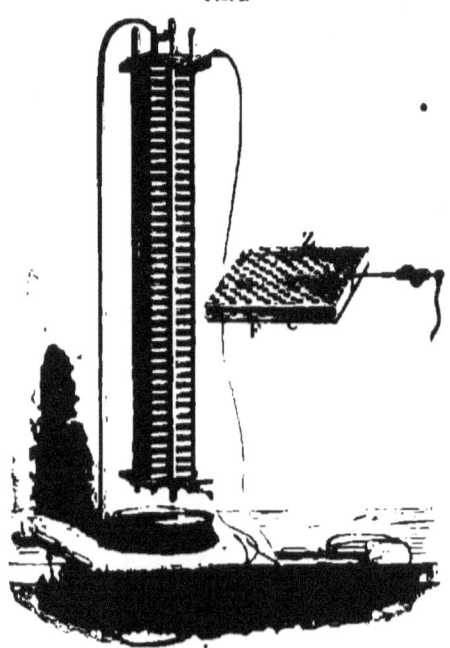

FIG. 2.

tion with the report of several cases of infantile paralysis, for the treatment of which I had devised the apparatus in question. In the QUARTERLY JOURNAL

But the working of all these apparatuses is entirely on the skin, and not on the deeper-lying tissues; it is accompanied with a chemical act—the oxidation of a metal, in fact, depends on this—and consequently comes to an end when complete oxidation has taken place. Nevertheless, such apparatuses are useful in certain cases, where we wish to awaken or diminish the sensibility of the skin, and many interesting cures of this kind are published by careful observers. Laennec[1] mentions a singultus of three years' stand-

of Psychological Medicine and Medical Jurisprudence, No. 1, July, 1867, p. 49, et seq., in a memoir entitled *The Pathology and Treatment of Organic Infantile Paralysis*, I described the instrument more in detail, and figured it as in the accompanying woodcut.

It consists of a series of elements formed of plates of perforated zinc and copper, as shown at F. These plates are soldered together, the copper being bent over at the ends, the zinc laid upon it, and the two securely fastened. A thin piece of wood is then placed between the plates, to prevent their being pressed together. The elements rest upon a plate of hard rubber, and are kept in place by four hard-rubber rods. Two other plates of hard rubber, having each a large hole in the centre and four holes for the rods, rest on top. These are kept in place by pins which pass through holes in the rods. The whole is hung to an iron or brass support, as shown in the figure, and a saucer underneath catches the vinegar used to set the instrument in action.

To arrange the apparatus, an element with a copper wire soldered to the copper plate is placed upon the lower piece of hard rubber; upon the element a piece of flannel or woollen cloth, the same size as the element, is placed; upon this, another element, then a piece of flannel, and so on. The elements are so placed, that the copper is always below. The last element has a piece of copper wire soldered to the zinc plate. Insulated wires are used to connect the poles with the electrodes.

To set the apparatus in action, strong vinegar is poured upon the top; it passes through the elements, and moistens the flannel. If the plates were not perforated, the flannel would only be moistened at the edges, and thus a great loss of power would be the result.

Copper gauze may be used instead of perforated copper plates.

This apparatus is easily made and kept in order, and is, therefore, admirably adapted to use in the country. The current is equable, and of a degree of intensity proportioned to the number of elements, and of quantity proportional to their size. I use from fifty to a hundred elements. Strong muscular contractions are induced by it in making or breaking of the circuit.—W. A. H.]

[1] Traité de l'auscultation médiate et des maladies des poumons et du cœur, 4 edit., Paris, 1837, t. iii., p. 498.

ing, which was cured by wearing two magnetic plates on the epigastrium and on the corresponding part of the vertebral column. After a lapse of six months the patient one day forgot to put on the plates, and the singultus returned and continued till they were again applied. Miguel[1] cured a case of epilepsy in the same way.

These pairs of plates are, however, much more powerful when they are placed on parts which have been previously deprived of the epidermis by means of blistering. Laennec[2] cured a case of angina pectoris by laying one plate over the pit of the stomach, the epidermis being removed, and the other on the back. Orioli and Cogevina[3] removed a cough of five years' standing, in a young girl, by placing a zinc and a copper plate, connected by a silver wire, on two positions, freed from their epidermis by means of a blister; finally, Spencer Wells[4] often healed ulcers which had withstood all other remedies, or threatened to become carcinomatous.[5]

Of the galvanic apparatuses, which are used specially for chirurgical purposes, we notice here:

1. The *Middeldorpf battery*,[6] which is constructed of the following dimensions:

A polished wooden chest, with two handles, that may be shut up, 12″ broad, 12″ deep, and with a cover 10″ 2‴ high, is divided by means of partitions, *b*, into four equal compartments, which receive four glass cylinders standing on pieces of felt. These are 6½″ high and 4½″ in diameter. They contain the 6″ high and 4″ wide strongly-amalgamated zinc cylin-

[1] Deutsche Klinik vom 1 October, 1856.
[2] *L. c.*, p. 497.
[3] Gaz. des Hôpitaux, 1847, p. 204.
[4] Bemerkungen über Heilwirkungen des Galvanismus aus der Praxis des Dr. Cogevina in Corfu. Oppenheim's Zeitschrift, 1849. Schmidt's Jahrbücher, Band lxiv., p. 161.
[5] S. section ix., Surgery.
[6] Die Galvano-caustic, ein Beitrag zur operativen Medicin, Breslau, 1854.

ders d, which have a circumference of 13″, so that each of them presents 78 □ ″, and all four, 312 □ ″. Within these there stand, on pedestals of stone, the clay cells e, 4½″ high and 3¼″ in diameter, into which the platinum stars f dip, which are furnished with glass covers, and have attached to their upper portion (as the zinc) a small copper piece for connecting with the conducting wires. Each platinum star consists of three plates, 3′ 10‴ high, 2′ 9‴ broad, united by means of a platinum clamp, and bent in such a way as to form a six-rayed star, having a working surface of about 250 □ ″.

Fig. 2.

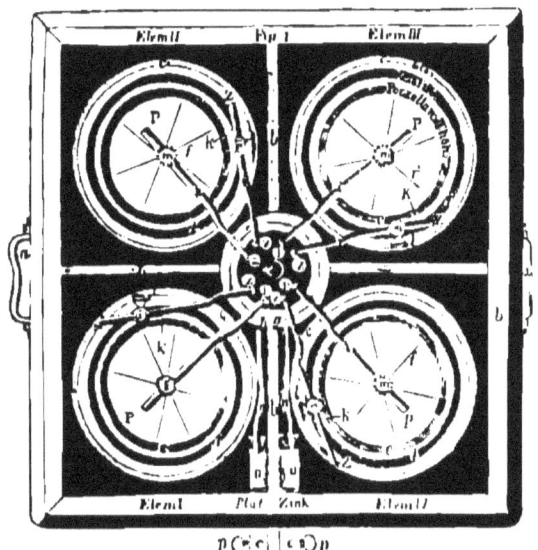

At the crossing of the partitions of the chest is placed the commutator A. This consists of a wooden column having on its upper slightly concave end eight little cups, 4‴ broad, namely PPPP in an inner circle, and ZZZZ in an outer for holding quicksilver. Into these little holes the copper conducting wires i, coming from the zinc and platinum, dip. On their way they pass to the $1\frac{1}{4}''$ high copper cylinder k, into which they are fastened by the screw m. The copper cylinders belonging to the zinc have a slit below, which allows them to be secured to the zinc cylinders, while those belonging to the platinum have a slit on the side so that the wires may be taken out, without removing the platinum from the acid. From the bottom of both sets of cups, which are connected with the platinum and zinc wires, there extend the wires n, which at p may be secured to the conducting wires of whatever kind.

In the commutator, as we have seen, all wires from the platinum plates come to the inner circle of cups, and all those from the zinc cylinders to the outer circle. In order to concentrate these to a simple chain or a chain of two pairs or to a pile, so-called commutating disks are used. These, which are made of wood, have a diameter of $2\frac{1}{4}''$, and carry copper wires furnished with feet, which are brought into connection with all the zinc cylinders, or all the platinum plates, or with each alternately, according to the combination desired. When setting the disks on the commutator, care must be taken that Ph always come in contact with the platinum of I. Zg with the zinc of the IV elements, and there are for this purpose on each disk two indications or mark-points. This battery is, as Grove's, filled with nitric and sulphuric acids, and continues of the same strength for hours.

Much cheaper, and answering the same purposes, is

2. *Stöhrer's large zinc-carbon battery*, which is placed in an oaken chest, and consists of six Bunsen's elements, which are filled with nitric and sulphuric acids (1 : 6). By means of stars of copper plate, which are marked Nos. 1, 2, and 6, and which can be laid in screw-stands so made as to receive the wires coming from the zincs and carbons, we can combine all the zincs and all the carbons into one pair, or into two pairs, or

into a pile, according as we wish to render incandescent a thick and short wire, one of middling strength, or one that is long and thin. In order to make a lessening of the current possible, Stöhrer has placed a moderator on the cover, which consists of a piece of tense silver wire, through which the current is conducted, and in this way diminished, before it passes into the apparatus containing the wire to be heated. On the foot of the moderator is a movable clamp, to regulate the amount of weakening of the current.

Less useful is

3. *Grenet's battery*.[1] This consists of nine amalgamated zinc plates and six copper plates covered with carbon, of which always three zinc plates combined with two carbon plates stand vertically on the base of the apparatus. The base is made of hard india-rubber; it has an excavation, and is furnished in its cover with five holes, through which the air, blown in by means of rubber tubes, in the excavation reaches the fluid into which the entire apparatus is dipped. This fluid is in a glass, wooden, or porcelain vessel, and consists of weak sulphuric acid, to which the bi-chromate of potash (in the proportions of 1 : 10) is added. After the battery is dipped into the fluid as high as the upper edge of the carbon plates, a Y-shaped tube is fastened to the rubber tube, and to this a pair of bellows; soon the fluid is thrown into considerable commotion, and after four or five seconds the platinum wire, which is secured to the conducting wires going from the zinc and carbon poles, glows. The current remains constant as long as the blowing is kept up. In Germany this battery has not met with the approval which Broca[2] has given it, because the rubber is easily destroyed, the bellows is not an exact regulator of the strength of the current, the apparatus is complicated, etc.

For galvano-caustic purposes, and in a still higher degree

[1] *Vide* Die Grenet'sche Batterie und ihre Bedeutung für die operative Heilanwendung des Galvanismus von Dr J. Samter, 1858.

[2] Bull. de l'Académie, xxiii, p. 75, Novbr., 1857.

as a means of producing the constant current, or that of Voltaic induction, the following are worthy of notice.

4. *The large zinc-carbon batteries* constructed by Stöhrer, because they consume, when not in use, neither zinc nor acids, though applicable in the same cases as the foregoing, and because they are furnished with a convenient regulator of the strength of the current. They consist of a greater or less number of zinc-carbon elements (without clay cells), which, secured to a beam in the middle of the battery, may be raised and lowered. In the cylindrical pieces of carbon is a deep hole with a diameter of about one-third of an inch, which is filled with sand and closed with a glass stopper, and serves for taking up nitric acid or concentrated chromic acid. Entire, well-amalgamated zinc cylinders encircle the carbon, and are prevented from coming in contact with this by means of glass isolators fastened to it. Glasses, which stand on the pedestal, and into which the elements may be lowered, serve for holding dilute sulphuric acid (1 : 6); according as the elements sink more or less deeply into this, the current is more or less strong. When not in use, the carbon and zinc are lifted so high, that the sulphuric acid no longer comes in contact with them, and, as the acid in this case takes up only the lower third of the glass, it may be transported without danger; besides, as there is no consumption of zinc, or decomposition of acid, the apparatus may stand for months without needing a new filling, and being always ready for use. Moreover, the elements may be united, as in the two following batteries, by means of clamps of copper plate, into one or several pairs.[1]

The most convenient apparatus for the application of the constant current to medical purposes is—

[1] [In an article on Organic Infantile Paralysis contained in the QUARTERLY JOURNAL OF PSYCHOLOGICAL MEDICINE AND MEDICAL JURISPRUDENCE for July, 1868, I have described Stöhrer's original battery at length. The accompanying woodcut (Fig. 4) will serve better than any additional description to give

REMAK'S BATTERY. 105

5. *Remak's zinc-carbon battery.* This generally consists of sixty elements, which have the following proportions:

an idea of its form. Stöhrer has recently greatly improved this battery by reducing its size, and altering the arrangement for getting the current from any number of cells.—See Appendix. W. A. H.]

Fig. 4.

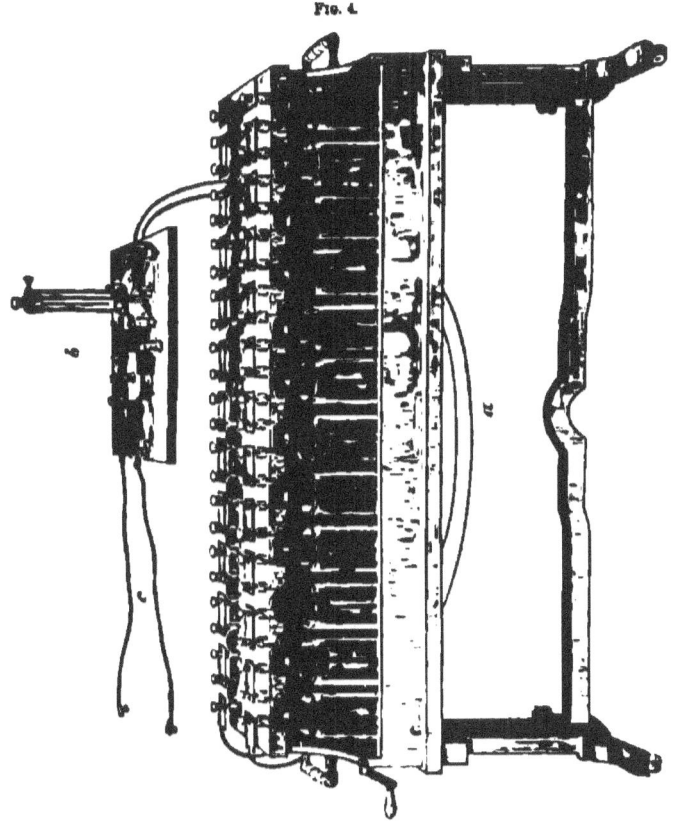

In a glass, 15 cm. high, and 11 cm. in diameter, there is a coil of one-inch-broad copper plate, to which there is soldered a copper wire which passes vertically upward through a glass cylinder, 2.5 cm. wide, and serves to connect with the next standing element. This glass cylinder, cemented into the bottom of a clay cell which covers the copper plate, is filled with water and pieces of blue vitriol up to its edge. At the upper part of the clay cell, surrounding it, and reaching to the bottom of the glass, there is a compressed layer of papier-mâché to the height of from 6 to 7 cm., on which, separated by a layer of fustian, rests a zinc cylinder, 1½ cm. thick and three times as high. This modification of Daniell's elements by Siemens and Halske has the advantage, through limiting the chemical process within the battery, of lengthening the durableness of the apparatus in this way, that the same may be used many months without repairs, if we only take care, every three or four weeks, to fill the glass cylinder with crystals of blue vitriol. It is advisable to clean the battery every three or four months, by which means the zinc is made more active; the security of the copper wire may then be tested, injuries may be repaired, and more acid water may be added, till the zinc is covered. These sixty elements, placed one behind another, are brought in connection with the current selector, rheotrope, and the galvanoscope, which three instruments are secured to a polished mahogany board.

The current selector, which has for its object the uniting for effect any number of elements, even as high as sixty, has the following construction: It has ten silver-plated buttons, arranged in opposite half-circles of fives, bearing the numbers 10, 8, 6, 4, 2, 10, 20, 30, 40, 50, which indicate the number of elements with which they are in combination. In the middle of each half-circle is a winch, which, moved from button to button, shuts off any desired number of elements. If we, for instance, need forty-two elements, we turn the winch B2 to 40, the winch B1 to 2; while, if we wish to use six elements, the winch B2 is moved to the nail O lying between the two half-circles, the winch B1 to 6. When both winches are at O, there is no current flowing.

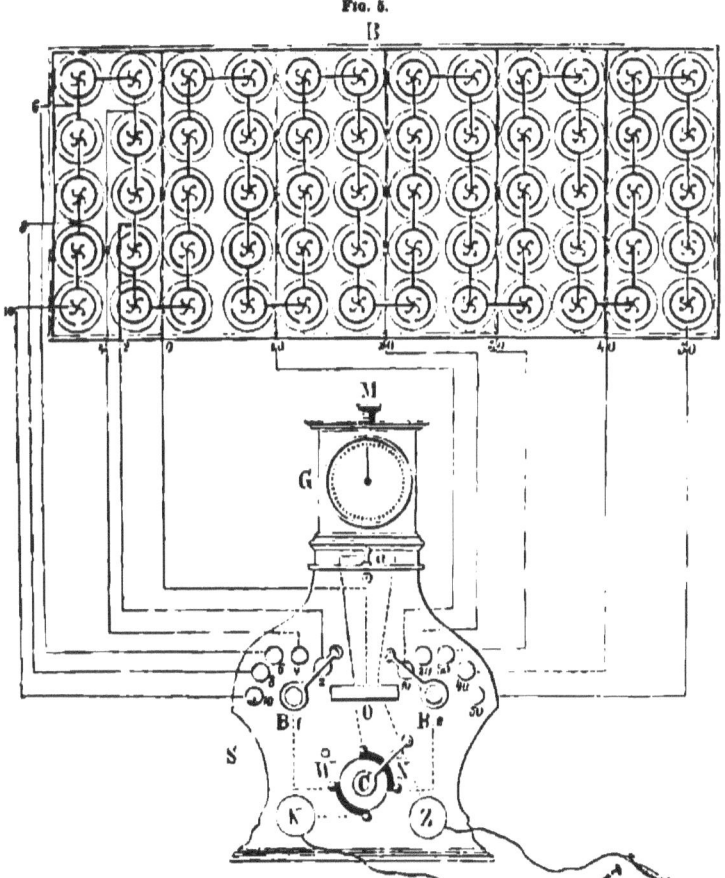

Fig. 5.

The change of the direction of the current is effected by means of the commutator C, in connection with the points

N (normal) and W (reversed). The conducting wires being secured by the binding-screws K (copper) and Z (zinc), the positive current passes, when the winch of the commutator is on N, through the clamp K and the conducting wire into the body, and through the other conducting wire to the zinc pole Z. If, on the contrary, the winch is on W, the positive current passes from the clamp Z through the body to K.

The *galvanoscope* G shows us, when the tips of the conducting wires are placed on any part of the body, and the stopper *a* is removed, how strong the current is, by means of the amount of deviation from the O point. On the brass button above the galvanoscope there is a small magnet-rod, by turning which to the left or the right we can place the needle on the O point, when this shows a deviation, the circuit being open.

The combination between the battery and the current selector is made in the following way: After the individual elements are arranged behind one another, and the zinc always connected with the copper, the first conducting wire of the copper pole of the first element is carried to the button 10 of the winch B1, and there secured by means of a screw. The second wire is fastened into the clamp which unites the second element with the third, and carried to the button 8. The same takes place between the elements 4 and 5, 6 and 7, 8 and 9, and the wires are united with the buttons 6, 4, 2, in a corresponding order. The wire between the tenth and eleventh elements is connected with the button O. From the eleventh element on, the enumeration is always by ten elements; the conducting wires are set on between the twentieth and twenty-first, the thirtieth and thirty-first, the fortieth and forty-first, and finally the fiftieth and fifty-first, and carried thence to the buttons 10, 20, 30, 40, of the winch B2. The last wire is carried from the zinc pole of the sixtieth element to button 50.

Remak's electrodes consist of wooden handles with brass

tips, which have the form either of buttons, from ¼ to 1 inch in diameter, or of segments of balls and plates, from 1¼ to 3 inches in diameter, or of square rods, from 1 to 3 inches long, and ¼ to 1 inch wide. These, to prevent oxidation, are covered with platinum plate, and then with a layer of flannel concealed by linen. The conductors are protected by cork coverings, from ¼ to ½ of an inch thick, which are secured to the metal plate by linen binding.

Lately, Fromhold has described an apparatus in a short paper,[1] which, so far as we can judge, is an improvement in the construction, since we can, by the use of it, not only obtain currents of a desired *intensity*, but of any *quantity*, for therapeutical purposes.

6. *Fromhold's apparatus* has the following construction: Its base has a length of 24″, and a breadth of 13″, and is furnished on each of its longer sides with a prominence for the reception of a wooden column, 21″ high, having a slit below, 3‴ wide. There is glued to the bottom, and secured by screws, a second board, pierced with 32 holes, which are for the reception of 32 battery-glasses. A similar board, serving as a point of support for the glasses, may be secured by means of two screws, which pass through the slits in the columns, at any height, even as far up as the edge of the glasses, and allow in this way an open view of these from all sides. (See Fig. 6.)

The 32 glasses, each of which has an outer diameter of about 2½ inches, and a height of 8 inches, are arranged in 4 rows, and serve for the reception of the zinc-lead-platinum elements already described. The electro-motor metals are secured to a wooden frame, of the dimensions of the bottom board, which is divided lengthwise into four parts, and carries on its middle cross-piece the dial (Remak's current selector) and the commutator. The four longitudinal divisions are so divided, by means of cross-sticks or saddles,

[1] Der constante galvanische Strom modificirbar in seinem Intensitäts- und Quantitätswerth, Pesth, 1867.

that each saddle comes exactly over the middle of a battery-glass. The entire frame is elevated when the metals are

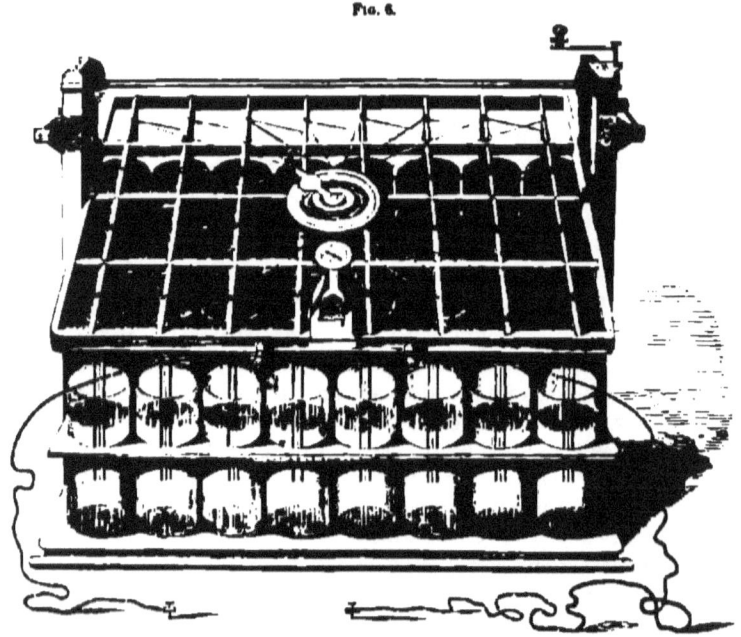

Fig. 6.

lifted from the fluid, and is lowered when these are allowed to sink into the fluid consisting of acid water, and this rising and sinking take place by means of a windlass. This consists of an iron rod passing from one column to the other, which holds on both of its inner ends a metallic disk of 3 inches diameter, and a cog-wheel where it passes at right angles through the column. This wheel is moved by means of an endless vertical screw, which turns it completely on its axis by 40 revolutions, and is held fast, through the friction, at any height. The *dial-plate*, which receives on its lower surface the conducting wires of all the positive poles, consists of a horizontal disk, 5 inches in diameter, of well-dried wood, which has on its surface 32 numbers, corresponding to the 32 elements, and of an indicator which can be moved without disturbing the apparatus from 1 to 32. Connected with this battery, as with Remak's, there is a commutator, and in place of the magnet-needle there is, separated from the apparatus, a tangent box-compass which is intercalated in the course of the current.

The power which this apparatus has of delivering currents of greater intensity and quantity, results from the possibility of introducing a greater or less number of elements, and of sinking them more or less deeply into the fluid: moreover, all possible modifications may be resorted to according to the various therapeutical indications or surgical demands. This battery also produces, by the slow sinking of the electro-motor metals into the fluid, a gradual increase of the *quantity*, and through the slow moving of the index from lower to higher numbers a gradual increase of the *intensity* —advantages which Fromhold considers of great service in therapeutics.

Deserving of special notice is

7. *Thomsen's Polarization Battery*,[1] because it has the advantage over all other batteries of producing sufficient electro-motor power by the use of one galvanic element, which takes up very little room, because, though the first cost is considerable, the expense of operating it is light, and because, with certain modifications, it may serve as a transportable battery for medicinal purposes. The theory which lies at the foundation of the construction of the apparatus is the following: When we touch the poles of a galvanic element to two platinum plates, which are dipped into dilute sulphuric acid, and then remove the element and con-

---

[1] Die Polarisations-Batterie, ein neuer Apparat zur Hervorbringen eines continuirlichen electrischen Stromes von hoher Spannung und constanter Starke mit Hülfe eines einzelnen galvanischen Elements von Julius Thomsen, Hamburg, 1863.

nect the platinum plates by means of a metallic wire, there arises an electric current, which runs in an opposite direction to the current which produced this condition—the platinum plates are then polarized; during the short time of contact there was formed an invisible film of the constituents of the water on the platinum plates—hydrogen on the plate which was in connection with the zinc pole, and oxygen on the plate in connection with the copper pole. The current has naturally only a short duration, since the hydrogen and oxygen quickly unite again, but we may, in a very short time, in this way charge a large number of plates, and obtain, if we unite these into a battery, an electrical current of very high tension. The strength of the current decreases, however, very quickly, unless we take care to charge the individual cells without breaking their connection with one another, and this is done by so arranging the platinum plates, as in a battery, and the connection of the polarizing element with each platinum pair, that the already present charge will be increased by the action of the charging current.

The *polarization-battery* consists of three principal parts: 1. The battery proper; 2. The galvanic element, which charges; 3. The distributing apparatus, through which the current produced by the element is conducted from one to another of the different cells of the battery. 1. The battery is formed of two open wooden chests, each of which is divided by means of 26 platinum plates secured in its walls, into 25 cells, so that—and this is a peculiarity of this battery—the plates themselves form partition walls between the cells, and the two sides of a plate belong to two different cells. 2. As the galvanic element must be able easily to decompose water, it is best to use a zinc-platinum or a zinc-carbon element with nitric or chromic acid. 3. The distributing apparatus consists of a flat ring, composed of insulating material, into which a number of short, radiating, metallic rods are secured, as many in number as the battery cells. Each of these is combined by means of a fine silver or copper wire with a platinum plate in the battery. Through the middle of the ring passes a vertical axis, which carries above two isolated arms alongside of one another, which stand in connection with two wooden clamps, serving for the reception of the conducting wires from the galvanic element. The two arms represent the two poles of the element; each is supplied with a spring, and they stand so far apart that, when one touches one metallic rod of the ring, the other is also in contact with the next. If the axis is now turned, which may be done by means of clock-work, a weight, or an electro-magnetic contrivance moved by a galvanic element (which causes a revolution in at most two or three seconds), each plate will become loaded one after the other with hydrogen on one side and oxygen on the other. After a single turning round of the axis all the plates are charged, and the battery is in a condition to begin its action. The intensity of the current is regulated through the polarizing element, and this again through the rheostat, i. e., an apparatus that enables us at pleasure to increase the conducting resistance by intercalating a longer or shorter metallic wire. The entire apparatus, exclusive of the galvanic element, is enclosed in a polished wooden chest 1½ feet long, 1 foot wide, and ½ foot high.

II. INDUCTION APPARATUS.

Among the magneto-electrical induction apparatuses we will mention:

8. *The apparatus of Pixii.* In this the electrical current is induced by means of a steel magnet rotating vertically on its axis, above the poles of which are two iron rods wound with connecting spirals. The magnet rotates, while the induction spirals remain immovable.

In all the later constructed apparatuses the magnet is immovable, and the horse-shoe shaped soft iron, either with the induction spiral or without it, is movable. To the induction apparatuses with movable spirals belong those of Saxton and Ettinghausen, Keil, Stöhrer, etc.; to those with immovable spirals, Duchenne's magneto-electrical apparatus, and that of the brothers Bréton.

9. *The Saxton-Ettinghausen apparatus* consists of a powful horse-shoe magnet, of five or seven plates, secured by means of screws to a wooden base. Between the arms of the magnet there is a small cylinder which may be set in motion by means of a turning wheel placed above the magnet. The cylinder, being of less diameter than the wheel, makes a correspondingly greater number of revolutions than the latter. With the cylinder the induction spirals turn and also the iron axle lying before these. On this axle are two steel rings, one of which, isolated by means of a covering of glass, wood, or ivory, receives one end of the induction spiral, the other end of this spiral is taken up by the second unisolated ring. This ring consists of two divisions, the front one of which is interrupted by two diametrically opposite indentations, while the hinder one has an unbroken surface. On each side of the axle is a small brass column, into which metallic springs are screwed; the right one supports two springs, one of which glides over the surface of the isolated ring, the other over the front division of the unisolated ring; the spring, secured to the left column, comes in contact with the other division of this latter ring. Finally, there is fastened to each brass column a metallic conducting wire, furnished with an application cylinder, between which the body to be electrized is intercalated. If the turning wheel, or with it the whole rotating system, is set in motion, each pole of the magnet produces an opposite polarity in the soft iron contained within the induction spirals, consequently with each half revolution of the axis the sides of the iron turned to the magnet change their polarity. Each magnetic iron rod produces an electric current in the spiral which surrounds it, according to the following law: if we excite, in an iron rod which lies in a spiral wound to the

right, magnetism in such a way, that on the active end a north pole is produced, then the positive electric current, induced through the magnetism, passes from this side into the spiral. The reverse follows with a winding of the spiral to the left. The brass columns on both sides of the axle have the office of conducting, by means of the metallic springs and wires, the induced current to the portion of the body to be affected, and this always takes place at the moment when the pole of the iron rod is moved away from that of the magnet, and the spring on the right side sinks into one of the indentations which are found on the front division of the unisolated ring. If we have to do with a spiral wound to the right, and at this moment the iron rod, whose wire end is connected with the isolated ring, leaves the north pole of the horse-shoe magnet, the positive current goes to the right column and (the conduction of the front right spring, which now stands in an indentation, being interrupted) thence through the conducting wires to the body operated on, and, passing through this from right to left, reaches the left

FIG. 7.

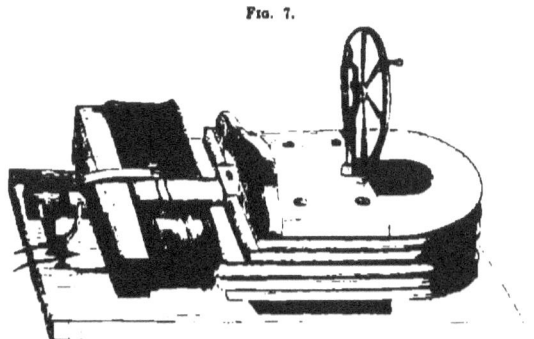

column, the spring of the left side, and finally the unisolated ring. After the next half revolution, when the iron rod, whose wire end is connected with the unisolated ring, comes under the influence of the south pole of the horse-shoe magnet, the positive current (the conduction of the front right spring being again interrupted) goes through the spring of the left side, the left column, the left conducting wire, into the electrized body, and, passing through this from left to right, returns by way of the conducting wire of the right side, the column, and the right hind spring, to the isolated ring. The current goes changing from right to left and from left to right, in an electrized arm, for instance: at one moment it passes from the hand to the shoulder, and at the next from the shoulder to the hand, and so on.

10. The same thing takes place with the *Saxton apparatus* modified by *Keil*, which has, in the place of the springs and steel rings, on the front end of the iron axle, a *gyrotrope* so arranged that it can be turned also by the wheel. It consists of four small half disks of German silver, covered

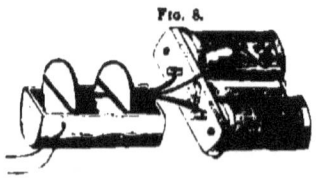

Fig. 8.

to within three lines of their edges with lac, which from their relative positions seem to form two round plates. Of these half-disks the upper and hinder stands in connection with the front and lower one, and lower and hinder is similarly united with the front and upper one, and each takes up an end of the induction spiral. The disks, which are separated by about one inch, dip into quicksilver, which, for the purpose of aiding the conduction, is placed in two furrows of a wooden vessel standing on an appropriate pedestal. In the quicksilver of each furrow there lies a metallic wire, to the outer ends of which the conducting wires are connected. Here also, with each half revolution, the direction of the current changes, which passes to the body to be electrized.

STÖHRER'S APPARATUS.

Stöhrer first succeeded, by means of his very ingenious commutator-contrivance, in changing the currents, flowing after each half revolution in opposite directions, into currents having the same direction and as such passing to the body.

11. *Stöhrer's apparatus* consists of a horizontally-lying horse-shoe magnet, of, at most, five equally long plates, and of an iron axle, between the arms of the magnet; to these

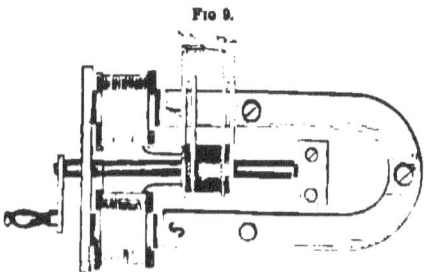

Fig 9.

are attached from behind forward: *a*. The commutator; *b*. The soft irons, wound with the induction spirals, which are secured to the ends of an iron bar at an angle of ninety degrees; *c*. A crank which, set in motion, turns the entire rotating system (axle, commutator, and induction spirals).

Here, as with the Saxton-Ettinghausen apparatus, each core of the induction coil, with each half revolution of the axle, is changed into a north pole and then again into a south pole; and yet, by means of the commutator, currents having the same direction pass over. The commutator consists of a shorter and broader, and of a longer and narrower brass cylinder, which, separated by means of a wooden tube, are placed one within the other, the shorter being outermost. On each end of each cylinder there is soldered a steel ring, so that we have four steel rings, which we will number from before backward, 1, 2, 3, and 4. The half of each steel ring projects beyond the other half by about ½ a line, in such a way that the prominent halves of 1 and 3 and of

2 and 4 correspond. One end of the induction spiral is connected with the ring 1, and this through the narrow brass tube with the ring 4, while the other end of the spiral is connected with the ring 2, and through this with 3. Finally, two steel springs are so secured to the wooden chest in which the apparatus is placed, that their free ends touch the steel rings lightly from above, and their fixed ends are furnished with conducting wires. If the apparatus is set in motion, during one-half revolution the steel rings 1 and 3, and during the other half the steel rings 2 and 4, are touched by the steel springs. The positive current from the one end of the wire goes through the ring 1, the corresponding spring and the anterior conducting wire to the human body, and then through the posterior conducting wire and steel spring to the ring 3, and so finishes its course, since it returns through the ring 2 into the spiral coil. By means of this commutator, currents having always the same direction are conducted through the body to be electrized. In order to increase the frequency of the interruptions, Stöhrer has recently attached to the axle a pair of toothed disks of copper, so that at each revolution of the wheel the current is frequently interrupted.

The so-called American apparatuses of Palmer and Hall, in Boston, and of Davis and Kidder, in New York, are worthy of notice, being small, compendious, cheap, and serving for many cases; they have, however, no commutator.

In regard to *volta-electrical induction apparatuses*, the earlier ones (Baumann's, Rauch's, etc.) consisted: *a*. Of a simple or of a constant chain; *b*. Of one or two wires, which encircled in numerous windings a high cylinder of paper or wood; *c*. Of a toothed turning wheel, which caused the interruption of the current; and, finally, *d*. Of conducting wires, which carried the interrupted currents to the body to be electrized. The intensity of the current was modified by means of iron rods, which in greater or less numbers were placed in the cylinder, as well as by a slower or faster turning of the wheel.

The *Neef-Wagner apparatus* is more complete than these, and may be considered as the foundation of all the more recent and more perfect volta-induction apparatuses which are furnished with a self-acting hammer.

12. The *Neef-Wagner apparatus*[1] consists of a constant chain, whose positive pole is connected, by means of the conducting wire *a*, with a little cup on the pedestal of the induction coil, filled with quicksilver, and whose negative pole, through the wire *g*, is connected with the beginning of the induction spiral *f*. The induction spiral, after numerous windings around a wooden cylinder, reaches the point *e*, and

Fig. 10.

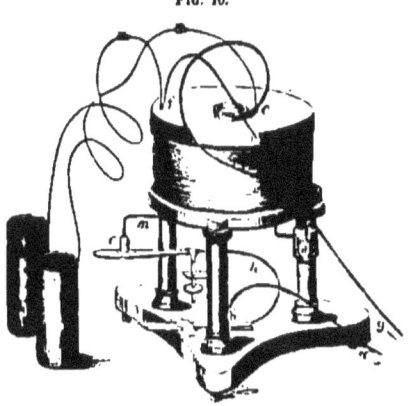

ends in a second quicksilver cup *d*. Between the cups *b* and *d* a connection is made in the following way: A copper wire *m*, which extends horizontally under the coil, ends in a small, light, movable platinum hammer *c*. This hammer rests on a platinum plate, which is soldered to the wire coming from *b*. Through the lifting up of the hammer *c*,

[1] Pouillet's Lehrbuch der Physik von Müller, ii. Auflage, Band ii., p. 232.

and through the resulting separation from the platinum plate which lies under it, the current is broken—through the falling of the same, the current is again formed. The apparatus, however, directs both operations. There is in the induction coil a cylinder of soft iron, which becomes magnetic as soon as the current runs through the induction wire. When magnetic, it attracts a small iron plate, which is soldered to the movable wire *m*, by which means both wire and platinum hammer are lifted and the current is interrupted. As soon, however, as the current is interrupted, the cylinder loses its magnetic power, the movable copper wire falls, and the circuit is again closed, in the next moment to be reopened, and so on. By means of the constant opening and closing of the circuit in the induction wire, currents are produced in a second wire running parallel with this, which can be used for physiological and therapeutical purposes. The rapidity with which the interruptions follow one another depends on the distance of the iron plate from the iron cylinder, and this may be regulated by means of a screw.

Klöpfer's, Gentsch's, Goldberger's apparatus, and others, are more or less compendious modifications of the above; they are mostly put in action by means of a Bunsen zinc-carbon element. Some, for the purpose of modifying the strength of the current, are furnished with a so-called *moderator*. This is a glass tube, filled with water, alcohol, or oil, into the upper and lower ends of which, closed by corks, the terminations of conducting wires enter. As we can at pleasure separate these from one another, and, consequently, shorten or lengthen the distance through which the current has to pass in the fluid, we possess a means of conducting a current of greater or less strength to the body to be electrized.

13. *Duchenne's volta-electrical apparatus*[1] is composed

[1] (Duchenne, de l'Électrisation localisée, etc., 1855 [p. 127, *et seq.*], 1861 [p. 184, *et seq.*].)

of two drawers in a wooden chest, and of a metallic covering placed above these. In the lower drawer, which is lined with cemented glass plates, so that the moisture may not affect the wood, is a Bunsen's element. The zinc has the

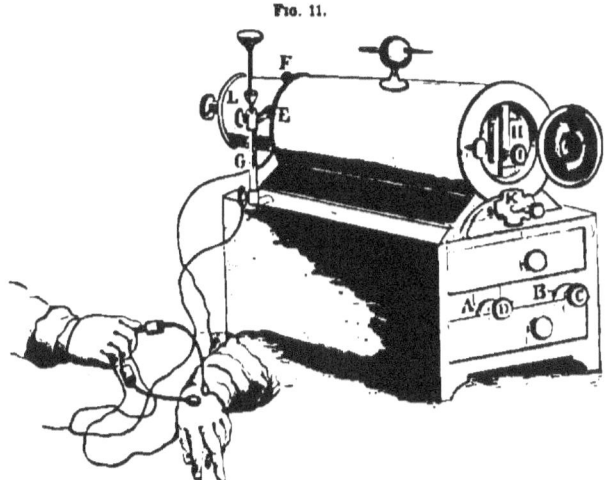

Fig. 11.

form of a flat box, in which the carbon without a diaphragm is placed. The carbon is flat, hollowed out in the middle, and filled with coke-dust. If the carbon is new, we saturate it with nitric acid and place it in the zinc vessel after we have moistened the whole surface of the latter with a saturated solution of salt. Lately Duchenne has changed the element: the carbon plate, saturated with water in an india-rubber box, is covered first with the sulphide of mercury and then with a layer of thin cloth; on these the zinc plate is placed.[1]

Two copper plates A and B, one of which is in connec-

[1] Such elements, lately come into use with the small volta-induction apparatuses in the hands mostly of the non-professional, have the advantage that they, firstly, need no acid, and secondly, that they are more lasting because they supply themselves the zinc amalgam.

tion with the zinc, and the other with the carbon of the element, communicate, by means of two platinum plates C, D, with the primary spiral, which, as the secondary, lies in the metallic covering on the upper part of the wooden chest. The primary or magnetizing spiral, consisting of a proportionably small number of windings of a 1 mm. thick wire, holds in its cavity a bundle of iron wires, and serves as a point of departure to the extra current, while, from the secondary or induction spiral, which is formed by a much larger number of windings of a $\frac{1}{2}$ mm. thick wire, the secondary current is carried off in E and F. Around this immovable spiral there is a closed, movable copper cylinder, which is furnished with a scale. If it is pushed entirely into the metallic covering, the currents have the lowest intensity; in order to gradually increase this, the cylinder must be drawn slowly out. As this lessening of intensity was not sufficient in powerful apparatuses, Duchenne placed another closed cylinder, holding a bundle of iron wires, within the magnetizing spiral, and obtained the least action when it was fully covered by the cylinder and spirals. The physical reason of this is, that closed conductors, near an induction current, having the form of metallic cylinders or of closed spirals, produce a weakening of the current, because currents are induced in themselves by coming and going, and at the expense of the induction current. So in this case, the current flowing in the spiral is weakened through the action of the outer copper cylinder, while through that of the inner the effect of the iron rods may be completely neutralized. As a third means of weakening the current, there is also attached to the apparatus a moderator G, which, on account of the greater or less depth of water through which the current has to pass, renders it possible to produce any desired lessening of the strength of the current. The interruptions may be made in two different ways: either through a, the hammer, which consists of a movable iron rod H and a screw I furnished with a platinum point, with which the soft iron of the iron-wire bundle, at a point covered with platinum plate, comes in contact; or *b*, through the cog-wheel immediately above the wooden chest, which is movable by means of a winch, and can be brought in connection with the spiral by a spring. We are thus able to vary the frequency of the interruptions at pleasure: by means of the hammer we may obtain four in a second, and through the turning wheel a still smaller number. In order to measure the strength of the current of the galvanic element, there is a so-called current-measurer in the upper drawer, a box-compass which indicates the degree of magnetism of the iron core. The disk of the box-compass is divided into four parts, and each part into 90 degrees. The current-measurer serves also to keep the primary current of the element of even strength. No pile is perfectly constant, and even Duchenne's element, after several hours of activity, loses a part of its strength; but we are able, when the compass shows a slackening of the current, by the addition of a few drops of nitric acid, to bring the magnet-needle back to its earlier stand-point, and we have the power, through the combined working of the current-measurer and the extinguisher, of ascertaining the degree of irritability, with great exactness, of any part of the body.

14. The *Baierlacher apparatus*[1] is a modification of Duchenne's, and differs from his in the following points: 1. It has, instead of two copper cylinders for regulating the strength of the current, only one, which, graduated to centimetres, can be moved in and out over the bundle of iron wires within the spiral. 2. Baierlacher lets his hammer, which has considerable weight, swing in a horizontal direction between an electro-magnet placed in the middle of the iron rod and a small platinum plate. The platinum plate itself may be made to approach, by means of a brass screw, a platinum pin in the middle of the spring which carries the hammer.

[1] Die Inductions-Electricität von Dr. E. Baierlacher, Nürnberg, 1857, p. 141, et seq.

15. *Stöhrer's transportable induction apparatus*, both the smaller and the greater, consist of a mahogany box which is divided into two parts by means of a partition. In the left side is a movable zinc-carbon element, already described, and in the other the induction apparatus. By means of the clamps which secure the zinc and coal to the partition, the battery current is conducted to the primary spiral and to the interrupter. This consists of a quadrangular iron rod fastened to an easily-moving spring, which may be attracted and set free from an electro-magnet composed of a bundle of iron wires, and allows of the motion of a hammer and the consequent induction of the secondary spiral. This latter can be lifted vertically by means of a graduated rod. A brass spring, having a screw, leans against the hammer, and serves to produce, through its greater or less action, a change in the strength and times of the induction shocks. Four screw-stands have the office of conducting the current to the body; those marked P give the primary current, and those marked S the secondary current. Modifications of the strength of the current can be produced: *a*. For both currents, by varying the arrangement of the battery-glasses and the action of the hammer-spring. *b*. We can further check the primary current by connecting the screw-stands of the secondary current by means of the attached wire bow, and by lifting the spiral by its rod. *c*. If in using the secondary current the wire bow is removed, the strength of the current is increased when the spiral is lifted. Various attachments are found in the drawer on the right side of the apparatus.

The larger apparatus differs from the smaller in that—
a. It has two battery-glasses; *b*. Its hammer is better constructed, consisting of an iron beam whose recoil is regulated by a spiral spring; *c*. As the primary current, even by complete lifting of the induction spiral, is not sufficiently weakened for certain cases, Stöhrer has lately added a copper tube in the interior of the induction apparatus, which, lifted

by a small graduated rod, slides over the primary spiral, and, in connection with the elevated closed induction spiral, reduces the primary current to a minimum.

16. *Du Bois-Reymond's apparatus* is most conveniently

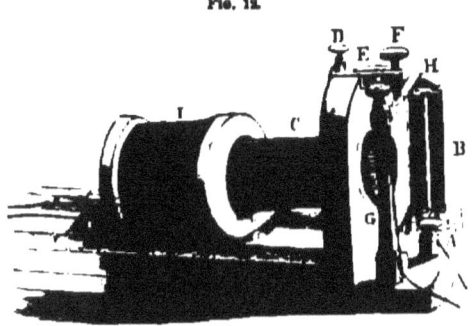

Fig. 12.

set in operation, when an intense current of no great duration is wanted, by means of a small Grove's element; when, on the other hand, a continuing strong current is needed, it is best to connect it with one or two Bunsen's elements, according to its size which are filled after Poggendorf's direction (see page 14), or with the chamber-battery of Stöhrer, described on page 104. In the latter case, it is also advisable to use the greater apparatus, with 5½-inches-long magnetizing and induction rolls, whose primary spiral consists of about 500 windings of a strong wire of 1.2 mm., and whose secondary of about 10,000 windings of wire of 0.25 mm.; while, when using Grove's element, the smaller apparatus, with 2¼-inches-long magnetizing and induction rolls, whose primary spiral consists of about 250 windings of a strong wire of 1.2 mm., and whose secondary of about 500 windings of 0.25 mm., is fully sufficient.

The wire going from the zinc pole of the element is secured in a standard on the front end of the apparatus, which at the same time is the starting-point of the magnetizing spiral. From A the wire passes to the horse-shoe B, around which it forms a spiral, and then goes to a horizontal wooden cylinder, C, filled with a movable bundle of iron wires, around which it also winds in a spiral form, and ends in the brass upright D. This latter is secured to a brass piece, E, which at its front end is pierced for the reception of the steel screw F. The conducting wire going from the carbon (or platinum) connects with a perpendicular column, G, which receives, above, the steel spring of an iron hammer, H, that, as soon as the apparatus is set in motion, strikes uninterruptedly on the steel screw F or on the horse-shoe B, and thus continues or breaks the connection between the wires. The positive current goes then from the carbon of the element to the brass column G, from this to the iron hammer H, as far as the point of contact with the steel screw F, thence through the brass piece E to the wire of the wooden cylinder C; it then passes to the horse-shoe B, and ends in the standard A, which receives the conducting wire coming from the zinc. Besides the wooden cylinder filled with iron rods already mentioned, the apparatus has a second, I, the so-called "sled," which, by means of a track on the pedestal, can be moved backward and forward over the small wooden cylinder, and may cover this more or less fully. The greater cylinder is, as has been mentioned, surrounded by a twenty times greater number of windings of a wire which has about one-fifth of the thickness of that of the primary wire; its beginning and end are taken up by standards placed on the posterior part of the apparatus, which serve also for receiving the conducting wires that carry the current of the second order to the body to be electrized. The extra-current is conducted from D, and from a standard near by, which is by means of a wire in connection with A.

The extra-current has its greatest intensity when the bundle of iron wires is shoved fully into the cylinder, the sled removed, and the action of the magnetizing spiral withdrawn; the more the wire bundle is pulled out and the sled pushed in, the weaker is the current. The current of the second order has, on the contrary, its greatest intensity when the sled fully covers both wooden cylinder and iron rods; the more the rods are drawn out, the sled removed, and the action of the magnetizing spiral diminished, the weaker is this current. The number of intermissions may be lessened or increased by the greater or less approximation of the steel screw F to a platinum plate placed on the middle of the hammer H.

Often the Du Bois apparatus is furnished with a measuring-rod, graduated to inches and lines, which is secured to the sled, so that comparative measurements of the contractility of different muscles at one time, or of the same muscle at different times, may be made. Yet this arrangement is mostly superfluous for the first purpose, and for the second insufficient, when the apparatus is not at the same time furnished, as is Duchenne's, with a compass, which measures the strength of the galvanic element, and, if necessary, regulates it. But even then the influence of the outer temperature of the dry and perspiring skin—not taking into account the variation which the apparatus shows through the deposition of coal on the platinum plate, through the greater or less approximation of the steel screw to the hammer, etc.—is so considerable, that the making of such measurements is not worth the loss of time required.[1]

We have, in the previous pages, described a number of magneto-electrical and volta-electrical induction apparatuses,

[1] [In the first edition of this work I gave it as my opinion that the induction batteries of Kidder were superior to all others made in this country. Since then, the instruments made by the Galvano-Faradic Manufacturing Company have been introduced, and are preferable in every respect to any heretofore constructed. They are fully described in the Appendix. Kidder's apparatus is, however, good of its kind. The galvanism is derived from either one or two Smee's cells, according to the size of the apparatus. The box contains the batteries, and also a bottle in which the dilute sulphuric acid employed may be kept when the apparatus is not in use.

128   AMERICAN APPARATUSES.

a consideration of which will give a tolerably complete idea of their gradual improvement. As to the first, we noticed those

Fig. 13 represents the galvanic cell, and Fig. 14 the whole arrangement. A full description of the apparatus is given in the published pamphlet of the inventor. Dr. Kidder also makes a very portable apparatus.

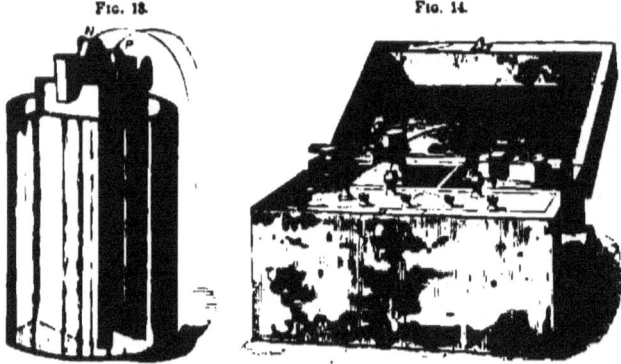

Fig. 13.   Fig. 14.

Fig. 15 shows the essential parts of a very convenient portable and sufficiently-powerful induction apparatus devised by Mr. Drescher, of New York.

Fig. 15.

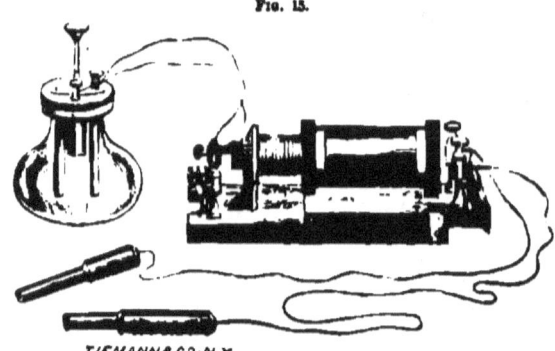

TIEMANN & CO. N.Y.

It is set in action by a Grenet's cell, a very convenient form of battery composed of a zinc and two carbon plates, which dip into a mixture of dilute sulphuric acid and bichromate of potash. The elements are contained in a glass

which have a movable and an immovable magnet; further, those which, with each half revolution of the induction spiral, conduct currents, having different directions, to the body to be electrized, and those which always transmit currents having the same direction. All deliver only currents of the first order. In most of these apparatuses the strength of the current is regulated by means of the greater or less approximation of the magnet to the induction spiral, through the action of a screw behind the magnet, and by a keeper placed on the magnet. As regards the first point, the iron is less strongly magnetized with its greater removal from the magnet, and accordingly produces less strong electrical currents in the copper wire, while the keeper, according to the extent of its surface and its nearness to the poles, participates in the magnetic power, and leaves, consequently, less for the production of the induction current.

Among the volta-electrical apparatuses we noticed first those which are excited through an inconstant series, and are set in motion by means of a turning wheel; we passed then to those with constant current and wheel, which both lack a means of turning the latter; next we considered the apparatuses which are self-moving, and first that of Neef and Wagner, which delivers only an induction current of the second order, the strength of which can only be modified through the use of more or less strong acid, or through the more or less frequent interruptions; and we closed with Duchenne's, Stöhrer's, and Du Bois-Reymond's apparatuses and their modifications, which deliver currents of the first and second order, and allow of different variations of the strength of the current in the most convenient way, by means of metal cylinders or sleds.

jar, tightly closed at the top, and so arranged that, when not in use, the zinc can be raised from the solution. The coil and its accessories, as seen in the cut, are contained in a mahogany box, eight inches long and four wide. This battery furnishes the secondary current only. The instruments of the Galvano-Faradic Manufacturing Company, described in the Appendix, are very great improvements on this arrangement.—W. A. H.]

ADVANTAGES OF DIFFERENT FORMS OF APPARATUS.

As to the preference which one class of induction apparatuses has over the other, we would say that, in general, the magneto-electrical have the advantage over the volta-electrical in that they need no preparation for use, and that their working, always, or at least for a very long time, remains regular. Through the frequent moving of the keeper it is true that the power of the magnet in the end suffers, but this is soon returned by the stroking movement. On the other hand, with the volta-electrical apparatus a chemical process must precede its action; moreover, the electrical current loses in intensity with the slackening of the power of the galvanic series, which necessarily takes place after some time; finally, this kind of apparatus when in use produces injurious gases, which, even when very inconsiderable, are disagreeable. The more-recently-constructed volta-electrical apparatuses have the advantage that in their working no assistance is required, that the intermissions are much more frequent, that these remain regular hour after hour, which is impossible with those apparatuses which have to be turned;[1] and that, finally, two kinds of currents may be obtained from them, one of which possesses a greater electro-motor power than the other.

As regards the last point, Duchenne has made the interesting observation that the current of the first order works especially on the contractility of the muscular fibres, the current of the second order on the sensory nerves of the skin, and he has, consequently, ascribed different

[1] Remak has constructed a sensitive apparatus for counting and for lessening at pleasure the number of shocks in a given time. This consists of a clockwork placed in connection with the conducting wires of a volta-electrical apparatus; the opening and closing of the circuit (the action of the spring being arrested) are brought about by the pendulum; at the moment when it reaches its highest point the spring is opened by the lifting of a small chain—at the moment when it leaves it, through the sinking of the same, it is again closed. By lengthening or shortening the pendulum we may produce few or many vibrations, and consequently few or many intermissions. By the same contrivance we can change any constant current into an interrupted one, with any desired frequency of interruption.

ADVANTAGES OF DIFFERENT FORMS OF APPARATUS. 131

actions to those two currents. But though the observation be correct, the explanation is unsatisfactory, for the reason that the difference in the action of the two currents is due to the difference between the two spirals in which the currents are developed, so that we have here before us a consequence of Ohm's law. The induced roll consists of very many windings of an exceedingly fine wire, the inducing of a much smaller number of windings of a thick wire, and the electro-motor power of a single winding of the inducing wire is stronger than that of a winding of the secondary wire. Now, it is true that the secondary spiral consists of a much greater number of windings, and the sum of the electro-motor power is, consequently, greater; but, as the resistance increases at the same rate, so the proportion remains the same, and the extra current in the inducing roll possesses a greater intensity than the current of the induction spiral. The proportion is easily changed with the addition of a new resistance. If this is small, as, for instance, when we, for irritating a superficial muscle lying under the skin, place moist conductors near one another on the moistened epidermis, the extra current is the most serviceable, because the quotient of the electro-motor power of the primary spiral through the sum of the conducting resistance of the wire and of the moist tissue is greater than that of the greater electro-motor power of the secondary spiral, through the still much greater resistance of the secondary wire together with that of the moist tissue. If we wish, on the contrary, to electrize the skin and to conquer the enormous conducting resistance of the dry epidermis, the proportion changes the other way, and we operate much more successfully with the secondary current. This is also the reason why the extra current often is not sufficient for irritating deeply-lying muscles, while the secondary current is able to overcome the resistance. For this reason we use, for physiological and pathological investigations, **exclusively the volta-induction apparatuses, which we** have more fully to notice in the seventh and eighth sections, while for therapeutical purposes the magneto-induction apparatuses take their place. Though these are not equally serviceable for exciting the nerves of the skin, Stöhrer's being, perhaps, the best for this purpose, they, nevertheless, are of advantage when we wish to produce not a constant tetanus, but a gradual contraction of the irritated muscles, as is sometimes advisable in obstetrical cases. Also, we cannot do without these in those cases where we, as, for instance, in the paralysis of certain muscles or the swelling of joints, etc., which often need much time for their curing, must leave the treatment in the hands of the unprofessional. In such instances the small apparatus of Palmer and Hall or of Davis and Kidder is to be recommended as well as on account of its cheapness.

In regard to the volta-induction apparatuses described under the numbers from 13 to 16, Duchenne's has the advantage over Du Bois's, when used for therapeutical purposes, that we can, by means of its hammer and turning wheel, to a much greater degree vary the frequency of the shocks—while through the greater or less approximation of the steel screw to the hammer of Du Bois's apparatus the number of intermissions, it is true, can be increased or diminished, yet this cannot be done to any desired degree. On the other hand, Du Bois's has the advantage that we can by the use of the sled alone regulate the strength of the current at any moment in the most convenient way and lessen it to a degree, which can only be accomplished in Duchenne's apparatus by the combined working of his extinguisher and moderator. Moreover, Du Bois's apparatus, the spring of which is not set in motion by means of the iron core of the spiral, but by a small horse-shoe magnet separated from it, allows of the possibility of being used with or without a greater or less number of iron rods, and so furnishes us with a ready mode of checking the strength of the current, which, especially when the rolls are near one another, increases very rapidly with their approximation. Both apparatuses have in common the failing that in many cases, in which the electro-muscular contractility is much reduced, their extra current is not sufficiently strong. Stöhrer's apparatus has the great advantage that it can be used at any moment without any chemical preparation, that it is free from all the inconveniences which are connected with the frequent filling of the element, and which, especially when using the most compendious and strongest Grove's element, are not to be considered slight—since they consist not only in a loss of time, but in unavoidable injury of the hands and of the clothing—on the other hand, especially in the small apparatus, the spring often stands still and its motion is not in all cases immediately recovered; moreover, the secondary current even of the greater apparatus has never the strength that it has in Du Bois's apparatus, and which is indicated, namely, in anæsthesia of a high degree, or where we wish to use the current as a diverting means. Finally, an addition is needed to the apparatus, by which the physician, who generally requires both his hands, for electrizing, can, without the assistance of others, gradually increase the strength of the current, since he would have thereby a means of rendering the application painless, as is desirable in all cases, especially with children and sensitive persons.

17. *Modified Du Bois's Apparatus* from the establishment of Siemens and Halske (now Krüger and Hirschmann).

In order to remove the above-noticed imperfections, I have, through our able mechanics Siemens and Halske, made the following alterations in Du Bois's apparatus, by which, it is true, the price is considerably raised (since it costs 60 thalers), yet it now answers all the purposes of physicians who occupy themselves especially with electrotherapeutics:

1. The hammer is made much heavier, and is so constructed that it can be almost doubled in length, by which

means, as with the increase in length of the pendulum the number of vibrations in a given time decreases, their frequency in a second may be greatly lessened. Also, in order to lessen the frequency of the shocks and with them the pain, a second metallic spring (similar to that in Erdmann's apparatus) is added to the first, which, in the moment when the stronger spring leaves the electro-magnet and the part of the body to be electrized receives the shock, can come into action to lengthen and consequently to blunt it.

2. In order to make the extra current stronger, the secondary spiral is so altered that it also can be used for lengthening the primary. For this purpose it is divided, by interrupted wooden rings, into four equal divisions, on each of which there is coiled, in numerous windings, a wire one-quarter as thick as that used for the extra current, and by means of a cylinder without the induction spiral it can be so arranged that, through simply turning the same and altering the commutators: a, all the four ends and beginnings of the thin wire may be connected with one another; the four wires may be disposed parallel with one another and thereby a wire as thick as that of the extra current may be produced; or b, the end of the wire of the first division may be connected with the beginning of that of the second, the end of the wire of the second with the beginning of the third, etc., the wires being thus disposed one after the other, and in this way a spiral perfectly analogous to the secondary spiral of the earlier apparatus, and four times as long and thin, is formed.

The figures 16 and 17 represent the course of the currents of the first and second orders, and in both figures the direct full battery-current is indicated by thick lines, the four-times-divided current in fig. 17 by thin lines, and the secondary current in fig. 16 by interrupted lines; the thin lines in fig. 16 indicate the wires, which, by this arrangement, are without action.

Let us follow the course of the current of the first order

(extra current). (See fig. 16.) After we have brought the apparatus, by properly arranging the commutators, into the

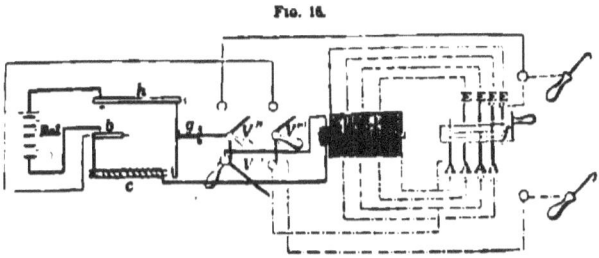

Fig. 16.

condition in which the current is lengthened by the induction spiral, the current coming from the zinc pole of the battery passes into the apparatus by b; from this it goes to the electro-magnet c, then to the magnetizing spiral d, then through the commutator V' to the secondary spiral. There the same, by arranging the cylinder, is brought into such a position, that the four wire-beginnings of the four divisions A' A'' A''' A'''', and the four ends of these, E' E'' E''' E'''', are united in a wire four times as thick, through which the current passes, and then takes its course, after entering the screw which serves at the same time for the reception of a conducting wire, through the commutator II (V'') to the steel screw g, to the platinum hammer, to the brass column h, and ends in the carbon of the battery. The screw serving for the taking up of the conducting wire of the second conductor is also placed on the hind end of the sled; between this and the point of entrance of the battery current in h, there is interposed a wire by means of the commutator III (V''').

In order to use the induction current, the commutator I (V') is rendered entirely inactive, as is shown in fig. 17, while the position of the two other commutators is changed. Through the change in position of V''', the cylinder f is at the same time brought into a position in which the wires of the four divisions of the induction spiral are arranged one after the other.

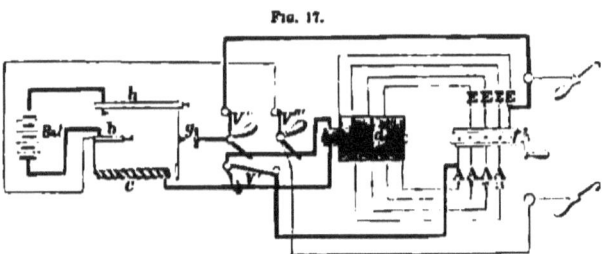

Fig. 17.

The current of the first order goes in this case from the zinc pole of the battery to the screw b, to the electro-magnet c, to the magnetizing spiral d, through this, and returns, in consequence of the change of position of V'', through the steel screw g and the brass column h to the carbon of the battery.

The induction current, on the contrary, goes from V''' to the beginning of the induction spiral A', passes through the first division to the end E', goes from here to the beginning of the second division A'', passes through this, and ends in E''; and so on to the wire end of the fourth division E'''', whence it enters the screw which receives the conducting wire of one of the conductors used for electrizing any portion of the body. After it has passed through the body, it returns by way of the second conductor, the screw and the track on the pedestal, to the commutator III (V''''). As is seen by this arrangement, a portion of the wire is inactive, which is indicated by the thin lines.

3. In order conveniently to regulate the strength of the current, I have attached to the front face of the chest on which my apparatus is secured a movable foot-board, which preserves whatever position is given it by the foot. From the front end of this board a strong brass wire rises perpendicularly, and passes into a perforated brass piece, in which

it moves with the foot-board here and there. The brass piece is also secured to the chest, and serves at the same time to take up a conducting wire which brings about the connection with the sled. On the perpendicular brass rod there is secured a horizontal one, from which a second vertical one dips into a glass tube (moderator) of about six inches length, which is held in place by a brass support. If I press with my heel on the hinder end of the foot-board, its front end is lifted, and with it the wire secured to it, as well as the one dipping into the water-tube; if I lower the point of my foot, the wire sinks in the same proportion into the water. Things are so arranged, that the current, before it passes into the body to be electrized, must traverse the water-column; hence, through the action of the foot, we have a convenient means of increasing the strength of the current slowly and gradually to any desired degree, and also almost imperceptibly. This simple contrivance, of the usefulness of which I have satisfied myself, can be attached to all volta-induction apparatuses.

The current-deliverers (electrodes, conductors, excitors) consist, in the most convenient form, of straight or a little curved metallic wires, with isolated handles, and tips of various kinds; sometimes these are rounded, sometimes they consist of small or large buttons, sometimes they are olive-shaped, and are covered with fine soft sponge. Frequently, a metallic cylinder adapted to receiving a small sponge is used, but oftener metallic tongs into which sponges of various sizes are secured; finally, small brushes of silver or gold wire often take the place of these. I have added to these an *interrupter*, by which we are able in certain cases, without removing the conductor from the skin, to produce single powerful shocks. For this purpose there is introduced, between the metallic cylinder, which receives the conducting wire, and the metallic rod, immediately above the handle, an isolator, three-quarters of an inch long, prepared of india-rubber or ivory, which comes into play only when we separate from this, by the pressure of the finger, the spring, which makes the connection between the handle and the metallic rod. Besides these, other contrivances are used for reaching certain organs — for instance, the bladder, the œsophagus, etc.—of which we will speak in the sixth section. In order to prevent the oxidation which after long use takes place on the points of the different tips, we cover them with thin platinum plate or use the so-called unpolarizable electrodes, which Stöhrer has made from prepared coal after the directions of Du Bois-Reymond. To diminish the conducting resistance of the skin, the conductors are placed in warm water (30° to 40° R.), or the skin itself is moistened therewith. The conducting wires, finally, which make the connection between the apparatus and the conductors, consist of metallic wire covered with silk, so as to prevent the escape of sparks, which, with a very strong current and moist wires, is sure to take place; these may be covered with thin rubber.

SIXTH SECTION.

METHODS OF USING INTERRUPTED AND CONSTANT CURRENTS.

Duchenne, De l'Électrisation localisée, 2e édit., 1861 (*l. c.*, pp. 47-102). Richters Bericht über die electro-physiologischen Arbeiten des Dr. Duchenne de Boulogne (in Schmidt's Jahrbüchern, Band LXXI., p. 258, *et seq*.). Dr. B. A. Erdmann, Die örtliche Anwendung der Electricität in Bezug auf Physiologie, Pathologie und Therapie, Leipzig, 1860, pp. 70-164. R. Remak, Ueber methodische Electrisirung gelähmter Muskeln, Berlin, 1856. Dr. H. Ziemssen, Die Electricität in der Medicin, 3. Aufl., Berlin, 1866. Prof. A. Fick, Einige Bemerkungen über die neuere Electrotherapie vom physikalisch-physiologischen Standpunkte, in der Wiener Medic. Wochenschrift, 1856, Nos. 48 und 49. Prof. A. Fick, Die medicinische Physik, Braunschweig, 1856, p. 454, *et seq.* J. Rosenthal, Physikalische und physiologische Bemerkungen über Electrotherapie, in der Deutschen Klinik, 1858, Nos. 3 und 4. J. Rosenthal, Electricitätslehre für Mediciner, Berlin, 1862, p. 158, *et seq.* Brenner, Versuche zur Begründung einer rationellen Methode in der Electrotherapie, genannt: die polare Methode (Petersb. Med. Zeitschrift, 1862, Band iii., p. 257, *et seq.*).

Though we have for a long time endeavored to direct the electrical current, for therapeutical purposes, into certain diseased organs, parts of organs, or tissues, and to avoid the neighboring parts as much as possible; though we have succeeded, for instance, in electrizing individual muscles, in conducting the electrical current into the bladder, etc., and have further, in order to avoid the burning of the skin, covered the excitors with soft moist leather, and, on the contrary, when we wished to irritate the skin, have placed the metallic plate on its dry surface—yet, to Duchenne is due the honor of having systematically introduced local galvanization or faradization, of having extended it, and of having given to it technical terms. It was reserved for German science and thoroughness, scientifically to maintain and establish what French practical tact without understanding had discovered.

Duchenne based his method on the following observations: 1. If we place two dry electrodes on a dry, hard skin, there appear, at the points of contact, sparks accompanied with a peculiar crackling. 2. If in such a case we moisten one electrode, a superficial sensation is perceived at the point which is in communication with the dry electrode. 3. If we moisten a little the skin, the epidermis of which is thick, under both electrodes, there follows a strong superficial sensation, but no sparks nor crackling. 4. If both skin and electrodes are considerably moistened, neither sparks, crackling, nor burning are perceived at the points of contact, but phenomena of contraction connected with a corresponding sensation.

We are thus able to allow the electrical current to act only on the skin or on the tissues lying under it. Duchenne discovered that the first-mentioned phenomena—sparks, crackling, and burning—are the result of irritating the skin alone, and that the last mentioned—the contractions and the accompanying sensation—are the result of the irritation of the muscles or nerves alone. Two pathological cases led him to these conclusions. He placed the dry electrodes on the exposed crureus muscle of a wounded person: there followed contraction, accompanied with a peculiar constricting sensation; the dry electrodes laid on a muscle covered with uninjured skin produced a sensation of burning, but no muscular contractions; the electrodes (covered with moist sponges) now placed on the same part of the skin induced again muscular contractions, with their accompanying sensation. A second wounded person had the radial nerve at the lower part of the forearm destroyed, and there followed loss of electrical contractility and sensibility in the muscles of the posterior part of the forearm, while the sensibility of the skin, its nerves not being injured, remained fully normal. In this case dry electrodes placed on different parts of the forearm always produced an intense burning, while moist sponges on the back part of the forearm excited neither contraction, nor the usually accompanying sensation.

In order to irritate the skin, Duchenne uses three different methods: 1, the electrical hand; 2, entire metallic electrodes; 3, metallic threads. In the first method, which is used only for the face, and in exceedingly irritable patients for other parts of the body, the physician places one moist sponge, connected with a polar wire, on a tolerably sensitive part of the patient, for instance on the sacro-lumbar region or on the sternum, and taking the other electrode in his hand passes his fingers slowly over the perfectly dry affected part of the skin. In order to irritate the skin or other parts of the body, entire metallic electrodes are used, and carried backward and forward over the dry, or, when it is very hard, somewhat moistened epidermis. If we wish to excite powerfully a small circumscribed spot, we hold on it for a long time the point of an olive-formed or round electrode. The metallic brush, with which we either strike the skin (electrical scourging), or act on the same spot as long as the patient can endure it (electrical moxa), we use for irritating the surfaces of the hands, the soles of the feet, and in very sensible parts of the skin, by drawing it over the surface. Later we will consider the special diseases, in which the electrical irritation of the skin is serviceable: here we will only remark, that the local effect at most remains local, and that we must consequently, when we wish to excite a considerable extent of the surface of the skin, subject it in all its parts to this treatment. In those points which, in the normal condition, possess a high degree of sensitiveness, it is well to begin with mild action, gradually increasing it, and as soon as a distinct sensation is produced (especially in the face) to return to the less irritating method.

In order to excite the motor nerves or the muscles, we place the moist electrodes as near to one another as possible on the parts of the skin immediately over these organs. As to the reason for this, we must first remark that the extent of local galvanization cannot be so well indicated as if the muscle or tissue were immediately in contact with the conductors, and were alone acted on by the electrical current. The current here directed from without to any part of the body is most intense at its points of entrance and exit, yet it nevertheless spreads itself throughout the whole body. "Not only does the current," says Du Bois-Reymond,[1] "pass through every molecule and part of a muscle, but also in its natural position through the bones, nerves, vessels, tendons, etc., in contact with it; when the thigh is bent upon the abdomen, the lower leg on the thigh, the current passes through each molecule of an abdominal or thigh muscle over the entire foot, lower leg, thigh, abdomen with all its viscera, and, if the leg is placed in water, or is brought in connection with a conducting arch, into the water or the conducting wire."

If Du Bois-Reymond could announce in its generality this proposition in regard to the current of the animal body which is appreciable only through a powerful multiplicator, how much more valid is it where palpable currents from without enter the body! Here the current spreads itself between its in- and out-going points in all directions and through all open paths. But the intensity of the current is not equal in all parts. This depends on different circumstances. 1. On the length of the way between the point of entrance and the point of exit. As the strength of the electrical current decreases according to the length of an intercalated metallic wire, so is its intensity lessened according to the distance between the poles; consequently, when the

[1] L. c., Bd. i., p. 687.

metallic conductors are placed on the dry skin one inch apart, they produce a much more powerful sensation than when they are applied at a distance of a foot from one another. 2. The current is strongest in the direct line which is the shortest distance between the conductors; its intensity decreases with the length of the curved way which we conceive to lie between the points of entrance and exit. Let us take an example, which Fick[1] has given and illustrated by a diagram, and lay one moist electrode on the top of the shoulder and the other on the forearm; all the curves, which the current, in order to reach from one point to another, can pass over, are of tolerably equal lengths, and consequently of tolerably equal resistance; the electricity in this case will distribute itself tolerably equally over the whole arm, and, moreover, when a not very strong current is used, the density will not be at any point so great as to excite muscular action. Had we, on the contrary, laid the two moist conductors near one another on the M. deltoideus, the ways, which the current could pass over, in order to go from one conductor to another, would be quite different as to their length, and the intensities of the current in the various curves would correspondingly differ: even with a weak current the intensity in the direct line between the conductors would be sufficient to produce a strong contraction of the deltoideus, while no disturbance of the neighboring muscles, the biceps and pectoralis, would be visible. Apparent exceptions to this law are found in the physics of the nerves—when, for instance, we excite a part of the N. ischiadicus, there follows a clonic or tonic spasm of the whole leg even to the point of the foot, and all the muscles supplied from the N. ischiadicus become contracted; contraction of the uterus, when one electrode is laid on the vaginal portion and the other on the foot, is to be attributed to the reflex action of the nerves of the neck of the womb, etc. 3. With different conductors the strength of the current is directly as

[1] L. c., 457.

their conducting power. On this law depends the use of moist sponges for electrizing the muscles, metallic plates or electrical brushes for exciting the skin. Let us first place the two electrodes armed with moist sponges on the well-moistened epidermis—the points covered by these are easily penetrated by the current which distributes itself to the parts lying under, and, when strong, to those in the direct line between the electrodes, and causes contraction of the muscles through acting on the sensory and motor nerves. If we now, on the contrary, hold two metallic plates, or better, two brushes of thin brass wire, on the same spots free from moisture, the dry epidermis presents so powerful a conducting resistance to the current that the same amount of electricity is not sufficient to cause contractions in the muscles lying under the skin. Yet, especially in using the brush, where the skin is touched only at certain small points, the intensity of the current is so great that, where it breaks through the skin, it excites the sensory nerve-fibres powerfully, and causes, by continued action, erythema, blistering, and in certain cases suggillation.

In order to obtain the greatest possible irritation of the nerves of the skin, we give one electrode the form of a plate covered with sponge and place this on the moistened skin, and apply the metallic brush as a second electrode on the dry skin; by this means we reduce the enormous conducting resistance of the epidermis, which the current by the use of two brushes has twice to overcome, almost to one-half, and thereby double the strength and intensity of the current. It is otherwise when acting on the muscles. Here Duchenne recognizes a direct and an indirect faradization, of which the first is produced through contact of the parts of the skin, over the muscle to be excited, with moist conductors; the second through irritation of the nerves supplying the muscle.

It did not escape the keen observation of Duchenne that, in direct muscular irritation, some muscles contract more energetically and promptly when acted on at certain points than at others, under apparently the same conditions. Remak found in his investigations that these points were the points of entrance of the motor nerves into the muscles, and set it down as a rule, that, in order to obtain with the weakest possible currents the strongest contractions possible, the point of one conductor must be placed on the entrance of the motor nerve into the muscle, the other in its immediate neighborhood—a law of the greatest importance for electro-therapeutics, because by following it we are able, with proportionably weak currents, to excite strong contractions in a less painful way. Remak called this method *extra-muscular* excitation, in distinction from intra-muscular (Duchenne's direct).

The cause of this lies, on the one hand, in the greater electrical irritability of the nerves compared with that of the muscles;[1] on the other hand, in the greater density of the current resulting from the application of small pointed conductors to the entrances of the nerves into the muscle, contrasted with the broad conductors which we place on the muscle. It yet remains to be proved that Remak's observation extends to all cases, that is, that all muscles are accessible to irritation at the points of entrance of the nerves, and then, through diagrams, to lighten for the physician the labor of finding the motor points.

Ziemssen has turned his attention to both these propositions in the before-cited paper. As regards the first, he found that the irritation of the points of entrance of the nerves was by no means practicable in all muscles, because on the one hand many irregularities occur in the course and ramifications of the nerves, as, for instance, in the N. facialis, again, in the shoulder and thorax nerves going

[1] Cl. Bernard found that the different organs required, for the exciting of their functional activity in the physiological condition, very different amounts of electricity, the muscles much more than the nerves. Of the nerves, the motory are more irritable than the sensory, etc. (Gaz. Méd. de Paris, 20 Fevrier, 1858.—Gaz. hebdomad., 20 Août, 1858, p. 596.)

out from the pars supraclavicularis of the plexus brachialis, finally and chiefly in the nerves of the lower extremities, which render the finding of the desired points very difficult. On the other hand, the nerves frequently enter the muscles at a considerable distance from the surface of the body, for instance in the interosseus, in the Mm. radialis, extern. long., splenius capitis, latissimus dorsi, teres major, semimembranosus, semitendinosus, etc., for the exciting of which we must always resort to intermuscular irritation. To satisfy the second proposition, Ziemssen has made tables to enable us easily to find the motor points on the living body. In order to ascertain these, after he had placed the conductor of the positive pole on the sternum, he sought to bring a fine-pointed conductor of the negative pole on the most superficial point of the motor nerve, which he marked with lunar caustic, and called, after he had found it again in the dead body on the corresponding spot, the *motor point*.

Especially for indirect (extra-muscular) faradization of the muscles is an exact anatomical knowledge of the course of the nerves and of their more or less superficial position in the different regions of their course necessary, in order to reach them at those points where the action of the current will be the most serviceable. We will mention the most important points, but must refer to Ziemssen's paper for the more exact study of the motor points.

The trunk of the N. facialis can be irritated, according to Duchenne, most conveniently from the outer ear-passage, by introducing one moist conical electrode into the ear-passage, and pressing it toward the lower side. This method is, however, injudicious, because it is painful and unsatisfactory, since powerful contractions, which Duchenne himself saw induced on the corresponding side of the face, are caused when the circuit is closed by placing the second electrode on the parotid gland. Less painful, but acting only with spare persons, is the irritation of the N. facialis after its exit from the for. stylomastoideum, by placing one thin electrode

close under the ear, between the proc. mastoideus and the angle of the lower jaw. The greater branches of the pes anserinus are easily acted on at their passage through the parotid, and cause contractions of the muscles supplied from the rami temporalis, or zygomatici, or buccales, etc.

The N. vagus must be faradized on the lower half of the neck, between the art. carotis commun. and vena jugularis; and the N. laryngeus inf. in the bifurcation between the oesophagus and trachea. The ramus extern. of the N. accessorius is in its entire course, from its exit from the M. sternocleido-mastoideus to its entrance into the M. trapezius, superficial and easily reached. The N. hypoglossus lies tolerably superficially directly under the cornu majus of the hyoid bone, between the M. stylohyoideus and hyoglossus.

In order to electrize the diaphragm, we find the anterior border of the M. scalenus ant. by pulling the skin inward with two fingers placed on the outer border of the M. sterno-cleido-mastoideus. Without discontinuing the action of the fingers, we separate them sufficiently to introduce between them a narrow moist conductor, which then presses directly on the N. phrenicus. After we have done the same thing to the other side, we allow the induction apparatus to work rapidly and powerfully. The two phrenici, in this way equally excited, cause immediately strong heavings of the chest, with rushing of air into the lungs. The plexus brachialis is to be acted on in the supra-clavicular region, between the M. scalenus ant. and med.

The thoracic and scapular nerves springing from the pl. brachialis allow of individual irritation when the integument is not too thick, but the frequent irregularity in their course must be taken into consideration; the N. dorsalis scap. may be electrized directly under the N. accessorius Willisii, on the edge of the M. trapezius; the Nn. thoracici posteriores, after their passage through the M. scalenus med., directly over the clavicle, and not far from the trapezius; the N. suprascapularis, frequently outward from the M.

omohyoideus, before the entrance into the incisura scapulæ; the Nn. thoracici anteriores are most easily reached under the clavicle on the upper edge of the M. pectoralis maj.

Among the nerves of the arm, the N. axillaris may be electrized at the upper part of the posterior border of the axilla; the N. musculo-cutaneus, after its passage through the M. coraco-brachialis, in the fork between this and the M. biceps. The N. medianus may be most surely excited on the lower third of the humerus, after it has passed to the inner side of the art. brachialis. Irritation of the medianus causes, besides the painful sensations in the region of the branches of the forearm and fingers, powerful pronation of the forearm, turning of the hand toward the radial side, and closing of the fingers. The N. ulnaris, electrized in the channel between the olecranon and the condylus int. humeri, produces, besides the sensations of pain in the region of the ram. palmaris longus (in the skin of the lower part of the inner surface of the forearm as far as the palm of the hand), a contraction of the M. flexor carpi ulnaris, of the M. flexor digitorum profundus, of the Mm. interossei, lumbricales tert. et quart., of the muscles of the little finger, and of the M. adductor pollicis. The N. radialis is most accessible to electrical irritation at the point of union of the middle and lower third of the upper arm, where it, appearing from under the M. triceps, passes to the outer side of the arm, which causes, in addition to the painful sensations on the outer side of the upper and forearm as far as the wrist, contractions of the Mm. sup. brevis, extensor carpi rad. and uln., extensor digit-comm., extensor indicis, extensor digiti minim. prop., extensor pollicis long. and brev., and abductor pollicis—finally, supination of the forearm, with complete extension of the hand and of the thumb, extension of the first phalanges of the fingers, and slight bending of the last phalanges.

The N. cruralis may be electrically reached after its passage under Poupart's ligament on the outer side of the art cruralis; then follows energetic extension of the lower leg, accompanied with painful sensations in the region of the N. saphenus major, minor, and cutaneus femoris ant. and med., also on the front and inner sides of the thigh, the knee, and of the inner surface of the lower leg as far as the great toe. The N. obturatorius may be excited at the for. obturatorium by placing the electrode perpendicularly against the horizontal branch of the os pubis and pressing hard on the skin and M. pectineus. The irritation causes a strong and painful adduction of the thigh. The N. ischiadicus may be electrized either at its origin in the pelvis through the hind wall of the rectum, or after its exit from the incisura ischiadica major behind the head of the thigh; there follows powerful bending of the lower leg, with painful sensations in the region of the sensory branches of the ischiadicus, also in the entire lower leg and foot. The Nn. peronæus and tibialis lie most superficially near the outer edge of the knee-pan; the first, accessible immediately on the hinder edge of the capitulum fibulæ, causes a contraction of the Mm. peronæi, tibialis anticus, extensor digitor. comm. long. and brevis, and extensor hallucis longus, with sensations in the skin-nerves of the back of the foot. The N. tibialis, irritated in the middle of the bend of the knee, produces energetic contractions of all the muscles on the hinder part of the lower leg, and on the sole of the foot, as well as painful sensations in the calf of the leg and sole of the foot.

On the above points, or, where we wish to excite an individual muscle, at the point of entrance of the motor nerve into the muscle, the negative pole is always placed, as acting the stronger both on the sensory and motor nerves, while the other electrode closes the circuit by being placed on the muscle itself. On the one hand, we thus make the weakening of the current between the two electrodes as slight as possible; and, on the other, we, moreover, act on, not only the motor nerve, but the branches running through the muscle, and thus produce with the smallest strength of current the greatest possible effect. It is advisable, however, when irritating the muscles of the face and neck, to close the circuit with one conductor on a distant part of the body, because otherwise irritation of the sensory trigeminal and cervical nerve-fibres is unavoidable.

When acting on such muscles as are supplied from two nerves, as, for instance, when electrizing the Mm. deltoideus, trapezius, biceps femoris, we place each conductor most advantageously on the point of entrance of one nerve into the muscle. Moreover, we may, in order to save time, in cases where there is muscular paralysis with marked diminution of the electro-muscular contractility, place the conductors on the motor points of two muscles, and can thus, since in such cases the difference between the irritating powers of the positive and negative poles is not considerable, excite two muscles at the same time. But, in more sensitive regions, where it is necessary to take notice of this difference, it is best to lay the negative pole on the motor point of the larger muscle; or, where there is a difference in the irritability of the two muscles, on the less sensitive—the positive pole on the motor point of the smaller or more sensitive muscle.

Though the *indirect* muscular irritation is of great importance to electro-therapeutics, and used in so many different ways, yet it does not take the place of the *direct*. Not only must we resort to intra-muscular irritation for exciting those muscles whose motor points are inaccessible from without, but in many other cases, as, for instance, where the electro-muscular contractility is fully lost, and we are consequently uncertain whether we have hit the motor point or not, no contractions being manifest; in others where there is destruction of the power of motion, which results from great atrophy following disease of the substance of the muscle; and, finally, in cases of paralysis, where every irritation of the nerves should be avoided. As to *direct* faradization, the superficially-lying muscles of the body and extremities in the normal condition are easily thrown into contractions by it, when we place both moist conductors near one another, and in the direction of the fibres of the muscle. Where the muscles are very broad, the conductors must be moved one after the other to the different parts, in order to excite them. Also the deeper-lying muscles often present a point in the neighborhood of their origin or attachment where the direct action of the electric current may be made effectual. When this is not the case, we must use a more intense current, which, passing through the superficial tissues that we reduce by strong pressure of the electrodes to a single obstacle, reaches the deeper muscles—a fact, the possibility of which we can convince ourselves in those cases of lead-poisoning where the contractility of the superficially-lying muscles is extinguished, while that of those lying deeper is retained.

The electrization of the muscles of the eye is particularly difficult on account of their position in the interior of the orbit, which renders them inaccessible to local irritation. It is true that, with the eye open and the bulb fixed, the individual muscles may be acted on by a fine electrode; nevertheless, the irritability of the eye, the danger of inflammation, the painfulness of the experiment, finally, the frequent mismanagement of the assistants, forbid the use of this method in most cases; where it is allowable, only currents can be applied which are so weak, that their utility is doubtful. I, consequently, faradize the muscles of the eye in this way: Placing the conductor of the positive pole in the hand of the patient, I lay a thin electrode, which is covered with sponge and connected with the negative pole, in order to irritate the M. obliquus sup., against the spina or fovea trochlearis of the forehead; to irritate the M. obliquus inf., on the margo infraorbitalis of the upper jaw-bone, near the fossa lacrymalis; to irritate the M. rectus externus, on the outer angle of the eye; to irritate the M. rectus internus, on the inner angle; to irritate the M. rectus superior, on the upper surface of the eyeball; to irritate, finally, the M. rectus inferior, on the lower surface. We can in this way, if we use conductors with weak currents which we slowly increase, apply currents of great strength. That in fact contractions of the muscles of the eye in this way take place, I was able to observe in an individual having paralysis of the M. obliquus sup. and M. rectus int., whose eye, little sensitive on account of repeated paralysis of its muscles, could be opened during the operation, and allowed the effect of the irritation to be seen partly in the position of the eyeball, and partly in the greater approximation of the double image. Benedict[1] used the constant current in paralysis of the muscles of the eye, and has published the following: He placed the copper pole on the forehead, and stroked the cheek-bone with the zinc pole for several minutes, in a case of abducens paralysis; in paralysis of the M. rectus internus and M. obliquus inferior, the skin on the side of the nose near the inner angle of the eye; in ptosis, the upper eyelid; in paralysis of the M. rectus inferior, the lower border of the orbit; finally, in paralysis of the N. trochlearis, the inside of the nose in the neighborhood of the inner angle of the eye.

As to the muscles of the larynx, the M. cricothyroideus is easily excited to contraction by placing two small pointed conductors on both sides of the lig. conoideum; the thyroid and annular cartilages approach one another, and the tension of the vocal cords is increased. The electrical irritation of the other muscles of the larynx is effected only through the region of the pharynx; Ziemssen, who has perfected the method,[2] uses for this purpose an induction current that is just strong enough to excite the M. frontalis to contraction, or a galvanic current of from eight to twelve Siemen's elements. He unites the wire coming from the negative pole with a bent catheter-shaped sound covered almost to the

---

[1] Electrotherapeutische und physiologische Studien über Augenmuskel-Lähmungen, Archiv für Ophthalmologie, X. Jahrgang, 1864, pp. 97–122.
[2] L. c., p. 200, et seq.

point, passes it quickly with the right hand into the mouth, while he controls his movements by the aid of a laryngeal mirror held in the left hand, and then allows the circuit to be closed through the aid of an assistant who places the second electrode, covered with sponge, on any selected distant part of the body. The M. arytænoideus transv. is easy to excite by touching the posterior surface of the cart. arytænoidea with the electrode; both cartilages move strongly on one another. As to the electrical irritation of the Mm. crico-arytænoideus post. and lat., and of the M. thyreo-arytænoideus, the sinus pyriformis, the inlet which is between the hind border of the cart. thyreoidea and the plate of the cart. cricoidea, is the conducting point for the electrode. To act on the M. crico-arytænoideus post., on the dilatator glottidis, we pass from the sinus pyriformis directly backward and downward; the M. crico-arytænoideus lat. is to be reached in the sinus pyriformis on the outer border of the plate of the annular cartilage; irritation causes slight rotation of the cartilages of the larynx, so that the free edge of the vocal cord approaches the middle. The M. thyreo-arytænoideus lies immediately on the front upper border of the M. crico-arytænoideus lat.; under electrical excitement it draws the laryngeal cartilages forward and downward, and narrows the vocal cleft. We may cause the muscles of the epiglottis, the Mm. thyro- and ary-epiglottici, to contract by placing the electrode on the side of its base.

Since intra-laryngeal faradization is one of the most difficult things in the laryngoscopical art; since, further, a preparation of several months is often required for the purpose of rendering the mucous membrane of the larynx less sensitive, which also requires unusual patience, both on the part of the patient and physician; since, finally, the motions of the larynx sometimes render the use of the mirror and the electrode impossible, this method is consequently of service in proportionably few cases of paralysis of the vocal cords, while cutaneous faradization answers in most of them.

We have still two methods of electrical irritation of the muscles to notice, namely, the *reflex* irritation and the *sympathetic* irritation (*Miterregung*). The first rests on the peculiarity that sensory nerves, in the irritated condition, have of inducing activity, through uninjured paths in the motor nerves, and can be used for exciting the muscles through electrical irritation of the nerves of the skin. This method is indicated: 1. In paralysis with simultaneous anæsthesia of the skin over the muscle, namely, in hysterical paralysis, where frequently, with the disappearance of the anæsthesia, the power of motion returns. 2. In those cases where the suffering part is not very accessible to the local application of electricity, for instance, in disorders of menstruation, etc.[1] The method in such cases is, to excite electrically those parts of the skin whose nerves end in the central organ as high as those of the organ on which we wish to operate. 3. The reflex irritation is applicable in neuralgia where we wish to blunt the abnormally-increased sensitiveness of the sensory nerves of the muscles by an intense action on the skin.[2] *Sympathetic* irritation, which consists in an irritation acting on a muscle or a nerve, causing other muscles to contract by transmission through the spinal marrow, we may use in certain cases suited to electrical treatment, where the less-paralyzed muscles may be excited by acting on those in which there is still greater paralysis. As the excitability of the central organ for reflex movements is increased when the irritated sensory nerve owes its loss of conducting power to the brain; so its excitability for sympathetic movements seems to be increased under the same conditions. I, therefore, use with advantage this method of irritation in apoplectic paralysis and contractions; for instance, where both arm and leg are paralyzed—the former, however, more than the latter—I expect, simply by elec-

[1] Schulz, die Reflexwirkungen der Inductions-Electricität, etc., in der Wiener Med. Wochenschrift, 1855, No. 49.
[2] Behandlung der Neuralgieen im therapeutischen Theil.

trizing the muscles of the arm, that the paralyzed muscles of the leg will be reached.

As to the exciting of the nerves of special sense through the interrupted current, the sense of touch is acted upon by placing the fingers for a longer or shorter time in contact with a dry, metallic, and with a moist electrode. The sense of hearing is irritated by placing one metallic electrode in the ear-passage, filled with water, and the other moist electrode on the temple, or by introducing one well-isolated conductor through the nose into the tuba Eustachii, while the other is applied to the temple. The sense of smell is excited by placing one conductor on the neck, while we move the other dry electrode backward and forward over the membrana Schneideri. The sense of taste is awakened by frequent stroking of the tongue with the electrical brush.

The majority of the inner organs are with difficulty reached by electrical irritation; the most easily accessible of these are the rectum, the bladder, and the uterus. In order to electrize the rectum or its sphincter, we introduce a metallic, isolated electrode, having an olive-shaped tip, carefully avoiding the exceedingly sensitive border of the gut, into this organ, which has been cleaned by means of a clyster, and press it on the M. levator and sphincter ani; in this way a distinctly-perceptible contraction of the rectum is brought about; the other electrode, saturated with moisture, we place on the back. As the rectum, like the bladder, is little sensitive to the electrical irritation, we may use a powerful current. In order to excite the latter, we introduce into the rectum an electrode with a metal button or olive tip, into the bladder a sound covered with india-rubber, as far as the button-shaped termination, and bring it, according as we wish to irritate the neck of the bladder or its body, in contact with its different parts. In many cases it is sufficient to lay one moist conductor above the symphysis pubis, and the other on the back. For the more difficult cases, Duchenne has invented a so-called "excitateur vésical double." This consists of two flexible wires tipped with buttons, that, separated from one another, pass into an india-rubber tube. With their ends side by side, they have the appearance of a buttoned sound, and in this condition they are introduced into the bladder. By shoving them forward in this organ, they separate from one another, so that two different points of the bladder are touched by them. After each wire is set in connection with the battery, they are slowly moved about. We use a similar instrument, but with a different curve and a larger button, for the electrical irritation of the uterus, which is carried by means of the index-finger to the neck of the womb. We can indirectly excite the organs of the pelvis by pressing an olive-shaped conductor on the posterior wall of the rectum, where it strikes the plexus sacralis and hypogastricus.

In order to electrize the testicle, we secure it or the much more sensitive neighboring parts between two moist electrodes. As the operation is very painful and the sensation accompanying the compression of the testicle spreads into the loins, we can only use a weak current, otherwise a neuralgia is easily induced. The vesiculæ seminales are best reached through the anterior wall of the rectum. The irritation of the pharynx and œsophagus is accomplished by means of a throat-electrode. This, consisting of a curved metallic sound, tipped with an olive-shaped end, from 3 to 4 Mm. in diameter, and isolated by means of an india-rubber tube as far as the end, is connected with the negative pole of the induction apparatus and carried to the desired organ, while the moist conductor of the positive pole is placed on the sternum. In irritating the pharynx we must avoid touching with the olive the sides, where the trunks of the N. vagus, glossopharyngeus and accessorius lie, while in ex citing the œsophagus we avoid the Nn. recurrens and vagus which are found behind the trachea. The heart and lungs, which are inaccessible to the electrical current on account of the thickness of the walls of the thorax, may be exposed to the electrical action by irritating the vagus in the lower part of the neck between the art. carotis comm. and vena jugularis.

In regard to the therapeutical value of quick or slow consecutive interruptions of the current, the first are indicated—1. Where it is desired to irritate the sensory nerves of the skin or muscles. 2. Where we wish to improve the tone and recuperative power of relaxed or atrophied muscles. 3. Where for physiological or diagnostical purposes we wish to test the functions or electrical irritability of certain muscles.[1] The interruptions slowly following one another, on the other hand, are indicated in those cases—1. Where the electro-muscular contractility is greatly diminished. 2. Where the will is unable to act on the normally-retained muscular irritability, as in apoplectic paralysis. Single strong shocks, which may be conveniently produced by using the induction apparatus with the before-described interruptor, or more intensely by the battery current, frequently changing the direction of the current by means of Remak's commutator, are in place—1. In many cases, in which we desire to diminish the irritability of the spinal marrow, increased through disease and manifesting itself through abnormal muscular movements. 2. Where we wish to increase the muscular contractility. 3. In those surgical cases complicated with powerful muscular action, as, for instance, in rigidity of the joints after the healing of a broken bone, or in anchylosis after rheumatic or traumatic inflammation of the joints, etc.

Generally a daily sitting, or on every other day, of from five to fifteen minutes is sufficient for realizing the beneficial effects; longer or more frequently-repeated sittings are apt

[1] See Sections vii. and viii.

to be followed by fatigue and pain of the muscles. There are, however, very sensitive individuals, in whom electrical irritation, by means of a weak current lasting for only a few minutes, produces clonic cramps; while, on the other hand, torpid individuals may be electrized by means of an intense current for half an hour without perceiving the least relaxation. The amount of time which we should devote to a single muscle depends on the irritability of the patient, the cause of the disease, and on the grade of the electro-muscular contractility; so that, where this last is retained, a short but frequently-repeated irritation is advisable, while, in those cases where it is considerably diminished, as in traumatic paralysis, an excitement lasting for many minutes is necessary. One or even a few sittings are very seldom sufficient to produce a cure; most cases need a treatment lasting for many weeks or months. Sometimes the process of recovery comes to a stand-still, or even an apparent relapse sets in; in such instances it is good to interrupt the treatment and to allow the muscles rest—on resuming the electrical applications the progress is often more rapid.

In the therapeutical use of the *constant* current naturally the same physical laws hold as in that of the induction current: we have here also on the one hand to concentrate the greatest intensity of current on the structure on which we wish to operate, on the other hand to diminish as much as possible the conducting resistance of the parts lying over this. The motor nerves, the muscles and the organs furnished with contractile muscular fibres are especially excited by the interrupted current (and in a higher degree by means of the galvano-electrical than the magneto-electrical), and through the first a momentarily intense irritation of the skin is caused; on the contrary, the so-called electrotonic actions, the modifications of irritability, the effects on the brain, the spinal marrow, the sympathetic, etc., the purely chemical actions in part singly and alone, in part in an imperfect degree, are produced through the constant current. In using the first we should, as much as possible, in accordance with the above rules, consider the direction in which the current passes through the nerve—in using the latter we should strive to exactly differentiate the points of application of both poles. Brenner[1] has clearly shown that in the living body it is possible in but a few cases to conduct the galvanic current in a certain direction into a nerve, because the poles are almost always placed on points not having physiologically equal importance, and consequently their action is in accordance with their difference in position." According to him, not the direction of the current, but the poles, analogous to their physico-chemical action, are to be considered as indicators of the different physiological effects of the electrical current. Brenner has further attempted to bring these observations of his into harmony with the physical laws on electrical irritation of the nerves and electrotonus, and finds them almost entirely confirmed by Pflüger.[3] He bases on them his so-called *polar method*, which consists in giving to that pole, whose action is appropriate to the case in hand, such a position as is most favorable, in regard to conduction, for its working on the nerve. This method, and the assertions on which it rests, are in general correct: the electro-therapeutist is frequently in practice, namely, in those cases where it is desired to diminish the excessive irritability of a nerve, obliged to place the cathode on a position as distant from the effective anode as possible—because in the same nerve near the anelectrotonus there is always present catelectrotonus—nevertheless, it is necessary in most cases also to consider the direction of the current, and in this connection I would refer to page 55 and page 96, paragraphs 9, 10, and 11.

Moreover, we use the current, according to Remak, in

[1] *L. c.*   [2] *L. c.*, p. 275.
[3] Untersuchungen über die Physiologie des Electrotonus, 1859.

two forms, *stable* when we hold the electrodes for a longer or shorter time unmoved on the same spots, or *mobile* when we move one electrode slowly over the skin. Fromhold has added a third to these methods,[1] *the swelling of the intensity*, which is produced by the gradual increasing and the corresponding decreasing of the number of the effective elements—a method on the therapeutical efficiency of which we are at present unable to give any opinion.

At the present time we can no longer doubt the possibility of acting electrically upon the central portion of the nervous system, on the brain and spinal marrow. The known manifestations of dizziness, which appear frequently when using the galvanic current near the head, and tolerably constantly when a conductor is placed in the fossa auriculo-maxillaris, and, in a still higher degree, the metallic taste, caused sometimes in hysterical and tabetic patients by conducting a current through the pelvis, render the introduction of a constant current into the brain and spinal marrow probable; besides, the observations of Erb, given on page 78, have shown that for this purpose not even an intense current is necessary. Erb was able, by means of a tolerably strong induction current, the conductors of which were placed on both temples, to excite contractions in a frog preparation which was for only a few lines in contact with the brain: the constant current acts so effectually, partly through its considerably stronger chemical effect, which, in connection with the favorable conditions for conduction presented by the skull and dorsal column, together with their numerous canals, blood-vessels, sutures, openings, etc., makes an intense action on the brain and spinal marrow possible, and partly through its endurance and the gradual increase of its intensity, which favor its penetration into the deeply-lying

[1] Der constante galvan. Strom, modificirbar in seinem Intensitäts und Quantitätswerth, Pest, 1866.

parts, while the interrupted current, with its momentary endurance, spreads itself out superficially.

The method of galvanizing the brain consists in conducting a current[1] coming from 10 to 16 elements for two or three minutes from the occiput to the forehead. The possible consequences of this we will notice in Section IX. To electrize the spinal marrow we use generally a large conductor, in connection with the positive pole of the battery, which we place on that part of the dorsal column where we believe the disease has its origin, while the negative conductor is brought in contact with a point at some distance right or left from the dorsal column. Here also it is advisable to use the electric current for not more than five minutes.

The galvanization of the sympathetic is conducted in the following way: we place one conductor, having a length of one inch and a breadth of from one-third to one-half an inch, on the course of the inner side of the M. sterno-cleido-mastoideus—when we wish to excite the ganglion cerv. sup. in the direction toward the second and third cervical vertebra —to act on the ganglion cerv. med. opposite the fifth and sixth, finally to act on the ganglion cerv. inf. opposite the seventh cervical and first dorsal vertebra, while the second large conductor is placed above on the neck, or on the posterior ends of the ribs on the side of the vertebra (corresponding to the position of the ganglion thoracica and lumbalia), or is moved slowly over the above parts. For the efficacy of this method the following case has given me evidence, which un-

---

[1] To regulate the strength of the current, i. e., to prescribe the number of elements necessary for a certain operation, is for the constant current more difficult than for the interrupted. In addition to the difference in sensitiveness of different individuals to the same strength of current on corresponding parts of the body, and of the same individual at different times, we will seldom find two batteries of absolutely equal strength, and, moreover, these will not be constant; we must add also the difference in the conducting resistance of the conductors. In those respects we are obliged to be satisfied with tolerably unsettled conditions.

doubtedly proves the action of the irritation of the sympathetic of the neck on the vaso-motor nerves.

CASE 1.—A. S. Kaufmann, aged twenty-two years, two years ago was without any known disease. Sitting in a restaurant, he was seized with an apoplectic fit, which paralyzed the entire right portion of the body, and from which he only very slowly recovered, so that on the 7th March, 1867, when I saw him for the first time, locomotion was very difficult and also the movements of the arm and hand—their sensibility was lessened and contractions of the right half of the face were present, namely of the Mm. zygomaticus and levator ang. oris. The chief difficulties of the patient were a constant roaring in the right half of the head, and, above all, of a sensation of unendurable heat in the right ear, which showed itself objectively through a remarkable redness of the left ear and an increase of temperature in the neighboring parts. In his case the prescribed method, i. e., placing the negative conductor on a spot corresponding to the ganglion cerv. sup., and the positive conductor on the occiput, caused, in addition to the gradual disappearance of the roaring, an improvement in the appearances near the external ear, which was so perceptible, both subjectively and objectively, beginning even with the first sitting, that after eight or ten sittings the complaints of the patient in regard to the heat in the ear ceased, and the corresponding redness and increase of temperature vanished. In brief, I will state that, through the subsidence of the contraction of the right side of the face after thirty sittings, the facial expression and speech were markedly improved, and through the peripheric treatment of the extremities the gait became normal and the use of the arm and hand was comparatively free.

Still more interesting is the following case in the practice of Dr. Drissen, to whom I am obliged for its history:

CASE 2.—C. P., sculptor, thirty-five years of age, was in the war of 1866, and has suffered in the following ways since the beginning of July of the same year: both arms are somewhat emaciated and ice-cold, the hands anæsthetic, bloodless, resembling dead hands, and when deeply pierced with a needle no blood flows out; the movements are difficult and powerless. There is the same condition, in a less degree, in the lower extremities. Neuralgic pains are present neither in the legs nor in the arms; the patient complains only of a sensation of pricking in the fingers. In the hospital the most powerful diaphoretics were not sufficient to produce perspiration, and Russian baths, later used, were attended with no better success. Dr. D. directed the constant current on the sympathetic, by placing the positive pole on the position corresponding to the ganglion cerv. sup.; in the second sitting a strong perspiration set in, which, on the ends of the fingers, appeared in the form of large drops, while the hands at the same time reddened. Powerful contractions in the muscles of the upper and lower extremities also set in (the so-called *diplegic contractions*, of which we will soon speak). From this time on, the mobility improved with the increase of temperature from day to day, so that the patient after twelve sittings was again in a condition to return to his occupation. A peripheric treatment in this case was not resorted to.

In the use of the constant current, Remak and others have observed, in addition to the antagonistic galvanic contractions noticed on page 50, in certain pathological cases, still other forms of reflex contractions, and have considered their therapeutic value. To these belong:

1. The reflex contractions, which especially appear in progressive muscular atrophy and are caused by the irritation of two selected points far distant from the muscle to be excited—*diplegic reflex contractions*. As the point from which the reflex contractions start, and on which the small conductor of the positive pole should be held, Remak mentions the fossa auriculo-maxillaris of the opposite side corresponding to the height of the ganglion cerv. sup., while the greater conductor of the negative pole should be applied

on the sixth cervical vertebra of the corresponding side, or on a spot lying below this, which is often with difficulty found, and sometimes is as low down as the loins. Remak adds that sometimes the proper points of irritation lie on the same side with the diseased extremities, and affirms that diplegic contractions can never be produced by means of the induction current.[1]

Fieber[2] has confirmed the assertion that the ganglion cerv. sup. plays the chief part in exciting the diplegic contractions, and that the current must have the direction affirmed by Remak, also that the position given by him to the positive pole, and to the negative, below the fifth cervical vertebra, is necessary for the production of the contractions—on the other hand, he was able, contrary to the belief of Remak, to excite these contractions also by using the induction current. Moreover, Fieber observed similar contractions, as had Remak in the beginning of arthritis nodosa, in rheumatic paralysis of the arm, in lead paralysis, and in apoplectic paralysis: Drissen observed these, not only in the two noticed cases of vaso-motor paralysis of the extremities, but also in paralysis of the nerves of the arms following, probably, inflammatory irritation of the nerves; I myself saw them, among other instances, in a very animated young girl, having paralysis and atrophy of the upper extremities, consequent on chronic arsenic-poisoning, and they were induced as well by the use of the constant as by the interrupted current. Dr. Drissen and Dr. A. Eulenburg had an opportunity in this case to observe, with me, how the diplegic contractions were produced by irritating different points at a distance from one another: these set in, first, on placing the conductors on the customary places; secondly, on their application to the right or left side of the dorsal column, especially at the height of from the fourth to the

---

[1] See Remak: application du courant constant, etc., pp. 27 bis 31.

[2] Die diplegischen Contractionen nach Versuchen an Menschen und Thieren erläutert. Berlin Klin. Wochenschrift, 1866, Bd. iii., No. 23, 25, 26.

eighth thoracic vertebra; thirdly, by placing one conductor on the pit of the stomach and the other on the above region of the dorsal column, and during this last application the contractions reached their greatest intensity, while they were much less pronounced when the poles were on the customary parts—moreover, in this case the fixation of the ganglion cerv. sup. was not sufficient to produce the phenomena.

2. *The centripetal reflex movements* Remak[1] and Braun[2] have observed in old cases of apoplexy, and used therapeutically with success. These were caused, in Remak's case of thirty-eight years' standing, by strong contractions of the arm and leg muscles, as soon as a constant current was conducted through the nerves of the paralyzed arm or leg, and the contraction of the limbs was relaxed. In Braun's case the contraction of the fingers was loosened and the arm was lifted upward and backward by an ascending current through the N. peromeus of the paralyzed side—a phenomenon which did not appear under similar conditions on the healthy side. On the other hand, in the last case a centripetal action could not be produced through the N. medianus on the leg of the corresponding side.

To bring about galvanic irritation of the nerves of special sense, we seek to give the electrodes such a position that the intensity of the current shall have its maximum in the respective organ. In order, for instance, to act on the retina and the N. opticus, we place one conductor on the inner angle of the eye, and the other on the temple, avoiding, however, too strong a current, since in sensitive eyes the light produced by the galvanic action may excite retinitis. To affect the sense of taste, we place one conductor on the tongue and the other on the neck, etc.

For peripheric irritation by means of the constant cur-

[1] S. Galvanotherapie, p. 221.
[2] Berlin Klin. Wochenschrift, 1865, Bd. II., p. 123.

rent, with which Benedikt in Vienna especially has occupied himself,[1] we may use either the so-called spinal-marrow root-current, by placing one, generally the copper pole, on the vertebral column, and stroking the latter with the zinc pole; or the spinal-marrow plexus or spinal-marrow nerve-current, by placing one pole on the plexus of the nerve and the other on its origin at the vertebral column; or the plexus nerve-current, where one pole rests on a plexus and the other on one of its nerves; or the nerve muscle-current, where one pole rests on the nerve and the other on the muscle supplied by it. We may also, when a considerable portion of a nerve is accessible, place both poles on the same nerve, or finally one conductor on the muscle and the other on its motor point, and in regard to this last method we would refer to page 146, *et seq.* Naturally we may in all these operations allow the current to work either in an ascending or descending direction, and it may be stable or mobile.

[1] s. u. A. Allgem. Wiener Med. Zeitung, 1863.

SEVENTH SECTION.

ELECTRICITY IN ITS APPLICATION TO ANATOMY, PHYSIOLOGY, AND PATHOLOGY.

We have already shown how, through local faradization by means of a frequently-interrupted current, not only each individual muscle, but also each muscle-fasciculus, may be brought into immediate contraction. Duchenne used these methods to ascertain in an exact manner the mode of working of each muscle, and he thereby disproved many errors found in the anatomical text-books, and showed that most movements were caused by a single muscle and not by the simultaneous action of different muscles. Bérard has consequently remarked that Duchenne, through the local application of the electric current, has become the creator of 'an "anatomie vivante."

In the following pages we will give a short *résumé* of his interesting investigations, referring for a closer study to Duchenne's works or to Erdmann's.[1]

I. Of the face muscles we ascribe to both Mm. zygomatici the office of drawing the corner of the mouth outward and upward; Duchenne observed that the M. zygomaticus major, in consequence of its attachment to the angle of the mouth, is active in laughing and in the expressions of merriment; and the M. zygomaticus minor, lying more within and forward, in crying and in expressions of sadness. The electrized M. pyramidalis expresses anger and threatening, the

[1] iv. Aufl. pp. 94-164.

M. transversalis nasi derision and contempt; and the irritated M. triangularis nasi gives to the countenance the expression of lasciviousness. The M. subcutaneus colli is strained in wrath and terror, as well as in the expression of resignation. The M. frontalis draws the skin of the forehead, eyelids, and eyebrows upward—slightly contracted, it brightens the countenance—more strongly, it expresses doubt, and when most contracted it indicates, with the simultaneous action of other muscles, agreeable surprise or dread. The M. buccinator draws the commissure of the lips strongly outward and forms long furrows on the cheek, which give the appearance of age, while the united action of the M. buccinator and M. zygomaticus major in some persons produces the lovely dimples on the cheek. The muscles of the tragus and antitragus contract the outward part of the ear, and have the office of protecting the ear from too powerful impressions, and sharp tones, while the muscles of the helix appear to be used for expanding this organ.

II. In regard to the muscles of the hand and arm, Duchenne showed that, when in the flexed condition of the hand and fingers we electrize the extensors of the fingers, at first the last two phalanges, then the first phalanges stretch out, and at last extension of the carpus upon the forearm takes place. The last two phalanges remain extended till the metacarpus forms an angle with the forearm, then they become flexed, while the first phalanges extend themselves still more. At the same time, the extensors spread the phalanges apart, which in the flexed condition were near one another. By irritating the extensor indicis proprius, the index-finger approaches the middle-finger; by irritating the extensor digiti minimi proprius, the little finger separates from the fourth considerably more than when contraction of the fasciculi, going to it from the extensor digitorum comm., takes place. It follows from this, that the extensor digitorum comm. and the extensores proprii not only extend the first phalanges, but also separate the fingers from the middle-finger. On the contrary, the adductors and abductors of the fingers, the Mm. interossei, Mm. adductores et abductores pollicis et digiti minimi, finally, the Mm. lumbricales, have, besides their peculiar function of adduction, abduction, and of bending the fingers, the office of extending the second phalanx of the thumb, and the second and third of the other fingers. The M. flexor pollicis brevis is a flexor of the first phalanx of the thumb, and in a higher degree an extensor of the second; the M. opponens pollicis flexes the metacarpal bone of the thumb toward the wrist, and at the same time turns the thumb with its palmar surface toward the index-finger. Finally, the M. supinator longus is only a supinator when the forearm is strongly prone; when this is not the case, and the forearm has its usual resting position, it is drawn toward the upper arm in a direction between supination and pronation. Pathological facts confirm these observations: A person with paralysis of the extensor digit. comm. can still extend the second and third finger-joints, while the extension of the first is impossible; the sidewise movement and spreading of the fingers is difficult, and the bending of the last two phalanges is imperfect. In paralysis or atrophy of the abductor longus and extensor brevis pollicis, the metacarpal bone of the thumb is permanently adducted, and consequently the holding of small objects between the first three fingers is interfered with; while, in paralysis of the extensor longus pollicis, the thumb, it is true, bends toward the metacarpus; but, if the extensor brevis and abductor longus remain uninjured, its use is but little impaired. In paralysis of the muscles of the ball of the thumb, in consequence of the activity of the extensor longus pollicis, the metacarpal bone of the thumb is so much extended, that it forms a prominent angle with the wrist, and the patient is unable to extend the last thumb-joint without at the same time extending the metacarpal bone and the first phalanx of the thumb. Paralysis or atrophy of the flexor brevis pollicis renders it impossible to bring the thumb in opposition with the ring and little-finger; if, however, the abductor brevis and opponens is unaffected, the thumb can still touch the first two fingers, and the hand may be used in writing; if, finally, the adductor, in paralysis of the other muscles of the ball of the thumb, is unimpaired, the patient may hold a considerable weight between the thumb and index-finger.

III. Let us now pass to muscles which move the arm and shoulder. The M. pectoralis major is divided into two parts, of which the upper (consisting of the clavicular portion and the fibres which are attached to the upper part of the sternum) draws the arm and shoulder upward and forward. When excited on both arms, the elbows move forward, inward, and somewhat upward, and the arms press against the thorax. On the other hand, the lower portion of the M. pectoralis is an abductor of the arm. Irritation of the entire muscle causes rotation of the upper arm on its axis, with simultaneous pronation of the hand. The M. deltoideus produces, besides the lifting of the upper arm, a change of position of the shoulder-blade, and in such a way that the angulus ext. scap. is depressed, the ang. int. is somewhat elevated and carried toward the middle line; finally, the scapula is turned on its vertical axis, and consequently its posterior spinal border is removed for four or five centimetres from the wall of the chest. If the M. latissimus dorsi is irritated in its upper third, the arm hanging down, it draws the arm inward and backward, and the shoulder-blade toward the middle line; while irritation of the two lower thirds causes a sinking of the shoulders and inclination of the body toward the corresponding side. If both muscles are irritated at the same time in their upper third, both shoulder-blades approach one another, and the shoulders stand directed obliquely forward and inward; while simultaneous irritation of both in their lower portions causes sinking of the shoulders and extension of the back, and consequently the military position. In paralysis of the deltoideus, the upper arm hangs by the side of the chest almost immovable; if the patient tries to give any one the hand, he swings the arm forward by means of the serratus. If, of the three bundles of fibres of which the deltoideus is composed, only one is paralyzed, the lifting of the arm toward this side is prevented, while it is allowed toward the other; the greatest obstacle is the paralysis of the anterior bundle. If the latissimus dorsi is paralyzed, the carriage is rendered difficult, since the shoulder-blades are held in their position chiefly through the Mm. rhomboidei. In regard to the function of the muscles of the shoulder-blade, Duchenne found that, when of the three bundles of the M. trapezius *the uppermost* and anterior (portio clavicularis) was electrized, the head inclined strongly toward the irritated side, and turned somewhat backward, so that the chin was directed toward the opposite side; the middle bundle lifted the shoulder-blade, and approached it to the middle line; the lower, finally, depressed the inner angle of the shoulder-blade a little, and drew the spinal border toward the middle line. When the whole trapezius is at one time irritated, the shoulder-blade rises, the spinal border approaches the middle line, the shoulders sink backward and inward, finally, the head bends forward and toward the opposite side. The M. rhomboideus (Duchenne includes under this name the M. rhomboideus major and minor) holds at rest the posterior border of the shoulder-blade securely against the thorax; when all its fibres contract, it turns the shoulder-blade on its outer angle, and elevates it; in the most extreme degree, the spinal border is directed obliquely from above downward, and from without inward, so that the inner angle stands out more from the middle line than the lower. If we excite the M. serratus anticus major in its lower part, there follows a turning of the shoulder-blade on its lower angle, in consequence of which the acromion is lifted, and the lower angle directed outward and forward. If the middle portion is irritated, the shoulder-blade moves forward, outward, and upward.

Consequently, the spinal border removes from two to four centimetres from the middle line, presses against the wall of the thorax, and makes a deep furrow in the skin; the lower part of the serratus elevates the shoulder. When the entire serratus is simultaneously irritated (through faradization of the N. thoracicus lateralis), the scapula, through the lifting of its acromial angle, is carried so far forward and outward, that the space between the scapula and the spinal column has twice its usual size; the inner border is pressed against the thorax, while the remainder of the shoulder-blade stands out like a wing.

In paralysis of the lower part of the trapezius the basis scapulæ removes from ten to twelve centimetres from the spinous processes, and forms the so-called "broad back" which we so often meet with among workmen who always sit, on account of their occupation, bent over; if to this there is added a paralysis of the upper portion, the shoulder sinks, and the shoulder-blade takes such a position, that its lower angle approaches the middle line more, and its inner, on the contrary, less, than in the normal condition: consequently the movements suffer many disturbances. In paralysis of the lower part, the patient is still able to draw the shoulder somewhat backward; if he tries, however, to approach the shoulders to one another, the Mm. rhomboidei draw the shoulder-blades in their direction, i. e., they lift them, and turn them at the same time on their outer angle. If the middle part is also affected, the shoulder-blade appears to be loosened from the thorax, and there is no longer any secure support for the upper arm; the movements of the arm which require a certain muscular power are thereby rendered difficult and inconvenient. If the M. rhomboideus is paralyzed, the basis scap. moves from the wall of the thorax, shows itself clearly under the skin, and there arises a more considerable fold between it and the vertebral column; at the same time, on account of the consequent preponderance of the serratus ant. maj., the lower angle is drawn forward and outward. As to the disturbance connected with this, the combined movement—which is accomplished by bringing the basis scap. close to the wall of the chest, and by a strong contraction toward the middle line, namely, the movement of the arm backward—is restrained. A paralysis of the serratus ant. maj. shows, when the arm hangs down, but little sinking of the shoulder-blade; at the most, the under angle of the shoulder-blade stands directed somewhat more backward and upward, and springs out more. When, however, the patient moves the arm from the body, and turns with it the shoulder-blade on its vertical axis, the posterior border of the shoulder-blade moves from the thorax, and forms thereby a channel; at the same time the under angle lifts itself from the thorax, while the anterior approaches this more closely. The more this evil progresses, the more striking are the changes, so that in the highest degree the shoulder-blade stands off wing-like from the wall of the chest. The movements of the arm are very limited in complete paralysis of the serratus; it may be lifted by means of the deltoideus to a horizontal position; movement beyond this is impossible, when not aided by the upper portion of the trapezius and the levator ang. scap., and, with their help, its action is very incomplete.

IV. The conclusions to be drawn from Duchenne's investigations in regard to the functions of the muscles of the foot are even as interesting, in an anatomical point of view, as they are important in a therapeutical. He found, that direct extension and direct flexion of the foot were produced only through the simultaneous action of several muscles, since each extensor or flexor muscle of the foot causes at the same time an adduction or abduction. He therefore gave the individual muscles names corresponding to their functions, and called the combined Mm. gastrocnemius, soleus, and tibialis post., which extend and adduct the foot, *M. extensor adductor;* the Mm. peronæus longus and brevis, which extend and abduct the foot, *M. extensor abductor;* the

M. tibialis anticus, which flexes and adducts the foot, *M. flexor adductor;* the M. extensor digitorum communis longus and M. extensor hallucis, which flex and abduct the foot, *M. flexor abductor.* Direct extension arises also from the combined action of the Mm. gastrocnemii, soleus, and peronæus longus; direct flexing, through the simultaneous action of the Mm. tibialis ant. and extensor digit. comm. long.

Irritation of the extensor adductor (gastrocnemius, soleus, and tibialis post.) causes, besides the strong extension of the posterior part of the foot and of the outer border of the front part, a turning of the member, so that the point is directed inward and the heel outward. The outer border of the foot turns outward at the same time that the toes take on the form of claws by the extension of their first and the bending of their other phalanges. Irritation of the extensor abductor (peronæus longus and brevis) causes strong sinking of the inner side of the front part of the foot, as well as abduction of the foot, the outer border of which is lifted, and the malleolus internus is rendered prominent. Paralysis or atrophy of the extensor adductor leads to the following appearances: In attempting to extend the foot, it is, through the action of the extensor abductor which now alone works, strongly abducted; the front part of the foot is turned inward, in consequence of a sinking of the first metatarsal bones, the os naviculare, and the os cuneiforme; the plantar side is hollowed out more, and the dorsal side is more arched. At the same time, the dorsal arching increases; the heel, on the contrary, sinks more and more, till finally the astragalus takes the place of the calcaneus, and there results the "hollow foot of the peronæus longus," as Duchenne calls it. Secondarily, retractions of certain muscles of the foot set in—of the adductor hallucis, of the flexor brevis digit., etc. In consequence of the paralysis or atrophy of the extensor abductor, the arching of the foot disappears almost entirely; in standing, the foot takes the talipes-valgus position, and its inner border rests flat on the ground. If, on the contrary, in paralysis of the extensor abductor, an effort is made to extend the foot, it takes the position of talipes varus, for through the tonic power of the tibialis anticus the head of the first metatarsal bone is drawn upward. Gradually a flat foot is formed, which disappears with the paralysis of the peronœus.

In regard to the movements of the foot, when the flexor adductor (tibialis anticus) is irritated, the foot is strongly extended and adducted, and the inner border of its anterior portion is lifted. By irritating the flexor abductor (extensor digit. comm. long. and extensor hallucis), the foot is flexed and abducted. The four last toes are thereby slightly extended, the outer border of the foot is lifted, the sole is turned outward, and the great toe is bent. In consequence of atrophy or paralysis of the flexor adductor, the bending of the foot is always combined with abduction, the foot is turned more outward, and in walking is apt to strike the ground; at last the action of the extensors prevails, and pes equinus results. In paralysis or atrophy of the flexor abductor, the sidewise movements take place in an opposite direction; the foot cannot be flexed without being at the same time adducted, with the sole turned inward. The anterior part of the foot turns upward, so much so, that sometimes the astragalus and calcaneus become prominent.

Irritation of the tibialis posticus and of the peronæus brevis causes, independently of flexing and extending, sidewise movements of the foot; the tibialis posticus produces pure adduction, and the peronæus brevis pure abduction; both acting together prevent the turning of the foot inward and outward. In paralysis or atrophy of these muscles, the foot assumes either the varus or the valgus position.

V. Duchenne's investigations in regard to the function of the diaphragm, showed, that when we electrize both phrenici, in man or animals, powerful and rapid contractions of this muscle set in: in consequence of which, the abdominal walls being uninjured, the false ribs rise and move outward, the cavity of the chest extends itself downward, and an amount of air, corresponding to the increase in space, rushes into the lungs. This sudden entrance of air through the glottis into the air-tubes is accompanied with a peculiar sobbing, which, according to Ziemssen, is produced by the sudden vibrations of the vocal cords, that are not taken out of the way on account of the unexpected and deep inspiratory movements. If the entrails of the animal are removed beforehand, and consequently the resistance of the abdominal muscles lessened, contraction of the diaphragm causes the false ribs to be drawn inward. In this case we hear no loud inspiration sound; hence it follows that the diaphragm needs support from below in the production of its inspiratory action. In atrophy of the diaphragm, the epigastrium and the abdominal walls sink in during inspiration, instead of becoming prominent, while the walls of the thorax lift themselves and expand: the reverse takes place during expiration.

VI. Irritation of a single M. intercostalis externus, by means of a thin electrode pressed immediately on the origin of the M. serratus magnus against the lower border of the upper ribs, causes, according to Ziemssen, in quiet respiration, a powerful and distinctly visible lifting of the lower ribs outward and upward. This movement also extends to the two under ribs, whose change of position may be felt with the fingers as well as seen. If we increase the current gradually, so that the M. intercostalis int. is affected, there is perceptible, nevertheless, no change in the position of the ribs and in the intercostal spaces. So long as the irritation continues, the ribs stand directed obliquely outward and are stone-hard to the touch. Also forced inspirations and expirations, during the irritation, appear to produce no alterations in these positions. The electrized intercostal muscles remain unchanged and stand like a wall, while the sinking backward and arching forward of the remaining intercostal spaces are distinctly visible.

VII. As to the abdominal muscles, irritation of each nervus intercostalis abdom., which enters into one of the muscles, that together form the M. rectus abdominalis, causes a hard and stretched condition of the belly of the corresponding muscle: the upper portions of the muscles draw the abdominal wall upward, and those parts below the navel draw it downward; moreover, each for itself draws the abdominal wall inward, and seeks to produce a level between the sternum and symphysis. Irritation of the M. obliquus abdominalis ext. causes lateral expansion of the abdomen. If we electrize the outer fasciculi of the Mm. obliqui ext. of both sides with several electrodes, by subdividing the conducting wires, or by using several wires coming from each pole, the outer parts of each side form a level, while the middle of the abdominal wall becomes strongly and narrowly arched. If the M. transversus abdominis is electrized at the same time on both sides of the crista ossis ilei and near the outer border of the quadratus lumborum, and is excited in this way, which is not always the case, there follows transverse contraction of the abdomen, which with a strong current is as powerful as when it serves for the emptying of the rectum or of the bladder—a phenomenon which is often accompanied with the specific sounds due to the movement and escape of flatus. If we carry the electrode more forward, we can exercise a partial action on the M. obliquus abdom. internus by pressing strongly over the spina ilei ant. sup.

We will now pass to the consideration of the paralysis of the nerves which supply the skin and the muscles of the extremities, and present an imperfect picture of the changes which the most important complete paralysis brings about in the functions of the affected parts.

In the upper extremities paralysis of the N. radialis

causes the following complex symptoms: The patient is not able to lift the hand, to extend the first phalanges, to bring the hand into supination, to adduct or to abduct it. Abduction and extension of the thumb are also impossible. On the contrary, all the other movements, flexion and pronation of the arm, bending of the fingers, adduction of the thumb, etc., are possible. In most cases there are combined with these a feeling of numbness in the hand and anæsthesia of the dorsal side of the forearm and of the hand. If the N. ulnaris is paralyzed, the patient, though able to hold with the hand objects of large size, is unable to take hold of small objects. The power with which he holds an object between two fingers varies according as he seizes it with the thumb and index-finger, thumb and middle-finger, or thumb and ring or little finger. The last is absolutely impossible, while the other movements are more or less possible. If he attempts to shut the hand, the last two phalanges bend sufficiently, while the first, especially those of the ring and little finger, are unable to reach the palm of the hand. If the interossei are fully paralyzed, the fingers separate from one another for several lines, when the attempt is made to extend them, and it is absolutely impossible to cause them to approach one another in this position or to separate them more widely. If we approach them forcibly, the first phalanges bend. On the other hand, the movements of the thumb, with the exception of adduction, also bending of the first phalanx, opposition and adduction may be performed: the extension of the wrist, the bending of the forearm on the upper arm, supination, and pronation remain unhindered. The usual position of the hand does not differ from its normal position, but its inner half has lost its sensibility, and the fingers, especially the last two, their normal sense of touch. If the N. medianus is paralyzed, the bending of the arm at the elbow is free, but that of the wrist is prevented; the flexion of the second and third phalanges of the fingers, and the pronation of the hand, are impossible. The thumb, it is true, can be adducted, but not bent, nor brought in opposition; the extension of the wrist and of the fingers, and the supination of the arm, are not hindered; the middle finger is numb, cold, and sensationless.

In paralysis of the N. cruralis of the lower extremity, the flexion of the upper leg, and the extension of the lower leg, are more or less limited; the patient, since motion forward is much prevented in paralysis of the quadriceps muscle of the thigh, can only lift the leg a little from the ground and take but short steps: going up-stairs is difficult, and rising from the sitting position is often impossible. If the N. obturatorius is also paralyzed, besides the adduction of the leg, the rotation of the body and of the thigh outward is checked.

Paralysis of the N. peronæus presents the following diagnostic appearances: the movements of the thigh and leg are more or less unaffected, while those of the foot are very limited; the patient in walking is unable to support himself on the metatarsal head of the great toe, to turn the foot outward, or to extend the toes, and he steps with the outer border of the foot raised. The sensibility of the skin is generally lessened on the external surface of the leg and on the back of the foot. In paralysis of the N. tibialis the movements of the thigh, with the exception of the more or less difficult rotation outward, are not interfered with, but the flexion of the leg, the lifting of both thigh and leg backward, and the rotation of the latter inward and outward, are prevented; the heel cannot be raised, nor can the middle part of the foot or the toes be bent. The outer border of the dorsal side of the foot and the sole have lost their sensibility.

EIGHTH SECTION.

THE IMPORTANCE OF ELECTRICITY IN THE DIAGNOSIS AND PROGNOSIS OF PARALYTIC AFFECTIONS.

As by the use of the stethoscope and the plessimeter the diagnosis of pulmonary and heart diseases has attained a scientific certainty, and the therapeutic processes, based upon the physical examination of the organs affected, have become rational, in like manner the treatment of paralytic cases has had a more scientific basis ever since we have been able, by means of that delicate re-agent, the electric current, to examine the nervous and muscular irritability of the parts affected, and to measure their variation from the normal condition. As, however, the physical examination of the thoracic organs, without consideration of other indications, suffices in but very few cases the attainment of a sure diagnosis, and never for the establishment of a rational cure, so, too, the electric current is only an auxiliary, which, when we have fully considered all the symptoms peculiar to the individual, the etiological forces, etc., will in many obscure cases assist us to a surer diagnosis; in cases where the symptoms are seemingly contradictory it will determine our opinion, and in those that are free from doubt it will confirm the judgment already formed; finally, in its bearing upon the prognosis of peculiar forms of paralysis of the greatest importance, it will lead us to a scientific certainty, obtainable by no other means. As proof of these assertions, before

I proceed to the diagnostic criteria of the several forms of paralysis, I shall describe a few cases, in which, in the absence or the uncertainty of other indications, I was enabled, simply from the electric conditions of the muscles, to draw up diagnoses, the accuracy of which further developments established beyond a doubt.

Case 3.[1]—Hache, a master-furrier, who, up to his 38th year, had enjoyed good health, experienced, for about five months, a certain weakness and stiffness in both hands, which rendered the extension of them more and more difficult, and during the last three months of this period impossible. Whenever he attempted to grasp any thing, or to sew, or hold out his hand to any one, the three middle fingers closed, while the thumb and little finger remained extended. The effort to spread the hand, or to separate the thumb from the index-finger, was equally vain. With the exception of light, dragging pains in both shoulders, no abnormal or painful sensations of any kind preceded the attack, nor could the patient ascribe its gradual increase to any particular cause. In the course of an examination made on the 12th of March, 1854, I found that not even a very intense electric current, directed upon the Mm. extensores digit. comm. of the hand, was powerful enough to extend the first phalanges of the

[1] This case is especially interesting, because it is the first in which I discovered, as a cause of paralysis, the habitual use of the snuff which comes packed in lead (vide Med. Central Zeitung of Nov. 22, 1854, and Virchow's Archiv., 1857, p. 209, et seq.). Since the publication of this case so many instances of poisoning from the lead taken up in snuff have arisen, that in France, Belgium, Prussia, and other German states, strong laws have been passed against packing tobacco in lead. Without doubt very many cases of paralysis owe their origin to similar causes, such as the saturation of silk in vinegar of lead to increase its weight, the use of white lead in paint for the face and in the preparation of other cosmetic appliances, etc., etc. Similar causes, frequently remaining altogether hid from the physician, produce paralysis, which, in consequence of the continuance of the injurious action, defy all the efforts of medical skill. Duchenne mentions some cases in which, by the use of wine to which a salt of lead had been added, or of beer which had been led through leaden pipes from the casks in the tap-room, paralyses have been caused.

fingers. The electro-muscular sensibility, also, of the paralyzed muscles was lowered to such a degree, that a very strong current was only slightly felt by the patient. The remaining extensors (with the exception of the extensores indic. propr. and the abductors of the thumb, of which the electro-muscular contractility and sensibility were also more or less impaired), as well as the supinators, and all the flexors and pronators had in both arms a perfectly normal electric condition. The case, therefore, seemed to me to be one of lead-paralysis, although neither from the patient's occupation or mode of life, nor from any antecedent symptoms of illness, could a cause be adduced which justified this diagnosis.

After I had applied electricity for the thirty-seventh time almost without result, the patient went on a journey, and consequently passed out of my charge. I saw him again about two months later, on July 9, 1854. In addition to the paralytic effects above described, there was now a considerable protuberance of the bones of the wrist and of the second, third, and fourth bones of the metacarpus—a symptom which confirmed me more and more in the opinion previously conceived. After a fresh examination of all the circumstances which, in the case of my patient, could possibly explain his poisoning by lead, I resorted to a qualitative analysis of the tobacco which he had been in the habit of snuffing for many years, and which he had brought packed in lead. The analysis gave as a result so considerable an indication of this metal, that a quantitative analysis seemed to me unnecessary. After the patient had given up the habit of snuffing tobacco, the employment, for four weeks, of sulphur baths and of saline purgatives considerably reduced the swellings, particularly those of the right hand; as, however, the paralytic effects still remained unchanged, the electric treatment was resorted to, and in forty sittings was carried so far that the patient was able, November 6th, to extend both hands, to separate the fingers, to raise the forefinger with ease in writing, etc., and could sew and perform the other details of his business. A perfect cure gradually followed, without the further application of electricity, or the use of other agents. At the end of the year, however, although all the usual movements had for a long time been executed with ease, the electro-muscular contractility of the muscles, formerly paralyzed, still remained low; it was not till August, 1855, that they were found, on examination, to have recovered their normal power.

CASE 4.—Mr. Z——, a trumpeter, a man of forty-nine years, who had always been healthy, fell sick in October, 1852, of a nervous fever, from which he did not recover sufficiently to undertake his former employment, till February, 1853, and then he made the sad discovery that, while he was able, though with difficulty, to bring out the higher tones, the lower ones were beyond his power. Now, to produce the latter, it is necessary to hold the mouth-piece to the lips very lightly, while for the higher tones it is pressed close; the patient was, therefore, supposed to be affected with a local weakness of certain muscles, induced in part by his recent malady, in part by the lack of exercise, and he was accordingly recommended to a stimulating diet, spirituous liquors, and to a regular, but moderate practice upon his instrument. Yet, notwithstanding this treatment, though the patient felt in other respects perfectly well, many months passed without the least change being apparent in the local difficulties, and the patient at last, by the advice of his physician, applied to me, May 30, 1853, for an application of the electric treatment.

I found him a large, well-built, rather muscular man, who at each respiration expanded the thorax to its normal extent. His lungs, larynx, etc., presented no evidence of disease; he could move the muscles of the face with freedom in every direction, and felt very distinctly the touch of the hand upon any part of the face. When, however, I pinched between my fingers the skin of either cheek, I thought I discovered more solidity of tissue on the right than on the left side—a difference, however, too unimportant to be made the basis of a diagnosis. I now faradized the muscles of the face separately, and found that the electro-muscular contractility of the right side, as compared with the left, was considerably lowered; that, in particular, the M. zygomaticus major, the M. depressor labii superioris, the depressor anguli oris, and even the M. orbicularis oris of the right side, contracted with much less promptness and energy than the same muscles of the left, and that the sensation associated with the contraction of these muscles was much less distinct on the right side; a like variation, however, between the Mm. masseteres and temporales of the two cheeks was scarcely perceptible. I, accordingly, diagnosed an exudation in the muscular substance and the cellular tissue of the skin of the cheek, which seemed to extend upward to the lower rim of the cheek-bone, downward to the lower rim of the inferior jaw-bone, and outward to the processus coronoideus of the latter. The electric current was accordingly directed upon the suffering parts, and with such effect, that the patient, after thirty sittings, was able, though still with difficulty, to produce the deep tones. On subjecting him again, November 3, 1853, to an examination, I found the electro-muscular contractility and sensibility of the Mm. zygomatici, the M. depressor lab. sup., etc., perfectly normal on both sides.

CASE 5.—Julius C——, of Grüneberg, a small, weakly, misshapen, but apparently healthy boy, of twelve years, was born with a club-foot (pes varus), for the correction of which defect the tendon of the M. tibialis ant. had been cut by Dieffenbach in the first year of the boy's life. The parents were at the same time enjoined to support the foot of the child, as soon as it made its first efforts to walk, with a strong, thick shoe. Such a shoe the child continued to wear for seven months, when, on occasion of a light fever, lasting a fortnight, it was laid aside, and the child was allowed to run about in slippers. In the course of its play, probably in consequence of some trivial injury to the tendon of the tibialis ant., an inflamed condition of the part was brought on, manifesting itself at first by a local swelling, and by painfulness to the touch at the point where the tendon had been cut, and finally by a disturbed action, by which the right leg was bent back against the upper part of the thigh, while the foot was abducted and extended.

Every effort on the part of the patient to move the leg, and every attempt of the physician to give it another position, were without success. When, by leeches, embrocation of the ungt. neapolit., and poulticing, the inflammatory effects had been subdued, all spontaneous movement still remained impossible—the leg retaining the position already described. On every attempt at locomotion the point of the foot scarcely touched the ground, and the physicians were frustrated in their repeated efforts to bring the leg to its normal position. In the course of a period of inactivity lasting seven months, during which time the patient either was moved about in a hand-carriage or limped around on the left leg, the nutrition of the right leg, especially of the lower part of the thigh, became deficient, the muscles grew thin and shrivelled, and the extremity cold. When Geh. R. Langenbeck witnessed the condition of the child, he sent him to me, April 27, 1857, to ascertain the electric state of the paralyzed muscles. The sensibility of the affected parts was undisturbed. All the muscles of the lower part of the thigh and of the foot reacted very well, when subjected to a weak current, and only when the N. peronœus, the M. extensor digitorum comm., and the M. tibialis ant. were irritated at the spot formerly painful, was any pain experienced. Having thus become convinced that the case was one of traumatic paralysis in its lightest form, I irritated the extensor digit. comm. again, at first with a weak current, which, however, I progressively strengthened to such a degree, by gradually pushing in the bundle of wires, that in consequence of a powerful flexion of the foot both it and the whole leg resumed their normal position, and the boy was able, though at first slowly and timidly, to walk about. In the two ensuing weeks which the patient spent in Berlin, under the application of an intermittent current, the painful sensations, which extended along the tendon of the tibialis ant., and had their seat especially in the os naviculare, wholly disappeared; the muscles resumed their full size, the temperature of the leg became normal, and the boy could walk great distances without difficulty.

CASE 6.—M. L——, the son of a physician, of Flensburg, a hearty, corpulent boy, who had already passed through two attacks of pseudo-croup, fell sick in January, 1865, when he was one year and eight months old, in the following manner: On the very day on which his nurse was taken ill with diphtheria, he became fretful, had a hot head and a coated tongue, and threw up the food he had eaten. An inspection of his throat gave the following results: white exudations, about as large as the head of a pin, on the left tonsil, both tonsils inflamed and somewhat swollen. On the following day the exudations had disappeared; his ill-feelings, however, continued eight days longer. About four weeks later his father remarked that his child, who had hitherto been very nimble on his legs, had become uncertain in his steps, complained of pains in his legs, and frequently grasped both hips with his hands—symptoms which usually passed away in the course of the afternoon. Eight days later, he was unable to walk with safety, and frequently fell or sank on his knees, when he wanted to stand, while in his general health he remained perfectly well, and in particular showed no trace of any inflammation of the brain. By the end of February, the lower extremities were entirely paralyzed; they were incapable of the least active motion, and became ice-cold; their sensibility and susceptibility to reflex irritation were wholly gone; the bladder and the rectum were also in a state of paralysis. Neither paralysis of the soft palate nor disturbance of the accommodation of the eyes ensued. This condition lasted till June, when slight traces of motive power in the upper part of the thigh, which had not become atrophied, began to be perceptible. In September, he was able to stand for a short time on a chair; soon after he could raise himself upright by taking hold of some firm object. From this time on, the temperature of the leg increased. In March, 1866, when led by the hand, he could walk a few steps slowly, and the paralysis of the bladder and rectum was passing off.

It was on April 13, 1866, that I saw the patient for the first time. He was now an extraordinarily corpulent little fellow of three years. The muscular development of the leg had suffered very little, and was provided with a thick cushion of fat; the adductors and gastrocnemii of both legs were much contracted; their temperature was now normal, and reflex irritability was exhibited. The question now presented itself for our decision, whether the case was one of what is called diphtheritic paralysis, or of paralysis from other causes. The electro-muscular contractility in the quadriceps femoris, as well as in all the inferior femoral muscles of the N. peroneus of both legs, was so much reduced that, in view of the previous course of the disease, and of the fact that, in the outset of the paralysis, the electro-muscular contractility was raised to its full power, and that this force is never extinguished by a diphtheritic paralysis, we were compelled to found the diagnosis upon an exudation in the spinal canal, occasioned by a chronic inflammation of the pia mater. The further course of the disease confirmed this diagnosis. When, in May, 1867, I saw the boy again, he was able, without external support, to walk about the room; but, in consequence of the imperfect restoration of the functional power of the inferior femoral extensor, in conjunction with the existing paralysis of the sural muscles, the upper part of the body was bent backward, and the patient usually stepped only on the toes. In all the muscles that were otherwise brought into play, the reaction against the electric current had gradually improved, so that after the tenotomy of the tendon-achilles, which is probably necessary, a perfect cure may be anticipated.

Having become convinced of the importance of electricity in the diagnosis and prognosis of paralytic diseases in general, we now proceed to the consideration of special forms of paralysis, in order that, by observation of the varying relations of paralyzed muscles and nerves toward the electric current, we may arrive at diagnostic and prognostic criteria. We shall meet, after having conquered the technical difficulties of such an inquiry, many other facts, the careful consideration of which can alone save us from gross errors. Thus, for example, the condition of a muscle subjected to local faradization is the product of two factors: the motory excitability of the intra-muscular nerve-fibres and that of the muscle-fibres.[1] A feeble contraction under local muscular excitement may, therefore, indicate either a diminished irritability of the nerve-fibres, in connection with a normal condition of the muscle-fibres; or a diminished irritability of the muscle-fibres, in connection with a normal condition of the nerve-fibres; or, finally, the product of the diminished irritability of both the muscle and nerve fibres. Thus we are obliged to proceed to further examinations. If a muscle, excited by the force of the will or by the electric irritation of the nerve, which ramifies through it, contracts in a normal manner, it cannot be essentially diseased, and, if the expected reaction is wanting, the abnormal effect is connected with a diseased condition of the intra-muscular nerve-

[1] The independent irritability of the muscle-fibres has been proved not only by Bernard and Kölliker's experiments in poisoning with curarina, but also by the continued contraction of a muscle, while subjected to a constant current—a fact first observed by Wundt—as well as by the peculiar condition of a muscle in electrotonus.

fibres.[1] In paralyses of long standing, the affected muscles, nerves, and central parts develop secondary changes, which exert an influence upon the electric condition, and render the diagnosis difficult. Finally, peripheric and central paralyses may occur at one and the same time in the same individual, springing either from one and the same cause—as when a tumor, proceeding from the cortical substance of the brain, and gradually increasing in size, compresses special nerves at the base of the cranium—or from various causes, as is shown by the peripheric paralysis frequently occurring with those who are hysterically affected.

On the other hand, an examination by electricity not only furnishes us the means of distinguishing the various paralyses that proceed from the brain, the spinal marrow, the sympathetic, the nerves, or the muscles, but it also opens to us still wider views with reference, in the first place, to the special seat of these varieties, whether, for example, in a nervous plexus, a nervous trunk, a whole muscle, or any part of these, etc. If, in the case of a peripheric nervous paralysis, on application of the spinal marrow-plexus current, a normal reaction ensues, while such reaction fails on application of the spinal marrow-nerve current, we thus find that the chief difficulty resides in the conducting power of the nervous trunk. If in a case of muscular paralysis the anterior portion of the deltoideus reacts badly, while the middle and posterior portions contract according to the degree of excitement, we then assign the seat of the disease to the clavicular portion of the N. thorac. ant. Similar conclusions can be reached in the case of anæsthesia. If, for example, in an anæsthesia of the skin, affecting all the branches of a nerve, the normal sensation is felt along the remotest ramifications of the excited nerve, we then know that the brain, the spinal marrow, and the nervous trunk, are all intact, and that the suffering arises from an excessive

[1] *Vide* M. Benedikt on the method of the electric examination of the nervous system, Allgem. Wiener Medic. Zeitung, 1868.

excitability of the extremities of the nerves. A like inference of peripheric disorder is permissible when, in the case of the complete anæsthesia of a nervous extremity, the nervous plexus or posterior nervous roots show a normal reaction; the absence, however, of such reaction is not a sure proof of, on the other hand, a more central disorder, for in the latter case either excessive irritability, or interrupted communication, or some cerebral derangement, may occasion the anæsthesia.

An examination by electricity informs us, in the second place, concerning the origin of the malady. It enables us, for example, to distinguish between a paralysis of the extensors, caused by the poisonous action of lead, and a paralysis of the N. radialis arising from rheumatic causes.

In the third place, this mode of examination furnishes us insights concerning the degree of nutritive disturbance in the nerve or muscle affected. It has been long known that the degree in which a muscle is disordered may be measured by the degree to which its electro-muscular contractility is reduced, as shown by the induction current, and that results of great importance in prognosis may be thus reached. Benedikt and Brenner have, however, ascertained, by the application of the constant current, that the opening or closing of the circuit leads to no less important results.

Brenner has even [1] drawn up a definite scale, according to which, in neuropathic or myopathic paralysis, a muscle loses its physiological power of reaction.

1st stage: Influence of the will checked, but reaction under the induction and constant currents. 2d stage: Effect of the induction current lowered or raised; effect of the constant current exhibited, often to a high degree. 3d stage: No effect produced except by the opening of the ascending constant current. 4th stage: No effect except by the use of the metallic current-changer. 5th stage: Recurrence of the convulsive state. 6th stage: Disconnected

[1] L. c., p. 293, et seq.

convulsive effects by reflex action, and through the irritation of the nerves of the skin, by means of the secondary induction current. 7th stage: No degree of irritation produces reaction in the nerve, the function of the muscle is impaired or destroyed.

Brenner adds that the muscle, as the malady increases, descends to a lower and lower stage, often omitting intermediate ones, while, on the other hand, as it gradually improves, it rises from the lower numbers of the scale to the higher; and that, moreover, only in the seventh stage, in consideration of the occasional return of the executive power of a muscle, are the conditions unfavorable for a prognosis. These interesting observations, of special importance in their bearing upon prognosis, need the corroboration of additional and carefully-managed experiments.

Historically, Marshall Hall was the first to direct the attention of the physician to the value of galvanism in the diagnosis of paralytic conditions.[1] He asserted that the degree of nervous irritability could be made serviceable as a diagnostic means of distinguishing spinal and cerebral paralysis, since in the former the muscular irritability diminishes, and in the same degree the muscular contractions attendant upon electric excitement become weaker, or altogether cease; while in cerebral paralysis the muscular irritability actually increases, and for the reason that the will is not then able to exert its influence. But Marshall Hall, as Althaus[2] justly observes, understood by "cerebral paralysis" a paralysis of the motor power of the will, by which the muscles are deprived of the influence of the brain, a paralysis which, according to him, arises from disease of the brain, or from diseases of the dorsal region of the spinal column; by "spinal paralysis," on the other hand, he meant, not a paralysis occasioned by some affection of the spinal

[1] On the Condition of the Muscular Irritability in Paralytic Muscles; *Med. Chir. Transactions*, Series II., vol. iv.
[2] *L. c.*, p. 195.

marrow, but one in which the muscles are deprived of the influence of this organ, such as, for example, occurs when a motor nerve is divided.

These terms, which Dr. Hall thus employed in a sense quite different from that to which they have been hitherto applied, have led many writers, and in particular those of the Continent, to frequent misapprehension of his positions.

II.—CEREBRAL PARALYSIS.

By cerebral paralyses, in the wider sense of the term, are understood those which are occasioned by derangements within the cavity of the skull. Romberg has the great merit of having brought into prominence, in his standard text-book, "On the Diseases of the Nerves," the important diagnostic and prognostic distinction between paralyses which affect the nervous filaments that proceed from the brain and those which affect the motory filaments that have their course within the brain, since the filaments that proceed from the brain constitute simply the first station of the peripheric path; and consequently the paralyses which affect them should be called peripheric, while only those should be designated, in the stricter sense, cerebral, which attack the nerves in their course within the brain itself.

The exciting causes of peripheric paralyses of the cerebral nerves are of the most comprehensive character: collections of a dyscrasic nature upon the periosteum, or the bones at the base of the cerebrum; secondary growths, tubercles, aneurismatic formations at the base of the brain and skull, etc. But paralyses, in the stricter sense cerebral, are occasioned by the emission of blood or frequent inflammations in the substance of the brain, or by intumescences of a cancerous or tuberculous nature, or by atrophy or hyperemia of the brain. Romberg[1] has also drawn attention to similar cases, in which diseases of the brain have injured the nerves

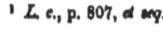
[1] *L. c.*, p. 807, *et seq.*

at their point of origin from the spinal marrow and the brain; and have consequently, without the addition of any cerebral affection, produced peripheric paralyses—cases, the diagnosis of which, while always extremely difficult, sometimes cannot, even with the most careful survey of all the symptoms, be made certain, unless, perhaps, the electric current, by nicely discriminating the muscles, whose electric condition is impaired, from those which, though paralyzed, remain in this respect perfectly sound, provide the means. But in this place we are only concerned with paralyses in the stricter sense cerebral. In paralyses of this kind, Marshall Hall affirmed, as already mentioned, that the irritability of the paralyzed muscles, in comparison with the healthy ones, is actually increased, a conclusion to which he was brought while conducting the electric current to the paralyzed members, in a series of cases, through two basins of water. Pereira, Copeland, and, in particular, Todd,[1] have disproved the universal validity of this assertion, for in many kinds of cerebral paralyses they found the irritability of the paralyzed muscles not only not heightened, but even reduced. Todd, after careful observations, was led to the following results:

1. In those cases in which the paralyzed muscles, when subjected to the electric excitement, exhibit stronger convulsions than the homonymous muscles of the unparalyzed members, a certain degree of contraction was apparent, corresponding in degree to the violence of the convulsion. There was thus in these cases, besides the paralysis, an irritable condition of the cerebral matter, such as is found in apoplexies where the brain is otherwise healthy, in tubercular formation, but especially in traumatic injuries accompanied with meningitis and meningeal apoplexy.

2. In those cases in which the electric excitement occasioned no convulsions, or but slight ones, the muscles were ordinarily weak, and in a condition of atrophy; the

[1] Clinical Lectures on Paralysis, London, 1856.

temperature and assimilative power of the affected parts were depressed; and the paralysis was attended with a structural modification of the cerebral substance, which arose either gradually, with an atheromatous deterioration of the arterial membranes, or suddenly, in cases where obstructions had occurred in the arteries.

3. In cases in which an apoplectic paralysis had attacked men who were not far advanced in years, and had always possessed good health, the paralysis being complete, no difference was perceived as regards irritability between the paralyzed and healthy muscles.

In opposition to the position of Hall, Duchenne claimed that in cerebral paralyses the electro-muscular contractility and sensibility of the paralyzed muscles remained perfectly normal, exhibiting no variations more important than are frequently found between the corresponding muscles of the two sides of the body when in a normal condition. I can, on the whole, assent to this proposition of Duchenne, so far, that is, as it affects cases that have recently occurred, and those paralyses which, as their effects show, proceed from the substance of the brain itself. The apparently violent movements, which in particular cases follow upon electric excitement, are, for the most part, reflex movements, which not only occur in experiments conducted like Marshall Hall's, but also when we direct upon the muscle under examination a sudden, intense current. These movements, however, are not perceived when we gradually increase the force of a current which in the outset was gentle and steady.

Case 7.—Mrs. H——, nineteen and a half years old, previously healthy, having been married three years, was suddenly attacked, in consequence of a change of residence, eight weeks after her second confinement, with a fit of apoplexy, and sank into unconsciousness. After remaining three days in this condition, she was found paralyzed in her left arm and left leg; her speech was difficult; the saliva flowed from her mouth, which was drawn to the left, and she could not see with the left eye. In February of the following year, she began to raise the arm at the shoulder, and to make the first attempts to walk.

On my first visit, April 11, 1857, she could, by dragging her leg, go up and down the room; the arm was somewhat emaciated, and its temperature lowered; she could raise the upper part to an angle of 75 degrees, but she could not stretch out her hand, the fingers of which were convulsively closed; the faculty of vision had returned, yet the traces of facial paralysis were still very apparent. In other respects, the patient presented (probably in consequence of the long continuance of an antiphlogistic treatment, and of too low a diet) all the symptoms of impoverished blood : a small pulse, pale face, attacks of dizziness, vomiting of food, etc. The electro-muscular contractility and sensibility of all the paralyzed muscles, even the extensors of the fingers, remained unimpaired.

CASE 8.—Louisa Kitzerom, a healthy child up to her fifth year, after having for several weeks showed signs of some extraordinary disturbance of her system, such as crying and screaming, unsteady movements of the arms and legs, convulsive movements of the tongue, etc., was seized, on New-Year's morning, 1849, after a night disturbed by fever and dreams, with a paralysis of the right side, affecting not only the right arm and leg, but even the right N. facialis. Upon the repeated employment of leeches, cupping-glasses, and other antiphlogistic agents, the child became more quiet, and the facial paralysis passed away ; but the signs of a generally disturbed condition still lasted, and it was half a year before she made the first attempts to walk or could use her arm a little. When I first saw the patient, February 16, 1857, eight years after the attack, she was able, though with much effort, to walk considerable distances ; she used the right arm comparatively little, although, even without aid, she could perform with it all the ordinary movements.

Not the slightest difference was perceptible between the right and left sides of the face; but the right arm and the right leg were shortened one inch, and the right foot about a quarter of an inch. The bones of the affected parts had not suffered in their transverse measurement, nor, though particular muscles were but little developed, was there any atrophy of the parts affected. The paralyzed extremities were a bluish red, and felt cold to the touch, but in the electric condition of their muscles they showed no variation. The mental faculties of the patient had not suffered in any respect.

On the other hand, in cases of cerebral paralysis of longer duration, Duchenne's proposition is subject to many exceptions. Thus cerebral paralyses sometimes occur which are peculiarly characterized by the sudden and great changes in the electric reaction of the parts affected; a reaction, in the outset, abnormally strong, will sink rapidly below the normal degree, or one which began feebly will quickly rise above the level. Cases of this kind are owing, for the most part, to intumescences in the cerebrum, which cause a pathological irritation of particular nerves. Benedikt[1] publishes the following case, which is appropriate here, and is of interest, on account of the annexed report of a dissection:

"Josefa Müller, a woman of the laboring class, aged forty years, having been operated upon in August, 1863, for a cancer of the breast, experienced in December, when convalescent, a pain in the head, cramps of the right lower extremities, tremblings of both the upper ones, strabismus, frequent dizziness, and vomiting, on which account she was removed, at the end of the year 1864, to the clinic of Oppolzer.

"The patient complained continually of pain in the occiput; her mental powers, with the exception of her memory for recent events, had not suffered; her speech was slow and

[1] Medicinisch-Chirurg. Rundschau, 1864; Vienna.

difficult, but her faculty of vision was unimpaired. She had cramps in the feet daily, continuous but slight tremblings of the hand; the action of her right leg was constrained; the extension of the knee-joint only partially possible; the movement of the ankle and the toes impossible; passive movements difficult; the left extremities were not affected. The paralytic symptoms underwent frequent changes; sometimes one, sometimes another ophthalmic muscle lost its power; sometimes the tongue was turned to the left; at times, slight numbness glided along the facial nerve; a similar alternation of paralysis and numbness, with normal motory power, affected the organs of speech and deglutition, and the right upper and lower extremities. On the 17th of February, amblyopia appeared; after that, in consequence of the increasing frequency and violence of the paroxysms of tremor, the patient lost consciousness; and on the 29th of February, dysentery, which then prevailed, put an end to her sufferings.

An electric examination by means of the induced current, frequently applied to the muscles of the paralyzed extremities, showed that either the electro-muscular contractility was reduced and rose quickly above the normal height, and, on continued faradization, soon fell again, or that it was normal and quickly (twice in about ten minutes) fell.

On dissection, a cancerous tumor, the size of a walnut, was found in the left hemisphere; the left corpus striatum and optic thalamus were congested slightly, and the right portion of the pons varolii and the right lobe of the cerebellum were in a condition of atrophy.

In paralyses of long standing of the kind in question, anatomical changes in the connective tissue and in the nerves and central parts frequently occur, which also disturb the results of an electric examination. Thus, for example, in old cases of apoplexy a destruction of the connective tissue of the paralyzed parts is produced, in consequence of which the resistance to the passage of the electric current is much diminished; it is, therefore, necessary to direct a relatively stronger current upon the muscle of the paralyzed than upon the corresponding one of the unparalyzed side; the former, consequently, will contract with correspondingly greater energy than the latter, and the sensation which accompanies the contraction will be felt with the more acuteness. On the other hand, a thick, hard epidermis, or an increase in the quantity of the connective tissue, arising from exudation, may considerably augment the resistance. Of this character is the case of a gardener, who, having had his leg paralyzed by a fit of apoplexy, caused it to be scourged with nettles one or two hours daily, during a period of two years, the result of which was that, in addition to the induration of the epidermis, an increase in the thickness of the connective tissue occurred to the extent of at least half an inch. In this instance the continued action of a strong current was necessary, in order to call forth in the muscles of the paralyzed side as energetic contractions as a current of moderate force produced in those of the healthy side. In other cases an anæsthesia of the skin or muscles of the paralyzed side affects the certainty of the results. Still another point of consideration is the organic changes which in paralyses of long continuance are effected in the nerves themselves, in both their peripheric and central distribution. Lastly, mention should be made of the destruction of the nervous fibres in the central organs, a fact which Türck[1] first observed. In cases where paralysis had been conditioned by old apoplectic attacks, he found in the corresponding spinal nerves of the opposite side a decrease, and, in parts, an entire disappearance, of the primitive fibres, their places being supplied by granulated and elementary cells. Half a year after the paralytic attack, the granulated cells were only visible here and there; at a later stage they appeared especially numerous above the origin of the ner-

[1] Zeitschrift der R. R. Gesellschaft der Aerzte zu Wien, 1853. Heft 10 und 11, p. 289, et seq.

vous plexus for the upper and lower extremities; at last they extended with the spinal marrow in still increasing numbers.

CASE 9.—Madame Heyer, a strong, healthy woman, in earlier life, now forty-one years old, married fourteen years, but childless, ceased to menstruate when she had only reached her thirty-sixth year, and from that time had complained of headache and vertigo. On the 21st of December, 1857, she was seized with a fit of apoplexy, by which the left half of the body was completely paralyzed. In the course of time the facial paralysis disappeared, but on the 20th of December, 1859, when I saw the patient for the first time, the paralysis of the left extremities remained unchanged. The patient had, besides, a contraction of the upper part of the left arm and of the left hand, and experienced pains in these parts whenever she attempted to move them or straighten them out. The left Mm. deltoideus, quadriceps femoris, and glutæi were emaciated; the glutæi were excessively relaxed and shrunken, as was also, though in less degree, the M. quadriceps femoris, while the M. deltoideus, notwithstanding its emaciation, felt tolerably firm. The sensibility of the skin to the touch seemed unimpaired. In their electric condition the paralyzed muscles constantly exhibited a great diversity; the left M. deltoideus reacted more promptly than that of the healthy side; the extensors of the left arm and hand displayed, notwithstanding their contraction, a normal electric condition. The reflex irritability of the leg, especially when the motor points of the M. vastus internus and rectus were touched by moistened conductors, was to a certain degree increased, so that the leg was immediately thrown up. As for the rest, the muscles that have been named, and in particular the glutæi, corresponding to their degree of relaxation, reacted very badly, while the muscles of the lower part of the thigh and those of the foot showed a normal electric condition. The electro-muscular sensibility in all the paralyzed muscles of the leg was lowered.

The patient had an old look, and her mental faculties had suffered under the depression of a settled melancholy.

In cerebral paralyses proceeding from other causes than those already named, the muscular irritability of the paralyzed muscles is also generally normal. Thus Brierre de Boismont,[1] in a case of general paralysis arising from mental disturbance, found the muscular irritability unimpaired. In corroboration of this result may be adduced the cases of three men suffering from progressive paralysis of the insane, whom, in company with Dr. Leubuscher, I examined, July 12, 1853, in the department for the insane of the workhouse.

Case 10.—Lary, an able-bodied man, forty-eight years old, had a heavy, irregular gait, an unintelligible, lisping mode of speech, a partial paralysis of the right arm, a contraction of the hand, the third and fourth finger, atrophy of the right forearm, and was imbecile in mind.

Case 11.—Broth, thirty years old, formerly a clerk, suffered under an incipient attack of dementia paralytica. His power of speech was still good, but his gait was unsettled, his movements uncertain, though he could hold out his hand without its trembling much. His body was very much emaciated, his skin shrunken.

Case 12.—Braunschweig, about thirty years old, suffered under a more advanced stage of dementia paralytica. His speech was broken and unintelligible, his movements awkward, with trembling of the arm when extended; digestion good; muscular development vigorous.

In all three cases the electro-muscular contractility of the muscles of the face, trunk, and extremities was perfectly normal; with Broth, who was emaciated, and whose skin was loose, the contractions proceeded with more precision

---

[1] Diagn. Untersuchungen verschiedener Arten der allgemeinen Lähmung mittelst der localisirten Galvanisation. Annal. Med. Phys. 1850; Schmidt's Jahrbücher, Band ix., p. 110.

and energy than with Braunschweig. In consequence of the torpidity and weak intelligence of the patients, the degree of electro-muscular sensibility could not be determined.

We shall refer to the distinguishing peculiarities of what are called the essential (spinal) and the cerebral paralyses of children, in the second part of this section.

The induction current should be resorted to, as the only sure and absolutely decisive diagnostic agent, in those recent cases, in which the question presents itself, whether a paralysis attended with cerebral symptoms (for example, a paralysis of the N. facialis) owes its origin to a pathological process in the substance of the brain itself, or is to be ascribed to an injury affecting the nerve in its course along the base of the skull through the canalis fallopii, or beyond the for. stylomastoideum. This current should also be employed in those cases in which we are in doubt whether a paralysis, accompanied with violent cerebral action, is connected, on the one hand, with an intermeningeal apoplexy, or a tumor at the base of the brain, or, on the other hand, with an extravasation or softening process in the substance of the brain. If the symptoms manifested are of peripheric origin, then the electro-muscular contractility, as we shall see, when we come to peripheric paralyses, begins to diminish with the second week, and, as the paralysis becomes complete, is, in the second or third week, wholly extinct, while in paralyses of a central origin this contractile power is found to continue unimpaired. Ziemssen[1] has published several interesting cases bearing upon this distinction; the first of these, the diagnosis of which was confirmed by a dissection, we shall here present in an abridged form:

Wilhelm Diest, a weaver, thirty-three years old, formerly uniformly healthy and vigorous, frequently suffered in the

---

[1] Ueber Lähmung von Gehirnerven durch Affectionen an der Basis cerebr. Virchow's Archiv., Band xiii., Heft ii. and iii., p. 213, 1858.

course of his twentieth year with an inflammation of the eyes. In the preceding year he had been attacked with an intermittent fever, which lasted six weeks. A short time after, a syphilitic ulcer broke out on the prepuce, which, having been only locally treated, left quite a large scar. Intumescences of the inguinal glands followed; three months later nodes and red spots appeared on the head, especially the forehead; and, finally, condylomata around the anus.

At the end of another three months the patient was suddenly attacked with diplopia, to which ptosis of the left upper eyelid was added. After still another period of three months, acute pains in the head, and singing in the ears, came on, followed by distortion of the face, particularly of the mouth, to the left, difficulty of speech, and lastly, paralysis of the muscles of deglutition, which made it impossible to swallow fluids in any quantity. After the paralysis of one side of his face, Diest complained of headache. At last, soon after his admittance into the hospital, August 10, 1856, a remarkable falling off of his strength became apparent; his step was heavy and uncertain, rendering change of place without support impossible. His mental power exhibited no signs of yielding.

A closer examination showed a complete paralysis of Nn. facialis dexter, oculomotorius sinister, trochlearis dexter, and both abducentes; an incomplete paralysis of the Nn. facialis sinister and oculomotorius dexter; also an imperfect paralysis in most of the extensors, and all the flexors of the hand. An examination, by means of the faradic current, constantly showed the electro-muscular contractility of the completely paralyzed muscles extinct, that of those completely paralyzed considerably reduced. The electro-cutaneous sensibility was normal on both sides. In this case, supported by his generalization of the symptoms, and by the electric condition of the paralyzed muscles, Ziemssen felt qualified to infer with safety the central origin of the paralytic effects, and to assume a paralysis—one probably of syphilitic origin—the first force of which was spent upon the nerves distributed within the cranial cavity, depriving them in some places partially, and in a few wholly, of their conducting power. The dissection, which took place twenty hours after death—occurring August 18th, with symptoms of pulmonary tubercles—fully confirmed this diagnosis. Not only were tubercles and cavities found in the lungs, but the brain, which was in other respects healthy, showed traces of a chronic inflammation of the pia mater, with effusion of serum and the formation of connective tissue, through the shrinking of which the nerves were knotted together. The affected nerves themselves showed a degeneration of their peripheric parts corresponding to the intensity of the pressure, and the muscles, as they consecutively lost their functional capacity, had been changed to fat. In the short central portion of the affected nerves, regressive metamorphosis, characterized by an enormous accumulation of concreted fatty granules, was discovered.

With cerebral paralyses must be associated the hysterical paralyses, inasmuch as in the majority of cases their immediate cause is a morbidly obstructed action of the will, though the spinal marrow and the sympathetic and peripheric nervous system are not without effect in producing them. That these paralyses are not grounded in a more radical disease of the parts named, is proved: first, by the remarkable alternation which frequently occurs between paralyses and the power of motion; secondly, by the effect of mental emotions upon them, since unexpected joy, fright, an impending peril, will often temporarily or permanently remove them; thirdly, by the absence of any considerable disturbance of the assimilative function of muscles that have been paralyzed by them for many years. The sexual functions, in the widest extension of the term, exercise the most important influence upon the development of hysteria in general, and, in particular, of hysterical paralysis, for which reason it is of most frequent occurrence with the female sex, and during the period of puberty; and we must probably look for its cause in the reaction of the excited condition of the sensitive fibres of the sexual organs upon the central organ. The characteristic signs of paralysis of this kind are: 1. The coincidence of the actual paralysis with anæsthesia of the skin, muscles, and bones; 2. The frequent transition, as the case proceeds, from anæsthesia to hyperæsthesia, and from a low to a high degree of motor irritability; 3. The insignificance of the operating cause compared with the frequently serious nature of the effects.

Except in cases in which the hysterical is united with peripheric paralysis, the electro-muscular contractility of the muscles, whose motions are not under the command of the will, is perfectly preserved, although their sensibility is lessened, or entirely gone.

CASE 13.—Miss Von S——, twenty-six years old, had repeatedly suffered from paralysis of one or the other arm or leg, which was generally quickly removed by the application of the induced current. In September, 1866, she was seized with a paralysis of both legs, and at the same time with a disagreeable sensation of swimming in both eyes, effects which on this occasion were so severe that the patient, on my first visit, November 28, 1866, could not rise from her couch or lift her leg. When lying on her back, she could not move either leg, more particularly the left, from its position on the bed. The movements of the left ankle and toes were limited; the outer side of the upper part of the left thigh was insensible to the touch, or when pricked with a pin. The electro-muscular contractility of all the muscles of both legs, when subjected to a direct or indirect irritation, perfectly normal, but the sensibility of the skin over the left M. vastus externus, and that of the muscle itself, so entirely extinct, that the addition of a moist and dry conductor (the latter the wire-brush) to a current of maximum force, applied one minute, was not felt. However, the patient, after the induction apparatus had been applied ten times, could walk a few steps in her room, and notwithstanding the continuance of the swimming sensation, she could stand when her eyes were closed, without the least wavering. The anæsthesia passed away very slowly; its domain was confined within narrower and narrower limits from above downward; but it was not entirely removed till after seventy sittings. As the swimming sensation still continued in both eyes, particularly in the left, and for the most part occasioned the patient's uncertainty of step, and as she was fatigued by a few minutes' walking, the use of the ordinary bath was recommended.

As respects the prognosis of hysterical paralyses, with a view to curative processes in general, and to the use, in particular, of faradization, no fixed data, as the extensive practice of Duchenne shows, can be given; for many paralyses, and those apparently of the most severe character, disappear with astonishing quickness under the influence of electricity, while others, frequently seeming to be very light cases, defy this as well as every other remedial agent. It is the paraplegic form of hysterical paralysis, in which electricity has shown the least favorable results. But, in general terms, half the cases of hysterical paralysis which were submitted to Duchenne—and they were for the most part cases in which the most diverse means of cure had been in vain employed—were successfully treated by him through the aid of electricity.

We extract from Duchenne's work[1] the following case:

"Marie Picard, forty-two years old, perfectly healthy till her thirty-eighth year, was seized, in consequence of long-continued anxiety of mind, with an hysterical attack, which began with an extension and stiffening of the toes, upon which convulsions, loss of consciousness, and finally a sleep, lasting three hours, followed; she woke from her sleep feel-

[1] L. c., p. 382.

ing perfectly well. During the first five or six months ensuing, similar attacks occurred three or four times daily; they then became less frequent, and, during the last years, intervals of four or five months intervened. About a year and a half preceding the examination of her case, she was affected with pains in the loins, itching, difficulty of evacuation, and paralysis of the bladder. Later, her arms became heavy; their power of motion was enfeebled. The paralysis of the arms lasted from five to six months; was more thorough on the left than on the right side, and on the left side was united also with a complete anæsthesia. During the past ten months, the movement of the arms was again unrestrained; during the last five months the paralysis also of the legs had improved, until, without any known incidental cause, two months prior to her admission into the "Charité" Hospital, the weakness in the legs again sensibly increased. The last hysterical attack had occurred fourteen days before. At the time of her admission, the following symptoms were manifested: some agitation of mind, but without pains in the head; weakness of sight in the left eye; diminution of the sensibility of the left conjunctiva, the skin of the left half of the face and the left hand; perfect insensibility of the left half of the body, with loss of the senses of smell and taste, and enfeebled hearing on the same side; anæsthesia, which, apparently affecting only the skin, extended exactly to the middle-line; muscular power in the left, upper extremity somewhat lessened; weakness in the left, and complete paralysis in the right lower extremities. The patient had kept her bed for five months; the application, twice repeated, of the actual cautery, and frequent vesication, had had no effect. Duchenne faradized the skin of the upper and lower extremities a single time, and after a few minutes the patient was able to walk about with ease. Duchenne had just before faradized the muscles, whose electro-muscular contractility was perfectly preserved, but without producing any improvement. On the next day, the sensibility was, in almost all parts, normal, perhaps a little lowered on the left side; the power of motion was unchecked, and five days after the patient left the hospital cured."

On the other hand, in the following case, the treatment of Duchenne was without results, though in the end the restoration of the patient's health came of itself:

A young girl, in consequence of a fright, had been paralyzed, a year before, in the lower extremities, and at the time had been treated by very severe remedial agents, including moxas. Duchenne found the electro-muscular contractility of the paralyzed muscles perfectly preserved; but the sensibility of the skin and muscles was lowered so much, that the highest degree of electric excitement did not produce the least effect. Duchenne undertook the cure of this case of hysterical paralysis with great confidence, and conducted it in the same manner as the preceding case; but found himself compelled, after thirty sittings, which were followed by no result, except, at the most, a slight improvement in the sensibility of the skin, to give up his efforts. Suddenly, however, after the electric treatment had been for some time discontinued, nothing in the mean time having been attempted, the paralysis disappeared, and the patient was perfectly restored.

Benedikt[1] describes the following case of hysterical paralysis, which attacked a person hysterically disposed on occasion of a wound received:

"P. M., a woman of the laboring class, thirty years old, who had led a toilsome, sorrowful life, five months before the examination of her case, was struck on the elbow with a piece of wood. For three weeks she was afflicted with cramps, but experienced no pains; then suddenly her whole arm, including the shoulder, was paralyzed. On her appearance at the clinic (May 4th), the patient, who was much de-

[1] Beobachtungen über Hysterie. Zeitschrift für pract. Heilkunde. Wien, 1861.

bilitated, experienced an exceedingly acute sensation of pain in the sound arm and in the upper part of the wounded one. In the upper part of this arm, when touched, the patient felt only a dull sensation, and in the forearm and hand none at all; nor could any sensation be excited by passive movements, or by electric contractions in the elbow, carpus, and phalangeal bones. The electro-muscular contractility of the paralyzed muscles was full; subjected to the spinal-nerve current, the motor irritability of the medianus was lowered, that of the radialis and ulnaris about normal; the sensibility of the nerve-trunks was increased; the hand exhibited a passive flexibility. By means of galvanization, some power of motion was restored to the fingers and wrist in six weeks; as, however, on the application of the spinal marrow, plexus, and nerve currents, the sensitive and motor irritability increased so constantly that a vigorous galvanic treatment became impossible; and as the faradization of the skin was of very transitory service, about the middle of June, galvanization—the patient being under the influence of chloroform—was performed. Immediately after the first sitting, the power of motion in the fingers and the wrist was fully normal, pronation and supination possible. After repeated applications, all the movements were restored by means of faradization in a few sittings, a series of them on each occasion. After the twentieth application, sensibility to passive movements was again revived, without, however, the power to feel electric contractions, or any improvement in the sensibility of the skin of the hand and forearm; on the other hand, the electro-muscular contractility was, to a considerable degree, restored. In the case of this patient, an interesting effect was manifested, which indicates a participation of the vaso-motor nerves, for on those parts of the forearm where electricity had been applied, and in particular the process of faradizing, scorbutic spots appeared."

We have in this case a peripheric united with an hysterical paralysis; hence the mixed nature of the symptoms—a heightened sensibility, corresponding to the usual course of hysterical paralyses, joined to an extinction of electro-muscular contractility in the paralyzed muscles.

II. SPINAL PARALYSES.

By spinal paralyses we understand such as proceed from the spinal marrow, such as are a result either of an injury done to the independent motor agency of the spinal marrow or to an interruption of its conducting power. Paralyses of the first kind are occasioned by fractures of the bones constituting the vertebral column, accompanied with injury to the spinal marrow, also by apoplexies of the spinal marrow, by myelitis, by tabetic processes, etc. Paralyses of the second kind are occasioned by pressure arising from bony tumors, exostoses, aneurisms, cancers, tuberculous disease of the vertebral bones, or by exudations and extravasations in the membranes of the spinal marrow.

A. *Paralyses arising from Injury to the Independent Motor Power of the Spinal Marrow.*

When all the parts that constitute the spinal marrow suffer an injury, the electro-muscular contractility and sensibility are entirely destroyed. According, of course, to the location of the injury, different groups of muscles are attacked, for all the motor and sensitive nerves that branch out from the affected spot are always paralyzed. According to the amount and depth of the injury, which may either extend quite across the spinal marrow or only affect individual cords, we find all the motor or sensitive nerves that branch out from the injured spot paralyzed either to an equal degree or in different degrees; or the one kind paralyzed while the other remains active. The loss of electro-muscular contractility and sensibility does not occur simultaneously with the injury; on the contrary, soon after the injury we find those muscles still susceptible of direct or indirect electric excitement, which do not fail to react till the fourth or fifth day, and sometimes not till the second or third week. The paralysis of the power of active motion, which in the outset is limited to the sphere of the nerves immediately affected, extends gradually to others not directly implicated in the injury—without, however, the muscles which these nerves supply losing, with their freedom of motion, their electro-muscular contractility and sensibility.

As to the prognosis of these paralyses, it is so dependent upon the degree to which the electro-muscular contractility and sensibility are depressed, that the more these two qualities have suffered, the more stubborn is the cure; while, moreover, as regards individual muscles, those whose contractility is least reduced suffer the least in their assimilative power, and upon application of electricity regain freedom of motion in a short time, whereas those whose electro-muscular contractility and sensibility are impaired, grow emaciated, and do not for a long time, if at all, become fit for use. If, in addition to the entire absence of electro-muscular contractility and sensibility, complete anæsthesia of the skin is present, the prognosis seems to be positively hopeless.

Mankopff (S. Berl. klin. Wochenschrift, 1864, No. 1) publishes the following case in point from the clinic of Professor Frerichs:

Kandal, a leather-dresser, forty-two years old, previously healthy, manifested about the middle of May, 1863, the following symptoms of a disordered condition, for which he could ascribe no other origin than his having twice saved himself from falling on a slippery sidewalk by a quick, energetic jerk of the spine. Soon after he experienced pretty severe pains between the shoulder-blades, which in a few days descended to the region of the loins, but which did not prevent him from continuing his daily work till May 29th.

Finally, however, when the pains had shot down to the points of his toes, and were accompanied with a feeling of great weakness in the legs, he was compelled to seek his bed. On the morning of May 30th the pains quite suddenly left his lower extremities, but in their place there was an entire loss of sensation and the power of movement, which was succeeded in a few days by weakness of the arms and paralysis of the bladder and rectum.

On his admission, June 6th, into the clinic of Professor Frerichs, the patient, in addition to great vital depression and corresponding fever, presented the following type of disease: The strength of his hand was below the normal point, his lower extremities were without the power of motion. While the action of the thorax was normal, the patient was unable to breathe with the abdominal muscles. The muscles of the upper and lower extremities contracted under an equal, and that a very slight, degree of electrical excitement. In the upper extremities the sensibility was a little reduced; in the lower extremities, as well as in the inferior and lateral abdominal regions, it was entirely extinct. He was sensible of pain only about the middle of the vertebral column, and this was increased by pressure upon the proc. spinosi of the lower dorsal vertebræ, which, however, were not displaced. The reflex irritability was in the lower extremities extinct, in the arms normal. In the further course of the disease, with the exception of the removal, by cupping, of the pains in the back, no change occurred in the symptoms affecting the nervous system, except that, ten days after the reception of the patient into the hospital, the electric irritability of the paralyzed muscles became utterly extinct. An ominous decline in the patient's vitality, which set in soon after his entrance, put an end to his sufferings, June 26th. The dissection revealed the existence of acute myelitis, softening of the cervical part of the medulla spinalis, and secondary neuritis at several nervous roots.

CASE 14.—G. L., a merchant, twenty years old, a man

of good health, and an experienced rider, was thrown with
such violence from an untamed horse, that he fell with great
force on his head and right shoulder, his head thus taking a
position inclined to the left shoulder. He immediately felt
an acute pain in the neck, a peculiar, warm sensation flowing
along the vertebral column, and he was paralyzed in both arms.
After he had been carried into a house, in the midst of inexpressible pains in the neck, and had been bled, the paralysis
extended, in the course of an hour, over both legs; a sensation of heavy pressure upon the breast rendered his breathing difficult; his consciousness went; and when the patient,
borne upon a stretcher, reached his home, he was, in the
most complete sense of the word, incapable of moving a single limb. The sensibility, too, of the skin and muscles had
entirely fled, so that the pricking of needles was not felt,
while the slightest touch upon the arm occasioned the
severest pains. An examination, made by Geh. R. Langenbeck and Dr. Schultz, gave a fracture of the right proc.
transversus of the fifth cervical vertebra, making the application of thirty leeches necessary. The general and local
symptoms demanded subsequently an energetic antiphlogistic treatment and frequent local bleedings; altogether, within six days, one hundred and twenty leeches had been applied to the right side of the neck. In the mean time the
paralysis had also attacked the bladder and the rectum, so
that, in addition to the administration of strong purgatives,
the catheter had to be employed two or three times daily.
About eight days after the unfortunate accident, when the
fever, with its disturbing dreams, had ceased, and the acute
pains in the affected parts were somewhat subdued, convulsive cramps attacked the legs, only excited at first by a tickling of the sole of the foot, but gradually afterward by the
lightest touch upon the leg, or even by the mere thought of
such a touch. So violent were the cramps that the thigh
was drawn up with great force against the abdomen, and the
knees near to the chin.

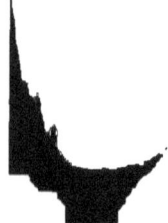

When, upon the request of the physicians above named, I visited the patient for the first time on July 19th, four weeks after his fall, he lay in his bed, utterly incapable of motion. At the seat of the wound, a considerable swelling was noticeable, which was painful to the touch, and only permitted a slight turning of the head. Respiration was superficial; evacuations and urination very inert, the former effected only by the use of strong purgatives, the latter by the introduction of the catheter; temperature of the skin, normal; appetite good; pulse small and quick. The electro-cutaneous and electro-muscular sensibility from the neck to the toes was depressed, but in different degrees at different points, so that while the arms showed some sensibility, the legs, and especially the left, reacted very feebly upon application of the electric wire-brush. Again, the buttocks had suffered an almost total, the lumbar region of the back only a partial, loss of sensibility. The electro-muscular contractility was in no one muscle wholly extinct; the right M. deltoideus, the left Mm. sacrolumbalis, longissimus dorsi and glutæi, both Mm. peronæi, the abdominal muscles and the muscles supplied by the N. radialis of both arms reacted with comparatively the most energy. The muscles, particularly of the left side, supplied by the ulnaris, reacted very badly, as did also both quadricipetes femoris, and the right glutæus maximus. The muscles of the lower part of the body were but little emaciated, while the emaciation of the lower arm and of the muscles of the hand was remarkable. Immediately after the first faradization, the patient was able to move at will the great toes of the right foot, and after the third sitting, the little finger of the right hand. Thus, from sitting to sitting, the power of free motion returned, though slowly. The patient was first able to raise the right arm; at a later period the left; the muscles of the back regained their power, and the sensibility of the skin and muscles of the left side returned simultaneously. On the other hand, the reflex movements increased in violence from week to week, and were in the night-time especially so severe that the legs were drawn with force against the upper part of the body, in consequence of which we were compelled, after the twenty-second sitting (September 3d), to pause for a period of ten days in the electrical treatment, though it had been applied as yet only about every other day, and in the outset, on account of the great excitability of the patient, with a current of little force. As, however, in this period of rest the reflex movements were rather increased than reduced in frequency and violence, and as upon a second such pause, from the 1st to the 19th of November, the same effect recurred, we continued the use of electricity without interruption, and without being troubled by these movements, and found in the end—a fact which I wish here to bring into prominence—that the strengthening of the muscles, produced by the continued application of electricity, was the most effective means of checking them. From the middle of August the phrenic muscles were from time to time irritated with a weak current, and soon the respiratory movement became more noticeable, the inspirations deeper. After the twenty-fifth sitting, the patient made his first efforts to write, and with fair success. After the fortieth sitting (November 23d), the sensibility of the skin and muscles had in great part returned, although the nates and the inner side of the left thigh were still exceedingly anaesthetic; the patient was no longer insensible to the flow of the urine, and evacuation of the faeces could be effected to a sufficient extent with the use of gentle purgative agents. The patient could move all his toes with freedom; the adduction of the upper part of the thigh was easy, the abduction was imperfectly accomplished; the legs could be extended and raised a little, although these movements were frequently hindered by movements of a reflex and emotional nature.

From the beginning of the new year (1859) the patient made more rapid progress in the use of the lower extremities. At the time of the sixtieth sitting (February 18th), he was able, when supported on both sides, to walk a few steps; the reflex movements were reduced in violence; the sensibility of the skin, especially on the left side, improved; reaction of the muscles, even of the right side, more free; respiratory power almost normal. By the employment of the iodide of potassium ointment, the pains and the swelling on the right side of the neck had been reduced, and the head could now be freely moved to the right or left. Potash-baths were now employed. After the eighty-fifth sitting, when we temporarily discontinued the electric treatment for the sake of a journey (May 19th) to the Teplitz baths, the patient could, when supported by the arm, walk about for a quarter-hour at a time, with a free and unconstrained movement of the limbs. The sensibility of the skin on the left side was normal. The extension of the fingers of the right hand with a simultaneous elevation of the wrist was not yet practicable; the left hand, too, could not yet be fully extended, nor the fingers spread apart; but the remaining movements of the hand were performed with tolerable ease, so that the patient was again able to write with freedom and to play on the pianoforte. The assimilative power of the muscles of the hand and arm had improved. The electro-muscular contractility and sensibility in the extensors of the fingers, and preëminently in the right extensor carpi radialis, and the left interossei ext. tertius and quartus, still remained depressed; a remarkable difference of condition was also noticeable between the Mm. sacrolumbales and longissimi dorsi of either side, those of the right reacting with much less power than those of the left. Evacuations occurred daily without artificial help; the urinary discharge was unobstructed, though the patient had often to strain a long time in the beginning, and a simple respiratory movement was sufficient to check it. The reflex movement still occurred at times with severity. The use of the baths at Teplitz for a period of six weeks, and the after-employment of the Waldwoll baths, in Liebenstein, added much to the patient's general strength, so that he was now able to walk great distances, but to go upstairs was still a difficult feat, and the elevation of the wrist with the simultaneous extension of the fingers was positively beyond his accomplishment. The urinary discharge was still troublesome, and the variations in the electric condition of the skin and muscles continued. Consequently, on the 5th of November, 1859, the electric treatment was again resumed, and was carried on for some time with tedious results. Many years were needed for the full restoration of the patient.

In those motor disorders which are occasioned by locomotor ataxia, and are attended with a reduction of sensibility — disorders which, as their nature indicates, can be traced to a diseased condition of the posterior columns of the spinal cord and posterior roots of the spinal nerves, extending thus only a relatively small part of the distance across the spinal marrow — the electro-muscular contractility and sensibility suffer comparatively little. In the electric condition, therefore, of the muscles of the lower extremities, no conspicuous departures from the normal standard are exhibited, even in those advanced cases in which the group of symptoms — consisting of paralysis of the ophthalmic muscles, peculiar walk of the patient, wavering motion when standing with closed eyes, sympathetic disorder of the bladder, etc., etc. — leave no room for diagnostic doubt. There are even special cases of this class, in which the electro-muscular contractility seems to be raised; they usually affect people of extraordinary excitability with the fearful excentric pains with which the disease arising from venereal excess is introduced. On the other hand, cases occur in which the irritability of the extremity which is more particularly attacked is lowered; this is made apparent by its weak contraction on application of the induction current, and by subsequent convulsions on application of the spinal marrow nerve-current.

CASE 15.—J. H., a merchant of Sommerfeld, who was much employed in a damp cellar, observed, about the beginning of December, 1866, a weakness in the toes, especially in the great toe, of both his feet, and a stiffness in their movement. The latter trouble increased so rapidly that, in consequence of it, as well as of a difficulty in raising the leg, his gait, particularly in a confined space, became unsteady. Disturbances in the urinary and intestinal discharges were added. When I visited the patient for the first time, March 23, 1867, his step was very uncertain; he trod heavily on the heels; he wavered when in a standing position, especially when his eyes were closed; he experienced a painful sensation in the lumbar region, particularly on the right side, and a feeling of tension in the calves, as well as stiffness of the fourth and fifth fingers, in particular those of the left hand. The lower extremities, from which, at an earlier stage there had been much perspiration, were cold; anæsthesia of the soles of the feet had gone so far, that the patient was insensible to pain when pricked deeply with the needle, and, when the soles were touched, gave very indefinite indications of sensibility. The reaction of the muscles, when irritated by the induction current, was normal.

CASE 16. — W., a merchant of this place, uniformly healthy up to his thirtieth year, addicted to the joys of love, perhaps to excess, was suddenly afflicted, without any known exciting cause, with an incontinence of the rectum and bladder, accompanied with constipation of a very stubborn nature, to which were soon added a feeling of weight, weakness, and cold in the left leg, an uncertain, heavy gait, and the sensation as of some foreign substance under the sole of the left foot. When the patient attempted to stand still with his eyes shut, he reeled to and fro. Erections failed him — he was impotent; but, at the same time, the urine was of normal character, and the vertebral column was in no part affected. By the repeated application of the induction current upon the N. ischiadicus and the skin of the suffering extremities, the condition of the patient was, in the course of four years, somewhat improved; the incontinence of the rectum and bladder was removed; evacuations became generally regular; the foot was warmer, the gait more settled, and the feeling as of some foreign substance under the sole of the foot was dissipated, but the ability to stand, with closed eyes without staggering about, was not restored; and this symptom, together with a sense of pressure in urinating, especially after long walks, and the inability to contract the sphincters ani et vesicæ, and, last of all, the impotence of the patient, plainly indicated the nature of the difficulty. The application of the electric current to the N. ischiadicus, or directly to the muscles of the legs, showed a reduction in the electro-muscular contractility and sensibility of the left leg as compared with the right.

To this place also belongs that species of paralysis which we frequently see occurring in children, a paralysis which is not of apoplectic origin, nor is occasioned by external injuries, but is produced by either a hyperæmia or an inflammation of the spinal cord. This is known as Infantile Spinal Paralysis.[1]

Although it is often a matter of great difficulty to indicate the lines of distinction between cases of apoplectic and of spinal paralysis in children—for the distinctions[2] given

---

[1] Heine's Paralysis infantilis spinalis; Rilliet's Paralysie essentielle; Duchenne's Paralysie atrophique graisseuse de l'enfance; W. Gull's Paralysis during Dentition.

[2] These symptomatic differences are, according to Heine, as follows: 1. In spinal paralysis, the lower extremities are paralyzed and contracted without a contemporaneous paralysis of the upper; in cerebral, the arm and leg of the same side are generally paralyzed and contracted at the same time. 2. In spinal paralysis, the functions of the mind and the senses are undisturbed;

by Heine, which we reproduce in the foot-note below, are not by any means always satisfactory; nevertheless, spinal paralysis, as occurring with children, has a stamp so peculiar to itself that the experienced practitioner, especially when he seeks the aid of an examination by electricity, can hardly be deceived.

Heine,[1] who has the great merit of having been the first to draw the attention of physicians to this form of paralysis, of so frequent occurrence in recent times, gives the following grouping of its symptoms, to the general accuracy of which the numerous cases falling within my own practice enable me to bear testimony:

It often happens that children, born with sound, healthy constitutions, at an age of from six to thirty-six months, exceptionally when older, with or without preceding indications of illness, fall suddenly sick, with exhibition of heat, congestive and irritable conditions, fever, frequent crying, and, where difficult teething is added, the further attendant effects thus induced; as well as sometimes with symptoms of the disturbed development of some exanthematic malady; or, finally, with those of a rheumatic fever. Soon after, convulsions of a light or severe form break out, and are repeated with shorter or longer intervals. In other cases, without any introductory symptoms, the disease suddenly appears with convulsions, foaming at the mouth and nose, blueness of face, etc. Often even these precursors are wanting, or show themselves in only a slight form, and

while in cerebral are exhibited a look of more or less simplicity, imperfect powers of speech, involuntary flow of saliva, weakened hearing and sight on the affected side, sparkles before the eye, strabismus, constant pains in the head. 3. In spinal paralysis, considerable atrophy and coldness of the paralyzed limbs are observable; while in cerebral these peculiarities are wanting, or exist but to a slight degree. 4. In spinal paralysis, great relaxation of the legs; in cerebral, great stiffness, and a spasmodic condition of the muscles and cords, are manifested.

[1] Beobachtungen über Lähmungszustände der untern Extremitäten und deren Behandlung · Stuttgart, 1840. Also Spinale Kinder Lahmung: Stuttgart, 1860.

paralysis comes on almost in a single night. After the malady has continued for a longer or shorter time, with greater or less violence, and with or without convulsions, a remission of the symptoms occurs; and the child, whose life was before in great danger, rests quietly, though pale and exhausted, and opens its eyes and looks around, as if it had just awakened from a deep sleep. Its parents begin to rejoice in the hope of its restoration, when they discover with alarm that their child is paralyzed, either in all its extremities or in one or both legs, or merely in a single arm or a single leg, etc.

Sometimes, the paralysis is still more extensive; in addition to the upper and lower extremities, the muscles of the back are paralyzed, so that the patient cannot sit upright, or certain lateral muscles of the body are included in the paralysis, as the sterno-cleido-mastoideus, etc., so that the head of the patient is turned to one side. The bladder and rectum generally remain untouched, or suffer but temporarily.

In the course of four to eight weeks, a reduction gradually occurs in the paralytic effects; if, in the outset, all the muscles of the extremities were paralyzed, at a later period only those of one side, or an arm and leg of different sides,[1] or the upper part of an arm or a thigh, or one only of these, or a calf and a foot, or the lower part of an arm and a hand, or the muscles of the back alone, remain paralyzed. However extensive the paralysis may have been in the beginning, in all the cases as yet observed, the little patients have still been able, in a reclining posture, to draw up the thigh a little distance, and again, though with greater difficulty, extend it. The sensibility of the paralyzed parts continues almost always normal; at the most, it is a little lowered, never raised. The temperature of the affected

---

[1] Heine, in his Monograph (*l. c.*, p. 15), says: "Cases of lumbar paralysis are in general very rare; none have fallen within my practice. In Case 18 I shall give an instance of lumbar paralysis."

members, after the first attack, soon sinks from the normal height lower and lower; the legs, particularly the thighs, become cold and bluish, and the Réaumur thermometer, held to them, falls sometimes to the 14th degree. While, as years are added, the longitudinal growth of the paralytic extremities generally proceeds with tolerable regularity, the atrophy of the affected parts, which soon follows the paralysis, increases. The trochanters, the knee-pans, and the scapula remain imperfectly developed; the tubular bones have a smaller circumference than in their normal condition; in some cases, the bones are also deficient in their longitudinal growth, and their ligaments are relaxed. Two or three years after the attack, when the little patients begin to put their paralyzed extremities again in motion, distortions arise, brought on by the use of the enfeebled muscles, such as pes varus, valgus, equinus, calcaneus paralyticus, genu recurvatum, inversum, eversum, paralyticum, etc. The physiological cause of their origin is as follows: Since all the muscles of the paralyzed parts have not lost their elasticity fully or to an equal degree, at every movement those muscles which still possess some vitality, having no opposition to overcome on the part of the antagonist muscles, undergo a gradual shrinkage; and thus, in the end, one or another, and sometimes several kinds of deformity are contracted by the same person. Thus, when the dorsal muscles are paralyzed, the continuance of a sitting posture induces lordosis; and when the lateral muscles are not equally paralyzed, scoliosis.

Upon the general health and the duration of life these paralyses exercise no detrimental influence; on the contrary, they frequently are attended with an inclination to a premature physical development, and with a certain immunity against other diseases, in particular, those of an epidemic character.

That the kind of paralysis here described belongs to the class of spinal paralysis is shown, in the absence of *post-*

mortem examinations, to which we refer by the following facts: 1. The perfect integrity of the functions of the brain. 2. The occurrence in special cases of a paralysis of the upper arm or thigh, without the contemporaneous paralysis of the lower arm and hand, or the leg and foot. 3. The quickly-following emaciation of the paralyzed parts, and the simultaneous check in growth. 4. The late origin and gradual increase of distortions in form, in contrast with the early occurrence of these in cases of cerebral paralysis. 5. The perfect correspondence of the electric condition of the paralyzed muscles to their condition in cases of spinal paralysis, as opposed to the fact that the electro-muscular contractility in the apoplectic paralysis of childhood is normal.

We find, accordingly, either that the muscles of the paralyzed parts have suffered but little as regards their electro-muscular contractility, or that some one smaller or larger member has suffered in this respect to a great degree. In the first case we are authorized to conclude that the paralysis will pass off in a comparatively short time, and may, therefore, make a favorable prognosis; while in the second case such radical disturbances in the nutritive processes are present, that even under the most hopeful conditions a treatment of long duration is frequently crowned with unsatisfactory results. If we examine such patients a short time after the paralysis has befallen them, we generally find a portion of the muscles of the paralyzed parts normal, another portion not so well off, and a third wholly without reacting power. Upon a later examination of these patients, those paralyzed muscles, whose electric contractility and sensibility were in the outset of the disease undisturbed, regain the power of active movement. Finally, the muscles which, after the lapse of a year, are still wholly deprived of electric contractility and sensibility, become utterly degenerate, and incapable of a restoration of function.

We find a very favorable case of this kind of paralysis, one, however, in which no mention is made of the electric condition of the paralyzed muscles, in Guy's Hospital Reports, vol. viii., Part I., 1852, p. 108, *et seq.*

A. E., a delicate child, with light hair and blue eyes, one year old, cut, in the course of six weeks, four upper and two lower incisor teeth, without any marked disturbance in the general health. During a subsequent period of about eight days a light fever and diarrhœa often came on. The mother observed one morning, after spending a sleepless night in watching, that her child could not raise its right arm, which hung loosely by its side. The muscles of the shoulder-blade, especially, had lost their tone. The paralysis continued, and the muscles began to dwindle in size. The child could move its fingers freely, but was not able to lift its arm. No indication of an irritation of the gums. Under an electric treatment of a very light character, a perfect cure was effected in six to eight weeks.

Of the numerous cases under this head which I myself have examined, I shall first, to prove the truth of the statements I have made, describe two of them, in which a favorable prognosis could be based upon the nearly normal electric condition of the affected muscles.

CASE 17.—Paul Jacoby, a small, lively, somewhat scrofulous boy of three years, in October, 1858, without any known occasion, became morose and inert, lost appetite, and was frequently feverish, especially toward evening. At the same time his parents observed that his head was held continually inclined to the left side, that he was loath to walk, and that in walking his left leg dragged. These indications gradually became more pronounced. The little patient could, at last, neither walk nor stand; the muscles of the lower extremities, especially of the thighs and buttocks, became thin, and felt lax and flabby. Cantharides along the spine, embrocations and baths, had so much improved the child's condition, that its head was less inclined to the left, and a slight increase in the strength of the lower extremities was observable. Nevertheless, when, at the request of Geh. Rath Romberg, I first visited the boy, April 6, 1859, six months after the beginning of the disease, he could neither stand nor raise the thigh; the movements of the tarsus and the toes were free; the head inclined to the left; the sensibility of the skin and muscles seemed normal to the touch and when pricked with a needle. An examination by electricity gave a tolerably good reaction of all the affected muscles as regards their contractility and sensibility, although a not inconsiderable difference manifested itself between the extension of the right leg and the right Mm. glutæi, and the muscles of the same name of the left side, the former reacting with much more power. The prognosis was consequently a favorable one, and in fact after the sixth sitting (April 18th), the child could already stand a few moments with the support of a chair. After the sixteenth sitting (May 23d), when led by the hand, it could walk about the room; the muscles had increased in strength and size; the head was less inclined to the left. On the twenty-sixth sitting, with which, June 1st, we ended the treatment, the little patient could walk several times up and down the room without assistance. The dragging of the left leg was no longer apparent; the muscles felt firm and elastic. A slight inclination of the head to the left was the only remaining trace of the disease, and this also disappeared upon the employment of the Sool bath at Rheme, from which the patient returned completely cured.

CASE 18.—Paul Allewelt was perfectly healthy till he was a year and a half old; in his sixteenth month he was able to walk, and had already at this time cut six teeth. About the middle of August, without known cause, he fell sick at the country-house of his parents; fever, light disorders of the stomach, and strong thirst, were manifested; on the other hand, all signs of cerebral irritation, cramps, etc., were absent. When the little patient, having been confined to his bed for eight days, rose, he could neither hold his head upright, nor sit, nor raise his arms or his feet. Within four weeks, by the use of invigorating baths, his condition was considerably improved. Paul could again hold his head straight, sit, and use his right arm and his left foot with freedom; on the other hand, the upper part of the left arm and the right thigh remained entirely paralyzed, while the movements of the left forearm and hand and the right leg and foot were perfectly free. When, at the desire of Dr. Abarbanell, Jr., I visited the patient, November 16, 1858, three months after the beginning of the malady, no essential change had taken place in his condition as above described; the left arm could not be moved from the side of the body, the M. deltoideus sinist. was lax, the right thigh could be only slightly raised, the leg could not be extended; standing and walking were impossible; the quadriceps fem. dext. and the glutæi were lax and shrunken. An examination of the electric condition of the paralyzed muscles showed the electro-muscular contractility and sensibility of the left deltoideus lowered, of the remaining muscles of the upper part of the arm normal; in the quadriceps fem. dext., however, this reduction of contractility and sensibility was found far greater; the right glutæi also reacted more poorly than the left. The temperature of the paralyzed arm and leg showed no remarkable variation. Accordingly, a favorable prognosis could be made, although a treatment of long duration, especially of the paralyzed leg, was to be anticipated. In point of fact, at the end of January—after twenty sittings—the little patient could already raise with ease and make use of the affected arm, though it was soon fatigued. From the middle of June—after forty-two sittings—he could stand upright when supported on both arms, and from the beginning of August—after fifty-four sittings—he could stand a longer time without support. After the sixty-eighth sitting—October 23d—Paul could walk, when led by the right arm, across the room, though in so doing he set down the right foot much out from the line of the body. After the seventy-fourth sitting—December 26th—whenever he fell he could rise without help, and could walk up and down the room alone, though still with uncertain steps; he set the right foot to the floor in a natural manner; he could raise the thigh freely and extend the leg with energy; the assimilative and reactive power of the muscles had improved. The few subsequent sittings served to give additional strength to the leg.

But other cases were not so fortunate in result as those above described. In many cases, where important muscles have suffered atrophy and a complete loss of electro-muscular contractility, all that can be hoped for is, at best, an improvement of condition by means of the electric irritation of the muscles still capable of reaction; in others not even so much as this can be attained.

CASE 19.—Clara S., a healthy, blooming child, from Russian Poland, when two years and a half old fell from a carriage and wounded the skin of her right thigh; the injury, however, was so insignificant that, a few days after, she was able to walk about without hinderance. About three weeks later, without known cause, a light fever appeared, which confined the child to her bed for eight days. When she was again able to rise, her parents remarked that the right leg was paralyzed. They ascribed this effect to her fall from the carriage, and hoped that with rest, invigorating washes, etc., the normal power of movement would return. Instead of this result following, the leg became more and more emaciated, grew cold, lax, and wholly useless. At the request of Geh. Rath Mitscherlish, on the 7th of September, 1858—about six months after the accident—I visited the child. The right leg was not shortened, but, in respect to temperature and assimilative power, differed very greatly from the left. The child could neither go nor stand alone, nor accomplish any movement of the leg except a slight elevation and adduction of the thigh. The knee-joint was relaxed, the leg and foot inclined outward; in a standing posture the right leg was depressed, and the vertebral column was bent somewhat to the right; when the patient lay face downward, the vertebral column was perfectly straight. As to the muscles, the Mm. sacrolumbalis and longissimus dorsi, and the glutæi of the right side acted with much less power than the homonymous ones of the left; the reaction of the M. quadriceps femoris was still worse, and it failed altogether in the extensors of the foot, the Mm. tibialis ant. and post., and the peronæus. A very unfavorable prognosis had, therefore, to be made, and, in fact, though the little patient, on December 31, 1858, after thirty-four sittings, could stand alone and could raise the thigh a little higher from the floor, and thus, when led, could walk with more ease, still not the least favorable change was observable in the leg; on the contrary, the leg and foot were blue and cold, and were covered with chilblains and deep ulcers, which, notwithstanding all applications, were not healed till the end of February. From this time, in order to use the muscles as much as possible, the patient wore on the joints of her hip, knee, and foot an adjustable apparatus adapted to the purpose, and, by the continued use of electricity—three times a-week—the use of the Waldwoll baths, and by rubbing of the skin, she improved so much that when, at the end of May, after ninety-six sittings, she went to Rehme, the reaction of the dorsal muscles, the glutæi, and the quadriceps femoris was greatly increased; these muscles had augmented in size, the temperature of the leg was higher, the walk more free and secure, and the elevation of the leg easier; the knee was still stiff, and the leg and foot bent considerably outward. The Sool baths of Rehme, which were employed for six weeks, and added to the general strength of the leg, had but little influence upon the power of motion, and thus, when, on the 4th of August, an examination was made, no observable contraction of the muscles of the leg and foot could be traced, even on the application of a strong current. When, at the end of September, after one hundred and twenty-five sittings, the patient left

Berlin, while all other movements were more developed, though the leg was thrown out less in walking, the foot much less inclined outward, and the variation of the temperature of the two legs much less marked, still the bend and turn of the foot outward or inward, or even to execute the slightest movement of the toes, was not yet practicable, and, on application of a strong current, only a very weak reaction of the affected muscles was perceptible.

CASE 20.—Richard G., a year and three-quarters old, was ill for about five months with light flushes of fever, which sometimes confined the little patient for a few days to his bed, but passed away without leaving any trace, until, a few weeks after, his parents observed that the child played with the right hand, but did not use the right arm. They soon also perceived a marked emaciation of this part, and (January 27, 1862) brought the child to me. The boy was strong and hearty; the right forearm and hand normal; the right arm somewhat emaciated; the deltoideus in a condition of complete atrophy; the ligaments were relaxed to such a degree that the humerus could be luxated in every direction. Upon direct excitement a slight reaction of the anterior part of the deltoideus was indeed still manifested, though an electric treatment, carried on for an unusually long time, had not the slightest result; and never in any similar case of great relaxation of the lig. capsulare humeri and its accessory ligaments, have I witnessed a favorable issue.

[ORGANIC INFANTILE PARALYSIS.—The subject of Infantile Paralysis is of very great importance both on account of the frequency with which cases occur, and the difficulty which attends their cure. In the generality of instances the disease is allowed to take its own course from a mistaken idea that nothing can be done toward its arrest. Several years ago, however, I pointed out the true method of treating the worst cases of the affection in question. The method consists in the use of the direct galvanic current.

In the *New York Medical Journal* for December, 1865, I reported the following cases:

CASE I.—H. J., male, aged five years, came under my care April 19th, 1865, to be treated for paralysis of both lower extremities. During the previous

SPINAL PARALYSIS OF ADULTS.

A similar paralysis of the lower extremities occurs in rare cases among adults, occasioned either by the influence of some exanthematic action, or other unknown cause. The

summer the child had suffered from whooping-cough, and when the disease was at its height motion and sensation were suddenly lost in both legs, from the hips down. Medical advice was at once obtained, and various measures were in consequence adopted, without any material benefit. Sea-bathing was then recommended, and this was faithfully persisted in for several months, with the result of restoring sensibility to both limbs, and motion to the muscles of the thighs. Since then strychnia had been administered, both by the stomach and by subcutaneous injections, without the least improvement being effected. Upon examination with the æsthesiometer I found the sensibility of both limbs tolerably good. The mercury of a delicate thermometer, the bulb of which was applied to the thigh, stood at 90°, while below the knees the temperature was but 82°. The child was able to flex, extend, rotate, abduct and adduct the thighs, and to flex and extend the legs. There was no power, however, over the feet, and upon careful examination I could not find that a single muscle situated below the knees was capable of contracting from strong induction currents. Both legs were atrophied. They were of the same size, being at the largest part six and a quarter inches in circumference.

Aside from the paralysis the child appeared to be in good health. Its appetite was good, there was no pain, and it slept well at night.

I directed that night and morning both legs should be put up to the knees in water of the temperature of 110°, and kept there for twenty minutes; that they should then be well rubbed for half an hour with a coarse towel, and the muscles kneaded for the same period; the child was also to be brought to me three times a week for faradisation.

This treatment was continued for three weeks with but little if any benefit. During this time I had continued to use very strong induction currents for fifteen minutes to each leg three times a week. The machine, which was very powerful, was put in action by a battery consisting of three Smee's cells. The current excited caused the most intense pain, but did not produce the slightest apparent contraction in any muscle. I then determined to make use of the constant current derived from a voltaic pile of one hundred pairs—and consequently possessed of great intensity. The poles were applied first to the tibialis anticus of the right leg. The instant the circuit was made the foot moved up. By continuing the experiment, I found that contractions could be induced in every muscle of both legs. I then had an arrangement constructed for making and breaking the circuit rapidly, and persevered with the treatment daily for a week. During the whole of this period, at every trial contractions were invariably induced in every muscle upon the circuit being made and broken. The warm water frictions and kneading were also continued. I now found that the temperature of the legs below the knees was 86°, and that the paralysis in such cases is, of course, subject to such modifications as the completed structure of the body would induce. Among these are the following: 1. "As the bones of the adult circumference was, at the former place of measurement, seven and one-eighth inches. The facts that the toes could now be slightly flexed and extended by voluntary efforts, and that there was some little power over the gastrocnemii muscles, assured me that the cure would ultimately be complete. In this hope I was not disappointed. Amendment continued, and on the 17th of August, when I saw the child for the last time professionally, power over all the muscles of both legs was almost completely restored. Very feeble induction currents now caused contraction. The tibialis anticus was still, however, weak; but I have no doubt that, by exercise, it, as well as all the rest, will become well nourished and strong. At this date the circumference of the legs was eight and a half inches, and the temperature 90°.

CASE II.—M. W., female, aged three years, was brought to me Dec. 6th, 1864, suffering under paralysis of the right lower extremity, the consequence of a fever with which she had been affected the previous summer. Upon examination, I found the temperature of the leg below the knee six degrees lower than that of the other limb. The circumference at the fullest part of the calf was an inch less; sensibility was obtuse, though not entirely abolished. With the exception of the flexor brevis digitorum, there was complete paralysis of all the muscles which act upon the foot and toes. There was not the slightest contraction produced in any other by strong induction currents.

Previous to my seeing the child, faradisation had been imperfectly used, and strychnia and stimulating liniments had been employed without any good effect. The opinion was expressed by several eminent physicians that a cure was impossible.

I determined to make use of very powerful induction currents, hot water, rubbing and kneading, as in the case described. I continued these measures, and by the 27th there was very considerable amendment. Faradisation had been employed at intervals of two or three days throughout the interval. The temperature of the leg had increased, and contractions of the extensor muscles of the foot and toes could be excited to a slight extent. There was no increase of voluntary power.

On the 20th of January I applied a battery to the limb, consisting of a plate of zinc and one of silver, connected by an insulated wire. The zinc plate was kept in contact with the thigh, while the silver plate was placed on the anterior part of the leg. The arrangement was worn constantly for several weeks, while the other measures were not discontinued. By the first of March there was a very decided improvement manifested in all the symptoms, and there was an undoubted increase of voluntary power. Still the contractions caused by the induced current were very feeble, and in some of the muscles, as the tibialis anticus and peronei, could not be excited at all. I therefore determined to

are fully developed, that retardation in the structural growth of the affected members, which may occur in cases of infantile spiral paralysis, has here, of course, no place. 2. In con-
make use of a more powerful continued current, and had the battery constructed which has been referred to in the history of the previous case. As soon as the poles were applied to the skin over the tibialis anticus, this muscle, and others in contact with it, contracted powerfully. The peronei also acted well under its influence. I continued to make and break the circuit over different points of the leg for fifteen minutes, every time causing strong muscular contractions. The treatment was carried on three times a week till the 1st of June, at which time voluntary power was restored to every muscle of the leg and foot. The tibialis anticus and peronei were still feeble; but, with all the others, had become responsive to induced currents. During the months of June, July, and August the child was sent to the coast, and sea-bathing was used every day. During this period no electricity was employed. It was resumed again on the 1st of September. By the 20th of October the little patient was almost well. The posterior muscles of the leg and those on the side of the foot were perfectly restored; the extensors of the toes were also quite powerful, and the peronei acted well; the tibialis anticus was the only one which was not entirely subject to the action of the will. The temperature of the leg was not appreciably below the other; it had not, however, regained its full size, though it gradually improved in this respect. The lameness, which at first was very well marked, was now scarcely perceptible, and was entirely obviated by a brace which prevented her dropping her shoulder—a habit she had acquired through the limbs being weak. Galvanism and faradisation were still continued once a week to the tibialis anticus.

Soon afterward I lost sight of the patient, in consequence of my going to Europe, and do not know what is her present condition.

CASE III.—W. S., male, aged four years, was placed under my care September 2d, 1865, with complete paralysis of the left deltoid muscle, which had persisted for over a year, and which had ensued upon an attack of measles, attended with great pain in the back. Originally the whole extremity had been paralyzed, but the other muscles recovered their contractile power in a few days. At the time I saw this child they all responded actively to induced currents except the deltoid, which was absolutely devoid of all irritability. The arm could not, therefore, be raised from the side. The muscle was shrunken, and the shoulder, in consequence, much flattened.

As I have said, induced currents failed to produce the slightest action in the muscle, and though I applied the full power of an induction apparatus of much greater strength than Duchenne's or Rhumkorf's, or any other I have ever seen used in medicine, no perceptible result followed. Upon applying the direct current of my voltaic pile, a strong contraction ensued, and similar actions followed on each formation and rupture of the circuit. This treatment was consequence of the adult's greater energy of will, impelling him to bring into action muscles which can be made to perform the duties of the paralyzed ones, as well as in consequence

tinued three times a week till the 24th. At this time slight movements could be accomplished by the exercise of the will. Induced currents were now used with the effect of causing strong contractions. Amendment continued to take place, and by the 10th of October, the muscle had acquired almost its full power. The child could raise the arm from the side with ease, and hold it in this position for half a minute. The atrophy had also nearly disappeared. The treatment was now discontinued, and gymnastic exercises recommended.

The voltaic pile used was the one figured and described on pages 98 and 99 of this treatise.

Now, this form of paralysis occurring in young children is that which Rilliet and Barthez[1] have described as the *Paralysie essentielle de l'enfance*, and to which Duchenne[2] has given the name of *Paralysie atrophique graisseuse de l'enfance*. Previous to the writings of these authors, the affection in question was not distinctly recognized as a separate disease, but was confounded with a much less serious disorder. Thus Dr. West[3] described it tolerably well in a paper on the paralysis of infants, but regarded it as a variety of disease which appeared under two other forms, one of which was congenital, and the other of subsequent origin. Both of these were not, in his opinion, of any serious character. The other, which was much more severe, occurred generally in debilitated children, and without exhibiting symptoms of any disorder of the brain. Recovery was often only partial, and though the general health sometimes became robust, the affected limb remained powerless and wasted away.

Dr. Kennedy[4] wrote two very excellent memoirs on a form of temporary paralysis, to which he had observed children to be liable. This came on very suddenly, and disappeared in a few days under appropriate treatment.

Dr. Handfield Jones[5] has recently related the details of several cases of this temporary paralysis, and a number of similar ones have been under my own charge. All recovered under the use of strychnia and iron, combined with mild faradaic currents applied to the affected limbs.

Duchenne, in the work to which reference has been made, describes the affection now under notice, with much minuteness, both as regards its symptoms and pathology. As the name he gives it indicates, he considers it to consist essentially in atrophy of the muscles, attended with fatty degeneration. That this latter is almost always the condition of the muscles, I am very sure;

---

[1] Traité clinique et pratique des Maladies de l'Enfance. Paris, 1853, t. II., p. 333.
[2] De l'Electrisation localisée, etc. Paris, 1861, p. 273.
[3] Medical Gazette, Sept. 8, 1843.
[4] "Dublin Medical Press," Sept. 29, 1841, and "Dublin Quarterly Journal of Medicine," February, 1650.
[5] Clinical Observations on Functional Nervous Disorders. Am. edition, 1867, p. 92.

of the greater firmness and resisting power of the ligaments of the adult, secondary deformities are not developed to the same extent as in the spinal paralyses of children. 3. As in at the same time, my experience leads me to the conclusion that the conversion of the muscular tissue into fat is not a necessary accompaniment. In the article from which I have quoted the foregoing cases, I stated that I was disposed to regard it as an affection in which the muscles become atrophied and lose their irritability without necessarily undergoing fatty degeneration. Further experience has confirmed me in this opinion. As a rule, however, there is no doubt of the correctness of Duchenne's view in relation to the pathology of the disease.

According to this author, the principal phenomena which characterize what I have designated organic infantile paralysis, are paralysis, atrophy, and in some muscles a more profound lesion—fatty degeneration, or substitution. The fact that Duchenne himself thus admits that this last condition is not invariable, is a serious objection, even if there were no others, to the term which he has applied to the disease. Its length and the difficulty of rendering it into ordinary English, have aided in inducing me to propose the name which stands at the head of this article.

Organic infantile paralysis is generally preceded by febrile excitement and pain in the back. This pain marks the seat of the disease of the spinal cord, to which the paralysis of the muscles is due. What the exact character of this spinal affection may be, cannot generally be determined. In one instance, when I had the opportunity of making a post-mortem examination and of inspecting the condition of the cord, I found a cicatrix partially filled with a very small clot. The paralysis in this case was situated in the left lower extremity, and had begun four years previously. The lesion existed in the lower part of the dorsal region, in the left anterior column.

In some cases, doubtless, the membranes of the cord, only, are affected, and the condition may be one of simple congestion or of inflammation, which generally appears in a chronic form. In others the substance of the cord is diseased. When the disease of the cord or its membranes wholly or in part disappears, so long a time has generally elapsed, that the contractile power of the muscles is lost, atrophy has begun, and fatty substitution is often going on. The affection is then entirely muscular. The nerves are not apparently impaired in the integrity of their functions; sensibility is not materially, if at all, lessened. There is simply mal-nutrition of the muscles, not due to any inability of the nerves to transmit impressions, but to the fact that, from central disease, the proper stimulus has not been sent through the nerves of the affected parts to the muscles, for so long a time, that the latter, having lost the power of being excited by their natural motor influence, are incapable of recovering their tone and healthy condition.

Very early in the course of the disease, the electric contractility of the lyzed ones, a striking hypertrophy of these muscles is induced.

Among other cases, the following have fallen under my observation:

ralysis for over two years. Oil-globules are seen along the course of the fibrillæ, these latter are irregular and torn, and the transverse striæ are becoming dim.

In figure 20 a still more advanced stage is shown. This cut represents a portion of the same muscle taken from the lower part. The transverse striæ have nearly disappeared, oil-globules are seen in large numbers, and fat-corpuscles are also abundant.

FIG. 20.

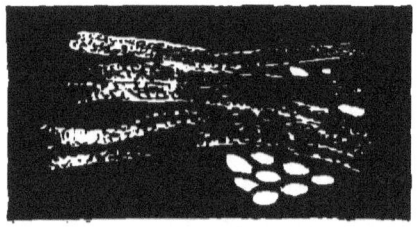

In figure 21 the progress of the disease is well shown. The lower margin of the specimen is a mass of fat-globules, and, throughout the whole, the transverse striæ are absent.

FIG. 21.

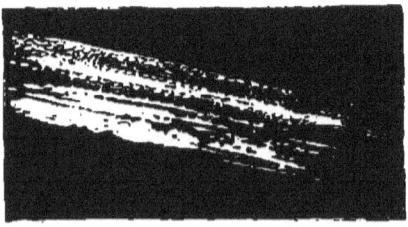

In figure 22 a portion taken from the same muscle one month after the preceding specimens were removed, is shown. The transverse striæ are entirely gone, and the muscle is a mass of oil-globules and fat-vesicles.

SPINAL PARALYSIS OF ADULTS.

CASE 21.—The two barons Von H., twin-brothers, well-built, fine, large men, uniformly healthy, in their eighteenth year, simultaneously fell sick with the measles. These, having run an apparently favorable course, were followed in

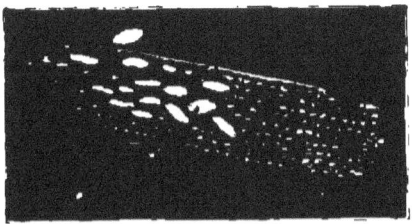

FIG. 22.

Figure 23 represents a piece of the same muscle six weeks later. It is now nothing more than a mass of connective tissue, the fat being almost entirely absorbed, no transverse or longitudinal striæ are to be perceived.

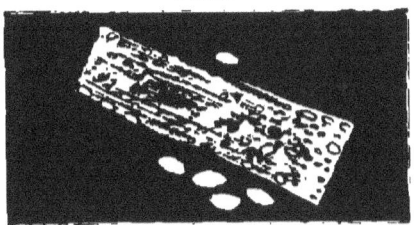

FIG. 23.

But, as I said, there is not this necessary degeneration in every case of organic infantile paralysis. In two cases, which had lasted over four years, and which were clearly due to spinal disease, I found the structure of the muscle unchanged. There were atrophy, loss of electric contractility, and reduction of temperature; but every specimen of the affected muscles that I examined showed no change from the normal character. In every other respect, the symptoms were similar to those observed in ordinary cases of the disease. Improvement was very slow, but finally every muscle, except the rectus femoris in one, and the tibialis anticus of the other, recovered, and the children were enabled to walk. The affection in both cases was confined to the left lower extremity.

I am hence led to the conclusion that fatty degeneration, though the ordinary result of organic infantile paralysis, is not an invariable consequence.

both with a paralysis of the legs, inducing a constantly increasing emaciation of those parts. When I visited them, which was not till they had reached their 24th year, the cir-

The treatment of the disease consists in the use of general and local means. Of these, the latter are of much the greater importance, especially after the spinal affection has in a manner subsided, and the disease is chiefly manifested in the paralyzed condition of certain muscles.

During the acute stage, there is nothing of so much efficiency as rest in bed. I know of no medicines which are capable of producing any specific action on the spinal cord at this time, and even after the spinal affection has become more chronic, the means mainly to be relied upon are those which are applicable to the local trouble of the muscles. It is to these, therefore, that I shall particularly ask attention.

Strychnia is useful, because it is capable of acting as a general stimulant to the nervous system, and is, moreover, a tonic to the muscles. I generally prescribe it in union with iron and phosphoric acid, according to the following formula: R. strychnia gr. 1; ferri pyrophosphatis ℨ ss, acidi phosphorici diluti ℨ ss, syrupus zingiberis ℨ iiiss. M. ft. mist

Of this a teaspoonful may be given three times a day to a child of four years old or over; half the quantity will be enough for a younger child.

The immediately local means of treatment are those which are calculated to promote the nutrition of the muscles, and restore or augment their contractile power. The first end is to be obtained by causing a greater amount of blood to flow through the diseased parts. The second is best effected by the persistent use of electricity and active and passive exercise.

Under the first head are embraced heat, frictions, and kneading.

Heat is best applied by means of hot water. A temperature of from 110° to 135° may be used, and the limb should be thoroughly immersed, and allowed to remain so for half an hour; salt may be added to the water, with the view of augmenting the stimulant effect. I think heat thus applied is more efficacious than when it is used dry. The pores of the skin are more thoroughly opened, and the tissues softened.

Frictions with a dry towel, a flesh-brush, or the hand, are also exceedingly useful. They should be practised several times in the course of the day, to the extent of reddening the skin.

Kneading the muscles affords a means of exercising them, and of increasing the amount of blood in the vessels. They should be pinched firmly between the fingers of both hands to the extent of producing some little pain. Under this operation, they often lose their flabbiness and become firm and hard. Half an hour, morning and evening, should be employed in this way. Under the second head are embraced the more effectual measures for restoring the diseased muscles to their normal condition, and electricity ranks first among them.

As generally used in this country, little or no benefit attends the use of

cumference of the thighs of each measured, respectively, 20 and 21 inches, the circumference of the calves 10 and 10½ inches; the latter dimension, if the normal relation of the

this agent. It is either applied in too weak a form, or it is employed in a manner not at all calculated to do service. I have seen the current from an induction apparatus passed through the body of the operator and brought to the affected limb by his fingers being lightly passed over the skin, and I have also witnessed what is called "galvanizing" the patient, performed by the poles of the machine being held in the hands. When the agent in question is to be used, the current should be applied in such a manner as to localize it in the affected muscles, after the manner so thoroughly elucidated by Duchenne. This requires an accurate knowledge of the anatomy of the parts concerned.

Wet sponges are to be fastened to the electrodes, the skin is to be well moistened, and the contact of the sponges with the skin is to be made over the points of origin and insertion of the paralyzed muscles, each being taken up in turn. In this way the current is made to pass through the diseased parts more effectually than it would otherwise do. To perform the operation with the necessary completeness, if an extremity is paralyzed, at least an hour is required for each séance, two or three times a week. When I employ the induced or faradaic current, I make use, generally, of Kidder's or Drescher's induction machine. I know of no other induction apparatus which is so convenient and so effectual as these. They are sufficiently powerful, are not liable to get out of order, and can readily be set in action.

But there are many cases of organic infantile paralysis in which the induced current fails altogether to cause the slightest contraction of the muscles, no matter what degree of power is employed. That these cases are not those in which the muscular tissue is entirely converted into fat, is very evident, both from microscopical examination and from the effects of the constant galvanic current in causing motion.

Before the introduction of the faradaic current into practice, the direct current was used with success by Humboldt, Aldini, Majendie, Nysten, and many others, and even after the discovery of the principle of induction, it was preferred by some practitioners. In this country, Dr. Dewees,[1] of this city, insisted upon its advantages.

Remak long contended for the superiority of the direct galvanic current over the induced or faradaic, but Duchenne, on the other hand, was equally strenuous for the latter, and appears, so far as England, France, and this country are concerned, to have carried a majority of the profession with him.

Stöhrer's zinc-carbon battery, an instrument which I described and figured in the Quarterly Journal of Psychological Medicine for July, 1868, and which is also represented on page 105 of this treatise, is the best form of constant current battery yet devised.

[1] New York Journal of Medicine, May and July, 1847.

thighs to the calves be as three to two, was accordingly four inches below the true standard. The glutei muscles on the contrary, as the patients made all locomotory

The employment of the galvanic current in cases of paralysis, in which the faradaic current is incapable of exciting contraction, is beginning to attract the notice which it deserves. Thus Dr. C. B. Radcliffe, in his article on Infantile Paralysis, published in the second volume of Reynolds's System of Medicine, says:

"There are certain forms of paralysis in which the paralyzed muscles do not react to the most powerful induced electric current, but react energetically to a galvanic current of low tension, slowly interrupted, the *petite courrent* of Remak. The diagnostic and therapeutic bearings of this fact have not yet been worked out, but so far the therapeutic promise is good. The phenomenon in question has been already observed in several very different cases; in facial palsy (first noted by Baierlacher); in certain cases of infantile paralysis, discovered by J. Netten Radcliffe, of London, and Hammond, of New York, independently of each other; in certain cases of local palsy, for example, palsy of the extensors of the forearm, and of other muscles, from lead poisoning (Bruckner and J. N. Radcliffe); in paralysis of the deltoid, not from lead (J. N. Radcliffe); in certain cases of muscular atrophy (J. N. Radcliffe); and in paralysis from traumatic injury of a nerve (Bruckner)."

It would be tedious to describe at length all the cases of infantile paralysis which I have treated with the direct galvanic current. If a contraction can be induced by it, recovery is merely a matter of time, but if no action of the paralyzed muscles can be brought about, the prognosis must be unfavorable. But even here there is hope, for in a case sent to me by my friend, Professor W. H. Van Buren, M. D., where, after the application of the current from Stöhrer's machine, no contraction could be caused in a paralyzed tibialis anticus muscle, I succeeded a few days afterward in producing very decided action by the same means.

In only four cases which have come under my notice was the disease so far advanced as to be in my opinion incurable. In twenty-seven no contractions of the paralyzed muscles could be effected by the strongest induced currents, while the direct current of feeble intensity caused strong contractions. As remarked by Dr. Radcliffe in the memoir already quoted, there appears to be no limit to the prospect of recovery if the electric contractility of the muscles is not utterly destroyed. But in most cases a long time is required to effect a cure, and even when the muscles are entirely restored, they must be reëducated to the performance of their functions. Few parents comparatively have the patience to wait and to devote the necessary time to doing their part of the work. Unless there is a reasonable assurance in regard to these points, it is better not to undertake the case. It is not, except in recent cases, a matter of days, or of weeks, but of months, and sometimes of years. But even when fatty

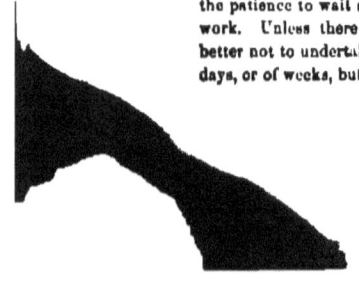

movements from the hip-joint, were developed to colossal proportions, contrasting strongly with the emaciated legs. Their walk was, therefore, very peculiar. As the degeneration is going on, the disease may be arrested by the proper use of the direct current.

Figure 24 shows the appearance of a portion of muscle as examined by the microscope, October 21st, 1860.

Fig. 24.

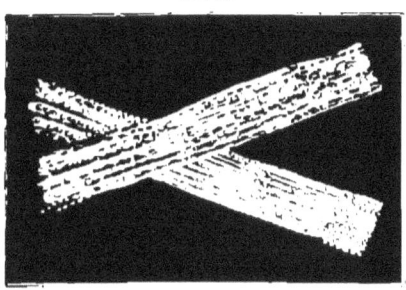

Figure 25 represents a piece of the same muscle from the same part on December 3d, six weeks after treatment. In the first, oil-globules are seen to have displaced the muscular tissue to a great extent; the transverse striæ have disappeared entirely from some parts, and are faintly seen even where they are present. In the second, the quantity of fat is perceived to be very much lessened, and the striæ are very much more numerous and distinct. This case, which was one of paralysis of the left leg and foot, entirely recovered.

Fig. 25.

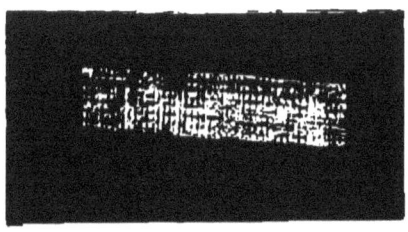

After the power of the will is to some extent restored over the muscles, the induced current may be used with more advantage than the direct.

legs could only be used as stilts, at every step of the right or left foot there occurred a rotary movement, from behind forward, of the right or left thigh, which communicated itself to the whole body, causing it to turn at every step toward the one or the other side. The extensor power of the leg was very limited; the dorsal flexion of the foot and the extension of the toes were not in the power of the patients, and but a slight adduction of the toes possible; the patients trod upon the outer borders of the feet, and in the Mm. tibiales, consequently, contorted forms were exhibited. The adductors of the thigh, as well as the muscles of the foot, were normally developed; on the other hand, the extensors of the knee-joint, and all the muscles of the leg, had suffered greatly in respect of assimilative power. The sensibility of the skin and muscles was perfectly preserved. The electromuscular contractility was reduced in the quadriceps femoris, and altogether wanting in the Mm. peronæi, the extensores digit. comm., the gastrocnemii, etc., but the adductors of the knee-joint and the toes showed a weak reaction. The rare occurrence of an affection of this kind as the result of measles, together with the simultaneousness of its appearance in the twins, who had, up to that time, enjoyed perfect health, gives good ground for the presumption of a fundamental anatomical predisposition to the disease. An electric and tonic gymnastic treatment, continued for a year, had no perceptible effect. At the present time, both the twins are incapacitated for any forward movement.

The intensity of the current generated by the instruments I have described, is very great. They should not, therefore, be applied to any part of the body to which the fifth pair of nerves is distributed, as the retina may be injuriously excited and even blindness be produced. The induced current has no such effect.

Along with the galvanism, passive motions of the joints should be made, and the child should be encouraged to direct the will to the affected muscles as often and as powerfully as possible.—W. A. H.]

B. *Paralysis caused by Interruption in the Conducting Power of the Spinal Cord.*

If the spinal cord is subject to a considerable pressure, produced by exostoses or periostoses, or by a gradually-forming curvature of the spine (as in Pott's disease), or by an affection of the fibrous and serous tissues, the electro-muscular contractility remains intact, notwithstanding the paralysis, and the affected muscles suffer but little in assimilative power. Of these paraplegias, there is a second and highly important diagnostic criterion — namely, the reflex movements, which occur in the paralyzed extremities whenever the lower part of the spinal cord is subjected to pressure or the skin is irritated, and sometimes through the influence of cold, etc.

Duchenne[1] gives the following case, falling under this head, with an accompanying dissection and report:

Pierre Bros, twenty-one years old, a robust, brawny water-carrier, experienced pains which centred in the lower part of the back, and radiated up to and embraced the lower ribs, preventing him from stooping. In the beginning of January, 1860, these were followed by weakness in the legs, and a staggering gait. On the 16th of February he was admitted into the Hospital Lariboisière. Both legs, and the trunk below the tenth rib, as well as the rectum and bladder, were deprived of all motor power and sensibility. The prick of a needle and cold were alike unfelt; both, however, as well as lying on the back, excited reflex movements, which the patient distinctly felt. He experienced also a sensation like that produced by the crawling of an insect. The proc. spin. of the sixth vertebra was evidently sprung outward, and was painful to the touch. Appetite, digestion, respiration, normal; both arms retaining their muscular power; the patient in good spirits. The only occasion of the attack was, as far as Bros was aware, the unusual exertions required

[1] *L. c.*, p. 253.

for the accomplishment of his regular work during the short winter days. On the sound leg and on both trochanters gangrenous spots appeared, which rapidly increased in size. The patient failed visibly; a nocturnal fever set in, followed by necrosis of the femur, and the swelling of the lower extremities; the paralysis extended up to the seventh rib, and on the 12th of April death ensued. Duchenne had satisfied himself that the muscles of the paralyzed extremities retained their electric irritability, and inferred from this the integrity of the spinal cord.

The dissection gave the following results: The vertebræ, when laid bare, presented to the touch a soft, fluctuating surface; in cutting through the ligt. vertebrale ant., an accumulation of purulent matter was found; the organization of the sixth and seventh dorsal vertebræ was for the most part destroyed; the adjacent ones, from the third to the tenth dorsal vertebra, were superficially disorganized; the proc. spin. of the sixth dorsal vertebra formed a sudden projection from the line. After removal of the posterior arches of the vertebræ, the dura mater and the cellular tissue were found red, flocky, and swollen. The spinal cord presented to the naked eye no perceptible alteration; its consistency was unmodified.

Case 22.—Ch. K., a woman of twenty-eight years, who had been for the last ten years the mistress of an old, impotent soldier, had experienced at times, in the course of several years, shooting pains in the legs, which frequently changed their place. For a year past reflex movements now and then occurred, which, when the patient lay on her back, shook her entire body, and, if she happened to be on her feet, jerked up the one or the other leg, and thus rendered walking unsafe. In September, 1866, a remarkable degree of weakness was felt in both legs; the pains became more persistent and rending. In November the weakness increased; the patient staggered in her walk, was apt to turn her ankle, most frequently the right one, and often fell.

After an injudicious application of cold bandages to the body, which excited no transpirations, there ensued a complete paralysis of both the lower extremities, as well as a paralysis of the bladder and the rectum, and a cutaneous and muscular anæsthesia of so intense a degree, that the patient did not feel the prick of a needle, and could give no account of the position of her legs. Upon the internal use of strychnine, the patient was, by the end of December, so far improved as to be able to extend the muscles of the thighs a little, and sometimes to feel the passage of urine. The menses were regular, and remained thus during the period of the disease.

When, at the request of Dr. O. Steinrück, I visited the patient, February 5, 1867, the evidences of paralysis were still all present; the patient could not move either the thighs, the legs, or the feet; the anæsthesia reached even to the navel, and was more intense on the right side than on the left. When the patient, held up on both sides, attempted to stand, her legs were so utterly incapable of giving support that they sank from under her, her feet slipping to the right and left; when lying on her back, her feet fell outward. The electro-muscular contractility of the paralyzed muscles, when directly or indirectly irritated, was found but little modified; on the right side, in consequence, probably, of the greater reflex irritability of this leg, it was even a little raised, so that the contractions, especially upon irritation of the right plexus cruralis, were somewhat convulsive, causing the leg to be thrown up. Tearing pains also were felt in the legs, accompanied in the left N. ulnaris with a dull sensation. The case thus presented was undoubtedly that of a slowly-progressing gray degeneration of the posterior roots of the spinal nerves, which had gone on for several years, united with an active exudation of serum, which, by inducing a pressure on the spinal cord, brought on the paralytic effects.

I employed the secondary induction-current and wet sponges to excite the nerves and the muscles, and the metallic brush for the excitement of the skin, and I had the satisfaction of watching the gradual improvement of the patient, as exhibited in the following stages: March 4th —eleven sittings: The patient, in a recumbent posture, could raise the extended legs a little, and could give some motion to the ankle-joint and all the toes. The distortion of the foot still remained; the urinary discharge was more frequently felt, at least in the daytime: March 23d—twenty-three sittings: The anæsthesia was very much reduced; a moderate pressure of the finger could be felt on every part except the soles of the feet, better in the thigh than in the leg, and better on the left side than on the right; the prick of a needle could be felt even in the soles of the feet, but not in the toes, and better also in the left than in the right foot. The heel could be raised four inches above the level. April 24th—thirty-nine sittings: The first attempts to walk were made, with success; the ankles, however, especially the right one, still frequently turned; the walk was like that of a tabetic invalid, the legs being kept wide apart. The prick of a needle in the toes of the left foot was very easily located. The electro-muscular contractility of the right leg was not heightened; reflex convulsive movements seldom occurred. May 24th—fifty sittings: The patient could go up and down her room without support, but, in turning, still displayed great insecurity of movement, especially in the use of the right foot, upon the heel of which she always first raised herself in the act of walking. The excentric pains in the legs and the ulnaris were entirely gone; fœcal and urinary discharges were normal. From this time the improvement of the patient progressed rapidly. About the middle of June she could walk for half an hour at a time in her garden, with only brief intervals of rest. The sensation of touch was felt on the toes of the right foot with considerable distinctness; not so well on those of the left. She had still the same peculiar waddle, and, when standing with closed eyes, exhibited an unsteady motion; in her treatment, therefore, the employment of the constant current was continued.

III. PARALYSIS OF THE SYMPATHETIC.

Since the discovery by Claude Bernard of the dependence of the arterial walls, as regards their vital tone, upon the sympathetic, and the success of this anatomist in showing experimentally that the section of the sympathetic effects a relaxation of the muscular fibres of the arteries; since, in the next place, within the most recent times, the anatomical and physiological relations of the vaso-motor nerves, their central origin and peripheric distribution,[1] and the effects of the irritation and section of them have been determined by Schiff, Budge, Ludwig, and others; since, finally, it has been shown by the accordant investigations of Bernard and Schiff, that the vaso-motor nerves of the extremities proceed collectively from the ganglia of the terminal branches of the sympathetic,—we are in a position to speak understandingly of the paralysis of this nerve and of the physiological conditions thus induced. The fact, however, of the distribution of the sympathetic nerves over the intestines,—into which they enter, partly in company with the blood-vessels, partly by themselves,—places it beyond the possibility of doubt that they exercise an important influence upon the functions of nutrition and excretion, which are independent of the consciousness and the will. That, therefore, the paralysis of the sympathetic may be accompanied with various disorders in these functions also, is very evident, though the strict physiological proofs are as yet wanting.

[1] The proof adduced by Claude Bernard (*Gaz. Hebd.*, 1852, No. 37), and by Schiff (in the same number), to show that the sympathetic fibres take their departure from the anterior roots of the spinal cord, explains the contemporaneous occurrence of disturbances of nutrition and the power of motion, which we so frequently meet with in cases of paralysis.

Disturbances in the vaso-motor nerves of the skin give rise to diseased modifications of this organ, such as appear in cases of herpes zoster and uticaria.[1] Primary arterial convulsions, and the consequent diminished supply of arterial blood, produce anæsthesia of the skin and secondary motory disturbances.[2] The direct participation of the sympathetic in apoplectic paralysis begets, in consequence of the enlargement of the blood-vessels, an increase of temperature, as shown in Case 1, page 162, of this work.

Continued disturbances of the nervous cords, with interruption of their conductive power, affect, at the same time, the vaso-motor nerves, and induce paleness, blueness, and gangrenous conditions, effects which we so frequently meet as the result of peripheric paralysis. A long-continued pressure, also, affecting the sympathetic, and especially its superior cervical ganglion, seems to have the power of exciting secondary disturbances in the power of motion, although we are not yet able to explain physiologically the manner of their origination; but, for the substantiation of this assertion, we may cite with confidence a case which occurred in the ophthalmic clinic of Von Graefe, in which a patient sufferring with a catarrhal inflammation of the eyes, subsequent upon a simple swelling of the sub-maxillary lymphatic glands, was attacked with, successively, a disturbance of the power of accommodation of the eye of the corresponding side, and a paralysis of the soft part of the palate.

To this division of our subject that species of paralysis also seems to belong which follows diphtheritis. Remak has not hesitated to connect paralytic attacks of this kind with the sympathetic; and this origination of them explains the fact that they often break out in places which are widely

---

[1] V. A. Eulenberg-Ueber Cutane Angioneurosen; Berl. klin. Wochenschift, 1867, Nos. 18, 19.
[2] V. Nothnagel-Ueber vasomotorische Neurosen. Deutsches Archiv. für klin. Medicin. Bd. ii., Heft ii.; p. 175, et seq., and p. 155 of this work, Case 2.

removed from the primary seat of the disease, as well as the fact that they sometimes follow the lightest cases of diphtheritic inflammation of the neck, and yet never succeed the severest of such cases.

As to the electric condition of the muscles affected by the paralysis that follows diphtheritis, in numerous cases which I have had the opportunity to examine, it is perfectly normal, and the prognosis, so far as concerns the paralysis, favorable. The application of the electric current always greatly accelerates the cure, and the electrization of the phrenicus will often rekindle the flickering spark of life.

Case 23.—Leopold Schmidt, in November, 1863, when ten years old, had passed through a light attack of diphtheritis, by which the tonsils, especially the left one, the uvula, and the gums of the left side, were affected, and which, under the internal employment of the chlorate of potash, with exclusion of all external applications, ran its course within eight days, without much exhausting the patient. But, about eight weeks afterward, disturbance in the accommodation of left eye returned, followed by paralysis of the soft part of the palate, with its accompanying symptoms of thick, muffled speech, regurgitation of fluids, etc. When (January 15, 1864, four weeks later) I first saw the little patient, the symptoms of paralysis of the velum had not reached the more violent stage. In uttering the letter "A," the left side of the velum remained unmoved, while the right was somewhat raised; the disturbance of the accommodation of the left eye had already begun to subside; a pressure on the left side behind the angle of the under-jaw occasioned sharp pain. Upon the second sitting, January 18th, a remarkable improvement appeared; and on the 25th of the same month, after seven sittings, the paralysis was fully subdued.

Case 24.—Richard K., seven years old, was attacked, January 11, 1861, with a diphtheritic inflammation of the throat, which by the 14th had increased so much in intensity that the left tonsil, which was much swollen, was covered with a foul, yellowish exudation, penetrating into the parenchyma, and the left side of the uvula was coated with a whitish substance. After treatment with the chlorate of potash and local cauterizations, the symptoms were so far subdued that on the tenth day the violent fever had disappeared, the exudations were checked, and the tonsils showed a wrinkled surface. The child slept well, ate little, but with good appetite, and seemed only to need a suitable dietetic regimen to regain his strength. But about ten days subsequently, a paralysis of the right soft palate set in, followed, in a few days, by strabismus convergens (more marked in the right eye than in the left), and at last by a weakness of both legs, which increased daily. At the same time, his general health deteriorated rapidly; his sleep became disturbed, respiration weak, expectorations thick and hard, and attacks of choking frequently threatened the life of the little patient. On the 4th of October, at the request of Dr. Abarbanell, Jr., I faradized the N. vagus and phrenicus, with evident good results; and after the third sitting, October 8th, all danger in this quarter seemed to be driven off. On the other hand, the paralytic effects now appeared in the arms, and with greater and daily increasing intensity in the legs, so that at last the boy could not move them. The electro-muscular contractility and sensibility were not lowered in any one of the paralyzed extremities; the sensibility of the patient, who was much emaciated, was so great that only a feeble current could be applied, and that but two or three times a week; and the treatment had consequently to be continued for nearly six weeks before the first attempts to walk could be made.

There is also another species of paralysis in which the sympathetic seems to be concerned—that species, namely, which is often induced by chlorotic and anæmic affections, and the origination of which is sought in the irritating action of impure blood. With this the hysterical form of paralysis should also be associated, although the peculiar disturbances of the sensibility which characterize it are in the former always absent, in which, on the contrary, as in the paralysis which follows on diphtheritis, the electric conditions of the paralyzed muscles suffer no remarkable variation from the normal state.

CASE 25.—Mrs. H., thirty-nine years old, had had in her sixteenth year a single slight menstrual discharge, married at twenty-five, but did not conceive, and in the fourteen years of her married life experienced only three or four times some weak traces of menstruation; on the other hand, she was continually subject to the fluor albus. An examination made by a competent person discovered the uterus rudimentary. Mrs. H. had, besides, suffered with a cough, accompanied by expectoration, and, seven years previously, with a light attack of hæmoptysis, and, finally, in November, 1865, with an iritis serosa of the right eye. About the middle of June, 1866, there occurred, without any premonitory signs, a severe hæmorrhagia pulmonum, from which, by the use of waters highly impregnated with salt, and of milk, at her country-house, the patient fully recovered. Having gone back to the city, Mrs. H., on returning from a short walk, on a fine, warm day, as she reached the last step of the second flight leading to her rooms, was suddenly attacked, immediately before her door, with a feeling of paralysis in both legs, and was unable to enter. Then, on the request of Prof. Traube and Dr. Schlochauer, I visited the patient, October 5, 1866; she was unable to make any movement with the thighs, legs, or feet, nor could she without help rise in her bed, or turn from one side to the other; the bladder and the rectum were not affected. There was no anæsthesia; the electro-muscular contractility and sensibility of all the paralyzed muscles were preserved, though those of the right side, when irritated by the induction current, reacted somewhat better than those of the left. By a few minutes' application of the induction current, the patient was at once enabled to make a slight abduction of the right leg. After the fifth sitting (October 10th), abduction was easier, the quadriceps femoris of either side could be extended, and the ankle-joint worked a little. On the twelfth sitting (October 18th), the patient could raise herself up in her bed, and, when lying on her back, could at times raise the extended leg from one to two inches, the right leg with more ease than the left. On the twentieth sitting (October 25th), the leg could be adducted and abducted, the extended thigh could be raised four or five inches, and the toes moved; the flexion of the thigh was readily executed. From this time the recovery of the patient progressed rapidly. After the twenty-sixth sitting (November 2d), the patient could stand almost half a minute without support, and, when led by the hand, made some attempts to walk. On November 8th, she could walk without aid across her room, and thus her improvement continued uninterruptedly till on the 17th of November the treatment was concluded with the thirty-fourth sitting. The patient could now walk up and down her room for a considerable time, but had still a feeling of weight, weakness, and tension in the left leg, which, however, under good nursing, gradually ceased.

Whether or not it be a fact that an affection of the sympathetic is the cause of progressive muscular atrophy, we must, for the present assume the affirmative view. The deficient nutrition of the muscles, which so frequently presents itself as the first symptom of this disease, the occurrence of the contractions[1] which Remak discovered on application of the constant current to the sympathetic and their undoubtedly favorable therapeutic effect in many cases, as well as the seemingly unaccountable wasting of particular muscles, supplied with various nerves, while others, supplied with the sympathetic, remain sound; all these considerations make this view not improbable. Schneevogt (*Niederlandsch. Lancet*, 1854, Nos. 3 and 4, p. 218) has even discovered by a *post-mortem* examination, in a case of mus-

---

[1] *V.* p. 168.

cular atrophy, a fatty degeneration of the sympathetic and its ganglion. Nevertheless we shall not treat of this disease, till we come to the subject of muscular paralysis, because, in the first place, in the present part of this work we are concerned simply with diagnosis, the criteria of which can only be obtained from an examination of the electric condition of the muscles attacked, and, in the second place, because a diseased condition of the muscular tissue has been proven in every case that has fallen under dissection, while in many of them, even under the most careful anatomical examination, no changes in the nervous system could be discovered.

We must here make mention of still another disease, which, as Remak has pointed out, is frequently associated with progressive muscular atrophy—the arthritis nodosa - a disease in which the swellings of the joints are often combined with the atrophy of the Mm. interossei. In this malady, particularly in its first febrile stage, the diplegic contractions, on irritation of the sympathetic in the manner above given, are excited in their most pronounced form. The therapeutic employment of them ought to result in a reduction of the pain and of the swelling at the joints, and in an increase of the volume of the muscles, as well as in diminished rapidity of the pulse in connection with a contemporaneous rise of temperature.[1]

I extract from the treatise of Dr. Drissen the following case, which I also, in association with him, had an opportunity of watching:

G. T., a brazier, twenty-four years old, reports that, when in bivouac a short time before the battle of Königgrätz, he was so chilled, that on the following day he could not move his arm. By the friction and passive movement of the suffering part this lameness was driven off, though from that time there were frequent returns of a feeling of stiffness in the left arm, which, however, was dissipated by

[1] *V.* Remak, Application du Courant Constant, etc., p. 81.

active movement of the limb. But the condition of the
patient had, a few weeks before the examination of the case,
grown much worse, and when, on the 12th of October, 1866,
he came under the treatment of Dr. Drissen, he exhibited the
following symptoms of disease: He could not raise the right
arm, and could raise the left only with great difficulty, and
with the experience of pains in the deltoideus, which felt
harder than was natural; he could not dress himself or shut
the door. The first and second phalangeal joints of the right
fore-finger were much swollen, and their movements were
reduced to a minimum; the same joints of the other fingers
also, with the exception of the little finger, were attacked,
though in slighter degree; the Mm. interossei were emaciated. On the left side about the same effects were presented,
though in a less marked form. The sympathetic being irritated by the application of the positive pole to the ganglion
cervicale sup. on the one hand, and of the negative pole to
the sixth dorsal vertebra on the other, diplegic contractions
occurred with evidently good results, especially in the first
days of the treatment. After fourteen days these reflex contractions could no longer be excited; on one occasion only, when
the patient, in consequence of a cold, had relapsed a little,
were slight indications of them traceable. Notwithstanding, however, the marked improvement of the patient in the
beginning, the treatment, which was directed exclusively
upon the sympathetic, had to be continued for almost three
months before the last remains of the affection were effaced;
the swelling of the right fore-finger opposed the most stubborn resistance to the course of the cure.

IV. NERVOUS PARALYSIS.

By nervous paralysis we understand that form of paralysis which is occasioned by any influences that affect
injuriously the conducting power of the nerves, at any point

in their course from the central organ to the muscles. Etiologically, paralyses of this kind are a result either of traumatic injuries, mechanical modifications, the severing of the connections by wounds, suppurations, etc., or of luxation or fracture, or of exudations (rheumatic, syphilitic, etc.), or of dislocations, aneurisms, swellings, etc., or, finally, of inflammation of or pressure on the nerves. The characteristic trait of nervous paralysis is, so far as concerns its diagnosis, the limitation of the disease to particular nervous cords or branches, in the domain of which active and reflected movements[1] are, in proportion to the intensity of the disease, restricted, while these movements remain unchecked in those regions which lie beyond the paralyzing influence. With this, generally occurs a modification of the conscious sensitive power, which varies greatly in degree, according as the sensitive nerves have suffered to a greater or less intensity or extent, sometimes being but slightly reduced, sometimes wholly lost. When the paralysis has continued to the second week, a disturbance in the electric condition of the paralyzed muscles arises, which varies in degree according to the severity of the attack, but is always associated with a depression of the electro-muscular contractile power. If the primitive fibres of a nerve are completely destroyed, the muscles with which it communicates lose their ability to contract. But the active motor power of all the muscles supplied by the nerve may be removed, without a single one

[1] A. Stech, in a brief paper published in the *Charité Annalen*, Band viii., Heft 1., has done good service in turning our attention to the importance of reflex movements as means of diagnosis in deciding the question concerning the central or peripheric origin of a paralysis. If, for example, in the case of a paralysis of an arm or a leg, in which this question presents itself, the medical attendant is able, by means of peripheric irritation, to evoke reflex movements, he then knows that the conducting power of the sensitive nerve, from its extremity to the spinal cord, is unbroken, that the central structure of the nerve within the spinal cord duly performs its function, that the contiguous motory part within the spinal cord is excitable, and that from this point back to the muscle no obstruction to the conducting power is present; that, consequently, the disease has a central origin.

having suffered in its electro-muscular contractility; from this it would seem that the disturbance in the assimilative function of the nerve has not been so thorough as to essentially injure its electric irritability. On the contrary, the active motor power of isolated muscles can be apparently preserved, while in fact this power is extinct, the movement being performed by other muscles of associated function; in such a case the diagnosis can only be determined by a local application of the electric current. Besides, the paralyzed muscles suffer more in their contractility than in their sensibility, and, again, generally regain the latter with more facility than the former.

The prognosis of nervous paralysis is dependent upon the depression of the electro-muscular contractility of the paralyzed muscles, with, however, this qualification, that the more frequently a muscle has previously suffered in its electro-muscular contractility, the less rapidly, under electric excitation, will it improve in the power of active movement.

CASE 26.—Mrs. Roy, a vigorous woman, forty-two years old, went to sleep with the outer side of her right forearm supported upon the sharp edge of a window-sill, her head resting upon the inner side of the arm. When, after the lapse of an hour, she woke, her right hand was paralyzed; the patient was unable to raise it, open it, or shut it. It was bent at a right angle to the arm; the fingers, particularly the thumb, middle finger, and forefinger, were turned inward by the superior weight of the flexors. The patient at the same time complained, as she presented herself before me—April 30, 1852, six days after the accident—of a dull sensation in the paralyzed hand and of a peculiar itching in the skin, extending along the outer side of the forearm to the thumb. She had been trying to excite the muscles of the arm by frequent rubbing, but without success. A closer examination discovered, besides the effects already mentioned, an insensibility of the skin along the outer side of the forearm and the thumb. The electro-muscular contractility of the paralyzed muscles—the extensores carpi radialis and ulnaris, the extensor digit. communis, the abductors and extensors of the thumb—was intact. In this case the twice-repeated faradization of the N. radialis and the paralyzed muscles sufficed to restore to the hand the ability for active movements. The torpid sensation lasted fourteen days longer, but was too unimportant to demand an additional application of electricity.

CASE 27.—Baron L. received in a duel a thrust on the inner side of the upper part of the right arm, at about the junction of the upper with the middle third, by which the N. ulnaris and N. cutaneus brachii med. were cut. The wound did not heal by the first intention, but formed a suppuration which discharged three inches lower down. In the course of a few weeks the patient was again able to execute the flexor movements of the hand; the sensibility of the inner side of the upper arm was restored; but the muscles supplied by the ulnaris still remained without the power of motion, and the corresponding parts of the skin were still anæsthetic. When—January 10, 1859, three years after the injury—I examined the patient, I found the following parts anæsthetic: on the inner surface, the ring-finger; on the ulnar side, the little finger completely, and the middle finger; on the dorsal surface, the little finger and the ring-finger; also the ulnar side of the hand, and, to a slight degree, the ulnar surface of the forearm. The hand was cold and emaciated; the falling away of the Mm. interossei, the opponens digit. min., and the adductor pollicis, was especially remarkable; the forearm, too, was thinner than the left. The hand had assumed a shape much like a claw; the second and third phalanges, especially of the last three fingers, could not be straightened, the fingers, particularly the last three, could not be brought near enough together to touch, and could only be separated a short distance, and the thumb could not be brought into contact with the little finger, or adducted in the least. The electro-muscular contractility and sensibility of all the muscles supplied with the ulnaris were extinct. A treatment lasting longer than a month increased the temperature, and partially restored the sensibility, but had no influence in exciting muscular activity.

CASE 28.—S., a goldsmith, the son of a tailor who had died of phthisis pulmonum, had suffered for two years with various pains in the breast, which, considered in connection with the results of a physical examination, indicated beyond doubt the development of phthisis pulmonum. Contrary to expectation, the condition of the patient gradually improved; expectoration and the sweating were lessened to such a degree that, when the results of auscultation and percussion were also taken into account, a favorable prognosis could be made. But, in January, 1853, tearing pains attacked both ears, followed by a copious discharge of matter and hardness of hearing, which ended in a complete deafness of the right and, later, of the left ear. Within about eight days after, an entire paralysis of the right N. facialis gradually came on. By repeated local bleedings, fomentations, injections, and the internal employment of antiphlogistic and, subsequently, narcotic agents, the pains were quieted and the secretion of pus lessened, but the deafness, united with a singing in the left ear, and a dull, beating sensation in the right, as well as the paralysis of the right side of the face, remained unchanged.

I visited the patient on the 12th of May, 1852, and found him a man of pale, cachectic appearance. All the muscles of the face supplied by the right N. facialis were paralyzed, the face being correspondingly distorted; the uvula, however, retained its normal direction. The tympanum was destroyed in both ears; the exterior auditory passage was contracted and filled by matter. Deafness of both ears; sensibility of the skin of the face normal on both sides; enfeebled sense of taste, joined with a sweet taste on the right half of the tongue. The direct application of the electric current upon the paralyzed muscles showed a loss of contractility and a great depression of electro-muscular sensibility. The case was accordingly a paralysis of the N. facialis in its course through the petrous bone; and, according to the investigations of Claude Bernard, the locale of the paralyzing action must have been situated above the point of exit of the chorda tympani.[1] In this case tuberculous caries of the temporal bone was the source of the malady. The treatment, which was, of course, of short duration, had no effect. The next year the patient died of phthisis pulmonum.

Case 29.—Julius Ritter, a mechanic, twenty-four years old, of weak constitution and relax muscular system, was attacked three weeks previously, in consequence of a cold, with a pain in the right temporal bone, which was followed by a trembling in the right facial muscles, ending in paralysis. To wrinkle the right half of the forehead or to close the right eye was impossible; swallowing was difficult; there was a constant trickling of tears; the right sulcus naso-labialis was closed; the face correspondingly distorted. After the patient had been treated by Dr. Abarbanell, first with antiphlogistic, then with purgative agents, he came to me, June 25, 1854, for electric treatment. So relaxed was the general muscular system of the patient, that the paralyzed half of the face scarcely exhibited a marked difference in this respect from the other; its sensibility was normal; the electro-muscular contractility and sensibility of the paralyzed muscles were not much reduced. Accordingly, both as regards the duration and the result of the treatment, the prognosis was a favorable one. In point of

---

[1] Bernard discovered (see his Leistungen auf dem Gebiete der Experimental-Physiologie von Laksch, Prager Vierteljahrschrift, 1853, Heft i, p. 180, *et seq.*) that the destruction of the chorda tympani effects a diminution in the sense of taste in that half of the tongue on which the cord is cut, while, however, the sense of touch in the affected part remains normal, and that accordingly, in cases of facial paralysis in which no reduction of the sense of taste is present, the nerve is diseased below the exit of the chorda tympani.

fact, the patient was able, July 27th, after only three sittings, to close the affected eye, and after the fifth sitting—July 29th—to wrinkle the forehead, and to eat and drink without difficulty. After the ninth sitting—August 4th—he could raise the corner of the mouth a little, and the sulcus naso-labialis began to be apparent. On August 10, 1854, after the thirteenth sitting, he was dismissed perfectly cured.

CASE 30.—The cure of a cabinet-maker, named Engelmann, was still more rapid. The patient, a man of thirty-five years, was attacked, August 10, 1854, without known cause, with a paralysis of the left side of the face, united with pricking pains in the left ear. After cupping-glasses had been applied to the nape and Russian baths had been employed a few times, the pains disappeared, but the paralytic effects remained unchanged, and on the 25th of August the patient was brought to me by Dr. Lode for electrical treatment. In this case also the forehead, on the affected side, could not be wrinkled, the lower eyelid hung down, tears flowed from the eye, the mouth was awry, and on the left side could not be opened, eating and drinking were difficult, etc., etc. The electro-muscular contractility and sensibility of the paralyzed muscles were not in the least affected. On the 26th of August, after only two sittings, the patient could wrinkle the forehead. August 29th—five sittings—he could distend the mouth a little, and close the eye, though with effort; his drink no longer flowed from his mouth. Having then to make a journey, I was compelled to discontinue the treatment; nevertheless, without further application of remedial agents, the improvement of the patient went on rapidly, so that on my return—September 17th—I found him perfectly recovered.

When electro-muscular contractility and sensibility are quite extinct, and to this condition anæsthesia of the skin is added—symptoms which in injuries of the nerves are often complicated with a loss of nervous substance—the prognosis takes a very unfavorable shape. But even in such cases we should not despair of the possibility of a cure, as the loss of substance may be repaired, and the muscles, even when, in consequence of interrupted innervation or mechanical conditions, they have for a long time lain altogether inactive, may, after the functional difficulties have been conquered and suitable nutritive conditions have been supplied, become again capable of action. In relation to the first point, Waller discovered[1] that, when the fibres of the peripheric extremity of an intersected nerve decay, a new formation of nervous fibres not only takes place at the point of intersection, but extends to the peripheric extremities. Having cut the N. vagus of a dog, twelve days after he found its peripheric extremity wholly disorganized, the nervous sheath almost entirely gone, and its contents disintegrated to a dark, granulated mass; a month later, in place of the destroyed fibres, new ones had formed—an observation which Schiff[2] has confirmed.[3] In agreement with this discovery, Duchenne found in certain cases, in which great injury to the nerves was united with a loss of substance, that the muscles which had altogether lost their contractile power, at a later period reacted under electric irritation and were functionally restored; he thence concluded that an absolute deficiency of electro-muscular irritability, though lasting for a long time, does not justify the assumption that the muscle is dead.

I shall, in this connection, reproduce the exceedingly interesting case which Duchenne publishes in his work.[4]

[1] Müller's Archiv., 1852, p. 392.
[2] Archiv. fur physiologische Heilkunde, 1852, p. 145.
[3] C. Bruch, of Basle, has pointed out (*vide* Archiv. des Vereins für gemeinschaftliche Arbeiten zur Förderung der wissenschaftlichen Heilkunde, Band ii., Heft iii., 1855, p. 409, *et seq.*) that the reunion of the parts of a divided nerve takes place in three ways. In favorable cases there is a direct concretion of the contiguous fibrous extremities; in other cases the fibres have to grow toward each other; but in the majority of cases the peripheric portion of the divided nerve wastes away, and its place is supplied by an extension of the central portion.
[4] *L. c.*, p. 252.

Albert Musset, a printer, nineteen years old, had his right hand caught, November 13, 1846, in a machine, by which the N. ulnaris, the Art. ulnaris, the tendons of the flexor sublimis and profundus, the M. palmaris brevis, etc., were so severely wounded that when, three months later, the patient left the hospital, the muscles of the hand were in a condition of complete paralysis and atrophy. The two last phalanges of all the fingers were constantly flexed, and the emaciated hand gradually assumed the form of a claw. When Duchenne first saw the unfortunate man (December 22, 1850), four years after the accident, the hand was emaciated to the bones, and on its inner surface the tendons of the flexors and the projections of the metacarpal bones were prominent. The two last phalanges of the fingers were permanently adducted, though they could be brought mechanically in the same line with the first phalanges, the articulations of which with the metacarpal bones were in a state of partial luxation. If an attempt was made to overcome this luxation, the tuberosities of the metacarpal bones, which were in a condition of hypertrophy, opposed insurmountable obstacles. If an attempt was made to straighten the fingers, the luxation was rendered complete; also the distention of the fingers and the adduction and abduction of the thumb were impossible. The forearm, which was somewhat emaciated, exhibited a straight scar, extending from above downward, and from the inside outward, and adhering to the tendons of the flexors. The flexion and extension of the wrist, the pronation and supination of the forearm could be accomplished with ordinary ease. The sensibility of the skin of the posterior half of the hand, and of the fifth finger, and upper side of the fourth, was weakened; the hand was the seat of constant pains, which were increased by every movement. Its color was a dull white; blue in the cold; its temperature, both to the feeling of the patient and to the touch, was considerably lowered; its veins were not visible. In all the muscles of the hand electro-muscular contractility was extinct; the skin of the posterior half of the upper surface of the hand, and of the little finger and the inner surface of the ring-finger, was wholly unsusceptible of electric irritation.

Duchenne, in his indefatigable zeal, did not lose courage in the presence of this seemingly hopeless case. He at once applied the electric current to the paralyzed muscles, and after only the tenth sitting—the sittings were continued, as a rule, from ten to fifteen minutes—Musset, instead of the pains which he had formerly experienced, felt in his hand a burning heat, though the fingers, as before, were affected with a painful and dull cold sensation. At the same time the nutrition of the muscles began to improve, and the depressions between the metacarpal bones to fill up; the luxation of the first phalanges diminished; the second phalanges assumed a more extended direction. At this stage, on account of the feverish condition of the patient, the treatment was remitted for three weeks. During this interval, not only was there no retrogression of the local evil, but, on the contrary, the warm feeling spread over the fingers, which now lost their dull sensation of pain. On recommencing the treatment, Duchenne united, with the faradization of the muscles, that also of the skin, using for this purpose the metallic wire-brush; the sensibility of the skin, thereupon, perceptibly increased, the veins in the back of the hand became distinct, the color of the skin normal.

The sittings being continued from day to day, the small muscles of the hand, which were not earlier noticeable, began, about the 15th of March, 1851, to develop distinctly, and the position of the index and middle fingers improved; the adduction of the first phalanges was now possible, the M. interossei reacted under electric excitement, but voluntary movements were not yet practicable. At this stage, the patient left the hospital and passed two months at large, with the intention of leaving to nature the completion of the cure. His hope, however, proved illusive; his hand did not increase in size, nor did the power of voluntary movement return; accordingly, he again had recourse to electric treatment, and from the beginning of June was subjected two or three times a week to faradization. In the outset the first phalanges of the first and second fingers assumed a position still more inclined toward the metacarpal bones; but the last two became more extended, and the active movement of the last members of the fingers, as well as the abduction and adduction of the fingers, became possible.

The improvement now progressed rapidly, so that, by the end of August, Musset could write and draw, and in February, 1852, notwithstanding an interruption of the treatment for more than a month, he could adduct the first phalanges of the index and middle fingers to a right angle with the metacarpal bones, and could fully extend the last phalanges. The position and motor power of the last two fingers had become better; the muscles of the thumb were almost perfectly developed, and were capable of all the movements; the tendons of the flexors were no longer prominent on the surface of the hand, and the muscles at the ball of the little finger were available for use. Musset now engages to transcribe manuscript; with the hand, formerly disabled, he copied for me the prize essay in which Duchenne published the report of this case.

But the most brilliant illustration of the extraordinary length of time during which muscles, that, in consequence of some mechanical obstruction, have lost their functional power, or in which this power has never been developed, can preserve their integrity, is furnished by cases of facial paralysis extant from both. In such cases the M. buccinator, which is provided with the motor roots of the trigeminus, is included in the paralysis. Here all that is necessary, in order to make it possible to move the mouth laterally, and hold it in a lateral position, is a faradization, once or twice, of the muscle named.

CASE 31.—L. H., a student, nineteen years old, was born with a paralysis of the right side of the face, which could be traced to no cause antecedent to birth. In addition to an absolute inability to perform any movement with the muscles of the right side of the face, to wrinkle the forehead, to close the eye, or to draw together the mouth, the sensation of taste was weakened in the right extremity of the tongue. In the position of the uvula there was, neither in this nor in the following case, any remarkable variation. After only the second sitting the patient was able to widen the mouth so much, that perpendicular wrinkles were formed in the cheeks. Thus a muscle which had lain dormant for nineteen years was, on a second application of the electric current, endowed with freedom of movement. The electric treatment, which was continued more than a month, and was then broken off by the departure of the patient, exercised also a decided influence upon the muscles provided with the facial nerve; thus after only six weeks the patient could whistle, wrinkle the forehead in both directions, and give energetic action to the M. levator lab. sup. alæque nasi.

CASE 32.—Margaret T., seven years old, besides being born with a paralysis of the left side of the face, was afflicted with the malformation here described: Though the left ear was present, the external auditory passage was absent, and the place of the external ear was occupied by a white fleshy prominence, of the size of a hazel-nut, provided with muscular fibres, and therefore movable, in which the proc. styloideus could be felt inclined abnormally outward. The entire left side of the face, particularly the left side of the lower jaw, was shortened; on the other hand, the left arch of the palate was broader than the right one. After only one sitting, the little patient was able to effect, by means of the M. buccinator, a lateral movement of the mouth; and in a few months, after twenty-eight sittings, all the muscles of the face were possessed of freedom of movement, though naturally, in laughing, the mouth was still considerably more drawn to the side originally sound; and in all spontaneous movements the preponderance of the muscles of the right side of the face was perceptible. In this case there was also a remarkable phenomenon presented, to which Duchenne has already drawn attention—namely, the continuous development of freedom of movement in the muscles of the left side of the face, though under neither direct nor indirect irritation did they display the least sign of reaction, a fact of which Professor Virchow, among others, was convinced. A difference in the sense of taste between the right and left sides of the tongue was not established in this case.

I have mentioned that in nervous paralysis a disturbance in the electric condition of the paralyzed muscles does not occur till the second week. I desire here to bring this fact once more into notice, in order to warn the practitioner against the prognostic errors, which easily arise, when, in view of the normal or but slightly-disordered electric condition which characterizes the first few days of such a paralysis, a favorable prognosis is made, without taking into account the fact that the disturbing action which affects the nerves has not yet extended to the muscles.

Case 33.—Carl II., a merchant, twenty-eight years of age, came to me (June 5, 1858) with a complete paralysis of the left side of the face, which he had contracted three days before, in consequence, as he believed, of a cold caught during the night. All the muscles provided with the N. facialis reacted equally well; but, after the second sitting, June 8th, the reaction was less strong; and on June 10th—that is, eight days after the beginning of the attack—it was fully extinct. From this time till the departure of the patient (July 16th), thirty-one electric sittings were had, but they were attended with only a slight result; so that, while some creases became apparent on the forehead, the eye could not be closed, nor the mouth be drawn up toward the left, or much contracted.

[NOTE.—No more interesting and valuable essay has yet been published upon injuries of the nerves, and the disorders consequent thereon, than the admirable monograph of Drs. Mitchell, Morehouse, and Keen (Gunshot Wounds and other Injuries of Nerves. Philadelphia: 1864). The student or practitioner, who desires to familiarize himself with the subject of paralysis in all its phases, cannot do so without an attentive study of this little book. Dr. Meyer does not appear to be aware of its existence. I would gladly transfer a portion of it to these pages, but it is all so much to the point that I must content myself with recommending its perusal to all who wish a full acquaintance with nervous pathology.—W. A. H.]

V. MUSCULAR PARALYSIS.

Dr. H. Friedberg, in his "Pathologie und Therapie der Muskellähmungen,"[1] has justly distinguished the paralysis of the muscles which arises from a disorder in the assimilative processes of the muscular substance, or myopathic paralysis—paralysis ex alienata musculorum nutritione—from that form of paralysis which is occasioned by an injury to the nervous centres or nervous cords, or neuropathic paralysis. In this connection, he has remarked that this disturbance in assimilative action may render a muscle incapable of obeying the will, even when the motor nerves are susceptible to the excitation emanating from the brain and spinal cord. In neuropathic paralysis the disturbed assimilative action of the muscle is the secondary cause; in myopathic it is the primary one, and therefore in the latter it appears earlier and runs a quicker course. On the other hand, in neuropathic paralysis the cessation of muscular contraction is the primary effect; in myopathic it is a secondary one. A disturbance in the nutrition of a muscle capable of inducing paralysis may be excited, according to Friedberg, by the following causes: 1. A similar disturbance in adjacent organs, communicating itself to the muscles; examples are, paralysis of the muscles covering the peritonæum, in consequence of peritonitis, paralysis of the intercostal muscles, in consequence of pleuritis, paralysis of the M. deltoideus, in consequence of inflammation of the

[1] Weimar, 1858.

shoulder-joint; 2. The effect of external force, a wound, a burn, laceration, excessive straining; 3. A sudden change of temperature; 4. Various diseases of the blood, as, for example, typhus, acute exanthemata, the action of certain poisons, as lead, disturbing the nutrition of the muscles; 5. Deficient supply of blood or repressed muscular movement, as in those nutritive disturbances in the muscles induced by diseased conditions of the vascular membranes and thrombosis, or those similar disturbances occasioned by the pressure of tumors; 6. Unknown causes, numerous cases of progressive muscular atrophy, etc.

The disturbance in the nutrition of the muscle which is effected by these various causes is, from a pathological and anatomical stand-point, always the same in essential character, namely, either a genuine inflammation of the muscle or a result of such inflammation. The structure of the muscle, abundantly supplied as it is with connective tissue which not only envelops the entire muscle, but the several muscular fibres and bundles of fibres, and through which the blood-vessels are abundantly distributed, is the seat of light inflammations, which arise sometimes from a direct influence brought to bear upon the muscle, sometimes by diffusion from contiguous tissues, and which, in consequence of the connection of the muscular integuments with the fascicles, extend more or less widely from the muscles primarily affected. The great quantity of blood-vessels with which the muscles are enriched supplies the conditions for the occurrence of one of two results: either, on the one hand, a speedy subjugation of the inflammation and a restoration of normal functions before the disorder has affected to any considerable degree the nutrition of the primitive fibres; or, on the other hand, if the inflammation be not subjugated, the formation of purulent granules, connective tissue, and fat, and the disintegration of the primitive fibres with their constituent tissues, or a fatty degeneration of them, the vessels and nerves becoming thus involved finally in the same diseased condition. The process thus described does not, however, necessarily embrace at once the entire muscle. The several fascicles of the same muscle may be affected in various degrees, some retaining their organization, others undergoing a fatty degeneration, etc. The muscular fibres may also—a result which cannot often be learned from an external examination—become deteriorated, without any appearance of atrophy in the muscle, which, in consequence of the new formation of fat or connective tissue, may seem much larger than it really is.

In harmony with this variety in the anatomical conditions of the paralyzed muscles, their reaction under the induced current is very various, every grade of electric condition being exhibited, from the normal one to that of a complete deprivation of electro-muscular contractility and sensibility—a diversity presented not simply by different muscles, but also sometimes by the various fascicles of the same muscle. By observing, however, the degree of depression in electro-muscular contractility and sensibility, we can at once determine: 1. Which muscles have primarily, and which have secondarily suffered, that is, which have been directly affected by the paralyzing influence, and which have been condemned to inactivity in consequence of a disturbance in their motor power unconnected with a condition of disease. 2. How deeply the muscles have suffered in their assimilative processes, and whether accordingly a speedy or a slow cure may be anticipated, or none at all. As regards the last contingency, even a complete loss of irritability under the induced current does not at all justify an unconditionally unfavorable prognosis, in confirmation of which I refer the reader to the experiments made by Brenner, mentioned on page 190.

CASE 34.—S., a merchant, twenty-eight years of age, had contracted, probably in consequence of the tightness of his boot, a paralysis of the M. extensor hallucis longus of the left foot, which, when the patient had drawn off his boot, prevented his raising his great toe from the floor. By the use of a strong sole, the inconvenience of this was but little lessened. The reactions of the paralyzed muscle showed only a slight loss of power, consequently the prognosis was favorable, and in fact the patient, who had come to me for treatment May 8, 1867, was able, after four sittings, to leave, May 17th, perfectly cured.

CASE 35.—Hauff, a merchant, fifty-two years old, having on a warm, spring afternoon, while working in his shirt-sleeves in his shop, exposed himself to a draught of air, was seized, toward evening, with violent, tearing pains in the right shoulder, which in the night increased in intensity, making every movement of the shoulder and the elevation of the arm impossible, and gradually spreading over the upper part of the arm, the forearm, and the hand, down to the finger-ends. Within about fourteen days, in consequence of frequent cupping about the shoulder-blade, and the employment of embrocations and Russian baths, the pains disappeared, but the power of voluntary movement in the shoulder was entirely abolished, and the muscles of the posterior region of the shoulder-blade and acromion, especially the M. deltoideus, became atrophied.

In this condition, about six weeks after the beginning of the disease, the patient, on the advice of his physician, Dr. L. Posner, applied to me for a trial of electric treatment. An examination, made May 22, 1852, gave the following results: The upper part of the right arm was wholly incapable of active movement, and lay rigid and motionless against the thorax. A limited passive movement could be made, but this was attended, especially on every attempt to raise the arm, with a severe sensation of pain. The right shoulder had lost its rotundity, the M. deltoideus being shrunken and relaxed to such a degree, that between the acromion scapulæ and the caput humeri there was an interval of about half an inch. The patient complained of an unpleasant sensation of dulness, itching and pricking in the forearm and hand, especially in the fourth and fifth fingers, causing him to seek its removal by repeatedly rubbing with the sound hand the parts thus affected. The electro-muscular contractility of the M. deltoideus was normal; the electro-muscular sensibility, however, especially of those fibres which take their rise from the acromion, was considerably heightened.[1] On June 11th, after only the ninth sitting, the patient was able to raise the arm, without pain, to a horizontal position. The caput humeri had approached to within two lines of the acromion; the M. deltoideus had increased in size. At this stage the patient interrupted the treatment with the intention of leaving the rest to nature, but, as his condition was rather deteriorated than improved, he applied again to me, August 18th, for a continuance of electric treatment. I accordingly subjected the patient fourteen times more to faradization, and dismissed him, October 2d, perfectly cured; the M. deltoideus had regained its power of movement, and the shoulders their fulness of form. The painful sensations in the arm and fingers had passed entirely away.

CASE 36.—C. L., a farmer, twenty-two years of age,

[1] This elevation of the electro-muscular sensibility, which Duchenne regards as an indication of what he terms rheumatic paralysis, that is, a paralysis arising from muscular rheumatism, neuralgia, or other rheumatic affection, is probably only the result of an accompanying hyperæsthesia of the affected muscles. It is no more a characteristic of rheumatic paralysis than the normal condition of the electro-muscular contractility is, which also Duchenne will have as a peculiarity of this form of paralysis. Froriep (Ueber die Heilwirkungen der Electricität. Erstes Heft: Die rheumatische Schwiele, Weimar, 1843) has assigned as the constant and distinctive feature of rheumatic forms of disease, the rheumatic callosity, an exudation which has its seat in the dermis, the connective tissue, the muscle, or the periosteum; but, on more careful observation, this, though frequently, is by no means always found in diseases of the kind named; when present, it occasions a corresponding reduction of the electro-muscular contractility. I myself have seen cases in which Duchenne's statements, and still more numerous cases, in which Froriep's held good; the distinction lies simply in this, that in the former there was no exudation, but probably a hyperæsthesia of the nerves of the muscle, while in the latter a greater or less degree of exudation was present, by which the muscular contractility was lowered in proportion to the increased resistance to conduction.

had been subject from his seventh to his seventeenth year to various kinds of nervous attacks; thus from his seventh to his twelfth year he had suffered paralysis of the lower extremities, alternating with intervals of relief, during which he was perfectly strong in the use of his legs. From his twelfth to his seventeenth year he had been subject to epileptic convulsions, which sometimes were excited merely by the brushing of his coat. From this time, he had grown physically so strong, that he could perform all the duties of an agriculturist, and was only inconvenienced occasionally by pains in the back of the head or spine, rendering necessary the application of leeches or cupping-glasses. He was, accordingly, notwithstanding his opposition, declared fit for military service, and was enlisted October 18, 1854.

So soon as October 21st, he experienced pains in both arms, especially the left, which, in consequence of continued military exercises, increased in intensity, being particularly severe in the region of the shoulder; these were accompanied with disturbances in motor power, disabling him from raising the left arm at the shoulder-joint with any freedom, or adducting it at the elbow. Being at last only able to hold the stock of his musket with the flexors of his fingers, he was received, November 16th, into the military hospital. But, notwithstanding the employment of douches and embrocations, a complete paralysis of the arm ensued, together with reduction of temperature, disturbance of sensibility, and a relaxation of the muscles of the shoulder and upper arm. The endermic application twice a day of strychnine, in doses gradually increased from $\frac{1}{8}$ to $\frac{1}{4}$ a grain, remained without favorable result, and the patient was at last, on December 22d, dismissed from the hospital as temporarily unfit for service. After an interval of several weeks, during which cuppings were applied to the nape of the neck, invigorating washes employed, and perfect rest for the arm enjoined, on the advice of Dr. Leubuscher, he came to me January 31, 1855. The upper arm could not be moved from the body; the elbow could not be bent, and the entire arm, therefore, hung lax by his side. The M. deltoideus and biceps brachii felt flabby. The sensibility of the skin on the upper arm was diminished. The action of the muscles of the forearm and hand was unimpeded. The patient complained of a feeling of coldness in the arm and hand; yet these parts did not feel cold to the touch. The electro-muscular contractility of the paralyzed muscles, the M. deltoideus, and biceps, was but little lowered, and accordingly a favorable prognosis could be made. In point of fact, after only the third sitting, the patient was able to raise the arm to the horizontal plane, the sensibility of the skin was increased, and the feeling of coldness subsided. After the ninth sitting (February 9, 1855), all the movements were performed without obstruction, the tone of the muscles was raised, the arm warm, the sensibility of the skin normal. A feeling of pain, however, aroused by repeated movements of the arm, and extending along the shoulder-blade to the spine, rendered an application of a gentle electric current two or three times a week still desirable. Under this treatment the muscles formerly paralyzed increased during February and March in volume. The pains were dissipated, and at the end of March the patient was again ready for active service.

CASE 37.—Hermann Schroeder, a boy of twelve years, who had been always healthy, having, while playing at ball, hurled the ball by a strong effort to a great distance, experienced a severe pain in the right shoulder, which lasted eight days. Two years later, about the beginning of the year 1854, his relatives remarked that the right shoulder was carried lower down and more to the front than the left, and that the thorax was fallen in on the right side. An examination (made August 26, 1854) gave the following results: If the patient was regarded posteriorly while assuming an unbent posture, his arms hanging by his side, the vertebral column, from the first to the seventh dorsal vertebra, showed a deviation to the left, which at its greatest distance was as much as half an inch. The distance of the superior angle of the shoulder-blade from the proc. spin. of the third dorsal vertebra measured, on the right side, four inches, and, on the left side, two inches; the distance of the inferior angle of the proc. spin. of the ninth dorsal vertebra measured, on the right side, three and a half inches, on the left side one and three-quarter inches. Consequently, the right shoulder-blade, especially at its inferior part, was but loosely connected with the thorax, while the superior free border of the latissimus dorsi, which in its normal position covers the inferior angle of the shoulder-blade, and is attached to the thorax, was here found, in consequence of the changed position of the scapula, underlying it; the right Mm. rhomboidei projected as a thick roll. When the patient held both arms horizontally to the front, so as to meet opposite the middle line, the deviation of the vertebral column disappeared; on the other hand, the distance of the superior angle of the shoulder-blade from the proc. spin. of the third dorsal vertebra measured on the right side four and a half inches, on the left side three inches; the distance of the inferior angle from the proc. spin. of the ninth dorsal vertebra measured on the right side four and a half inches, on the left, three inches and a half. If, now, he moved both arms at the same time from the front horizontally as far as possible behind him, though he succeeded in bringing the left scapula in contact with the vertebral column, the inferior angle of the right one remained, on the other hand, at a distance of three and a half inches, and the superior angle at a distance of two and a half inches; this nearer approximation of the latter was only effected by a powerful tension of the Mm. rhomboidei. The case thus presented was one of complete paralysis of the right M. trapezius, induced probably by a muscular laceration, as well as of apparently a secondary relaxation of the M. latissimus dorsi of the affected side. A treatment, continued for a considerable time, effected at the most only a greater tension of the latter, whose electro-muscular contractility was tolerably well preserved; but the irritation of the trapezius, whose electro-muscular contractility, in consequence, probably, of an insufficient union of the severed muscular fascicles, was entirely extinct, remained without result.

In the case which is here described we find, in addition to the paralysis of the M. trapezius, a hypertrophy of the Mm. rhomboidei of the corresponding side. A like muscular hypertrophy frequently occurs as a result of muscular paralysis, whenever the power of making a certain movement is not taken wholly away from the member attacked by the paralysis. If the movement particularized can be accomplished by other auxiliary muscles, working in the same direction as the paralyzed ones, the former, having now added to their own proper function that of the latter also, undergo an increase of volume corresponding to their increased activity.[1] As the paralyzed muscles gradually recover their freedom of movement, the hypertrophy subsides. Moreover, in cases of muscular paralysis, we often meet, either in addition to or without hypertrophy, certain muscular deformations developed in the antagonists of the paralyzed muscles, in consequence of the removal of the natural muscular equilibrium, and which, in like manner, gradually disappear with the restoration of executive power to the paralyzed muscles.

In the following case we find, as a result of the paralysis of the serratus ant. major, a hypertrophy of the upper part of the trapezius and the levator angul. scap., and at the same time a deformation of the Mm. rhomboidei.

CASE 38.—Sann, a journeyman tinman, nineteen years old, as a child scrofulous, but later in life always in good health, was a young man of weak build, without strength of muscle, and pale in the face. In the autumn of 1856 he was seized, without known cause, with violent tearing pains in the right shoulder, which, when warmth was sup-

[1] See Case 21.

plied, always soon disappeared, but returned at times, especially in the morning hours. Sann having, on one occasion, about Christmas-time, when he had been working very hard, supported his head for a long time in a bent position, suddenly felt a tearing pain which ran from the lowest cervical vertebra to the fossa supraspinata dextra, and, as soon as he raised his head, increased in violence. From this time Sann could not elevate his arm without pain, and though, after he had kept his bed several days, this pain diminished, still, up to January 14th, the patient could not take down his coat from the cross-bar of his bed without suffering severely. From this time until his admission into the Schoenlein department of the hospital, February 4, 1857, he was subjected eight times to the electric current, by which means the severity of his pains was much mitigated.

At this stage his case presented the following points: There was a slight curvature of the spine, in its dorsal region, toward the right, and the right shoulder stood correspondingly higher. When the arms hung down, it was observed, in the next place, that the interior border of the right shoulder-blade was inclined obliquely downward to the left and that its inferior angle stood farther from the thorax than the corresponding part of the left shoulder-blade. The region of the fossa supraspinata was more prominent on the right than on the left, a difference induced by the hypertrophy of the superior part of the trapezius and the levator ang. scapulæ; in like manner, the region lying between the upper dorsal vertebra and the upper part of the interior border of the scapula was more prominent on the right side than on the left, a difference induced by the shrinking of the Mm. rhomboidei. The patient could raise the extended arm to an angle of 120 degrees; but on every attempt to raise it higher he experienced pain, and at the same time involuntarily inclined the head to the right. If, in this effort, he was assisted by having the inferior angle of the scapula pushed outward, he could raise the arm conveniently to the head. On the elevation of the arm, the inner border of the scapula was removed so far from the spine, that the fist could easily be laid between the wall of the thorax and the inner surface of the scapula. When the right arm was thus raised to the head, the dentiform appendages of the M. serratus anticus major of the right side disappeared, while those on the left side, when a like position of the left arm was assumed, could be distinctly marked. When the shoulders were moved forward and downward, the Mm. rhomboidei dextri were much strained, and the ang. inferior scap. stood higher than that of the other side. When the arm hung down, Sann experienced no pain in any part; but a pressure upon the shrunken muscles was, on the other hand, painful. I first saw the patient on February 23d. At that time no considerable change in the symptoms had appeared, except that, in consequence of the increased hypertrophy of the superior part of the trapezius and of the levator ang. scap., Sann could raise the arm somewhat higher. The reaction of the serratus ant. mag. of the right side was so deficient that a treatment of very long duration was foreseen; this reaction was exhibited both upon intra-muscular irritation—which I excited by placing one conductor in the cavity occasioned by the paralysis between the thorax and scapula, the other in the neighborhood of the anterior insertions of the muscle in question, upon the ribs—and also, in an especial degree, by extra-muscular irritation, which was produced by the application of one conductor upon the N. thoracicus longus, immediately over the exterior border of the superior part of the trapezius, about one inch from the clavicular, the other upon the ribs. Not only the serratus, but also the trapezius, in its inferior part reacted with much less force on the right side than on the left. Thus, on May 2, 1857, after forty-eight sittings, when the patient stood erect, his arms hanging by his side, the inferior angle of the right shoulder-blade stood out more from the thorax than the corresponding one of the left. The region of the interior border of the scapula was also still prominent; the interior border of the shoulder-blade was still obliquely inclined, though in a less marked degree, from above downward to the left and inward; finally, the rhomboidei still displayed unusual tension, and the upper part of the trapezius and the levator anguli scapulæ were still in a condition of hypertrophy. When the arm was raised to the height of the shoulder, the right scapula was still considerably removed from the vertebral column, its inferior angle being four inches distant, while the corresponding angle of the left side was but one inch distant. On the other hand, the patient could now, without inconvenience or pain, bring the extended arm to the head; the insertions of the M. serratus were, when such movement was executed, marked with considerable distinctness; the reaction, if not yet quite normal, was still much improved. Sann now left the hospital to resume his work, while he continued the treatment at my house; but, after the second sitting, an attack of intermittens tertiana, a malady which so frequently affects patients of impoverished blood, interrupted the treatment for three weeks. After the fifty-fourth sitting—June 6th—the insertions of the serratus were distinctly perceptible; the depression between the spine and the interior border of the shoulder-blade was much shallower; the inferior angle of the scapula was more closely applied to the thorax. After the sixty-second sitting—July 15th—on the elevation of the arm to the height of the shoulder, the inferior angle of the shoulder-blade was only two inches distant from the spine; the inferior part of the trapezius was no longer relaxed, and the dorsal flexure of the spine no longer visible. About the end of August, when the patient again visited me, he could use his arm freely in his pursuits. The only remaining traces of the disease still observable were a scarcely perceptible prominence of the insertions of the serratus, a slight hypertrophy of the upper part of the trapezius and the levator ang. scapulæ, and, lastly, a somewhat deficient electro-muscular contractility of the once-paralyzed serratus anticus major. The deformation of the right Mm. rhomboidei was scarcely perceptible.

These deformations and hypertrophies, especially when they are combined in the same case, frequently make certain movements practicable, which, on the paralysis of the muscles specially designed for these movements, seemed impossible. Thus Sann, when the paralysis of the M. serrat. ant. was not yet complete, was able, in consequence of the hypertrophy of the superior part of the trapezius and the levator ang. scapulæ, and of the change in the position of the scapula brought on by the contraction of the Mm. rhomboidei, to raise the arm to an angle of 120 degrees. Thus, by progressive exercises and by the aid of electric excitement, the strength of the muscles undergoing hypertrophy may be increased to a point which shall qualify them to supply the place of the paralyzed ones.

If we had done this in the case above described, the usefulness of the arm would certainly have been earlier restored; but there would also have infallibly arisen a considerable curvature of the spine. Other cases, however, occur, in which, following the bent of nature, the operator can employ with advantage the process of faradization upon the muscles undergoing hypertrophy, without fearing similar results.

The secondary deformations, however, must be distinguished from the primary idiopathic ones, which are sometimes developed from rheumatic conditions, but in most cases are of unknown origin, and the diagnosis of which may be made with confidence in view of the unimpaired motor power and normal electric condition of the antagonist muscles. Duchenne has made observations upon such idiopathic deformations of the rhomboideus, trapezius, peronæus longus, the diaphragm, etc. We extract from his work[1] the following case:

Agloeé Prude, thirteen years of age, remarked for the

[1] Page 880.

first time in February, 1849, a pain, produced by some unknown cause, in the middle and posterior region of the neck, on the right side, which was increased both by pressure on the spot and by the inclination of the head to the left. For a year and a half no other symptom, except a slight difficulty in effecting certain movements of the head, was perceived, till accidentally in 1852 a deformity of the shoulder was discovered, when the patient was recommended by Bouvier to Duchenne, who gave the following synopsis of the case: When the arms hung down, the inferior angle of the right shoulder-blade was raised to an almost equal height with the exterior angle, and was pressed close to the middle line of the vertebral column. If the inferior angle of the shoulder-blade was pushed forcibly down, it immediately assumed, upon remission of the pressure, its former false position, and, at the same time, a distinct grating was heard between the shoulder-blade and the thorax. Over the spinal border of the shoulder-blade a marked prominence was observed, which seemed to be formed by a contraction of the rhomboideus and another such prominence on the neck, in the triangular space between the anterior border of the trapezius and the sterno-cleido-mastoideus, which was apparently formed by the levator ang. scap. The head was slightly inclined to the right, and could not be turned to the left without pain. Deformations of the rhomboideus and of the levator ang. scap. were undoubtedly present, and the question thus arose whether the primary cause of these deformations was a paralysis of the serratus magnus. That the latter was not the case could be inferred from this: that, when the patient extended the arms to the front, the shoulder-blade assumed a normal position, whereas, in the case of the primary paralysis of the M. serratus, it is by the anterior extension of the arms that this deformation is first clearly distinguished. Duchenne, however, by the faradization of the serratus anticus major with a quick, strong, painful current, overcame these muscular deformations, though they were of two years' standing, in three sittings, notwithstanding he had previously applied, for the space of a month, a constant, rarely-interrupted current, without the least effect.

Under the head of muscular paralysis we have still to include two forms of disease to which the substance of the muscle is subject, which are characterized by a very peculiar electric condition. These are: A. Paralysis from the poisonous effects of lead, a form of the disease which, in whatever way this mineral may attain to an oxidized molecular condition in the blood, always affects definite muscles in a definite manner: B. Progressive muscular atrophy, which probably depends upon an affection of the sympathetic nerve.

A. *Paralysis from the Poisonous Action of Lead.*

In the form of paralysis which is induced by the poisonous action of lead, the muscles attacked suffer in their electro-muscular contractility and sensibility; the first is considerably lowered, or often entirely removed, while the last is only a little weakened. The extensor muscles are always and in a preëminent degree the sufferers; in general, however, only those of the superior extremities, seldom those of the lower extremities in addition, and very rarely the latter alone. Of the extensor muscles, the extensor digit. comm. is the most liable to a modification of its electric condition, either in all or in isolated fascicles; the triceps and the deltoideus are the least liable to such modification, though in rare cases the deltoideus is the first and greatest sufferer. The supinators always retain their electro-muscular contractility in its normal degree, even when they have suffered in their motor power. Only those muscles, whose electro-muscular contractility has been affected, lapse into a condition of atrophy, and these resist for the longest time the ameliorating influence of the electric treatment. The M. interosseus ext. prim. sometimes offers an apparent exception, since it may exhibit a condition of atrophy, without a loss of contractility; but in this case the atrophy is one produced not by the poisonous action of lead, but by mechanical causes, such as, with house-painters, the pressure of the brush. In general those muscles seem to suffer most which are strained the most by the patient, or which either naturally or in consequence of preceding maladies are the least capable of resistance. Thus, for example, the muscles of the left arm less commonly suffer than those of the right, and among house-painters the thumb and middle-finger, with which they usually hold the brush, suffer in a higher degree than the remaining fingers. I had, however, occasion to treat a house-painter who was left-handed, and in whose case consequently the extensors of the left side were paralyzed the most; and again, another of the same craft who, in consequence of being hump-backed, was subject to a weakness of the lower extremities, by reason of which the paralysis had especially attacked the Mm. peronæi, the extensores digit. ped. long. and the extensores hallucium prop.

CASE 39.—Wilhelm Schultze, a house-painter, was seized, December, 1852, with an exceedingly violent painter's-colic, united with a constipation of three weeks' duration. At the same time a violent trembling was felt in both arms, especially in the right, accompanied with paralysis of the right forearm. When the patient applied to me, May 2, 1853, for a trial of electric treatment, the M. extensor digitorum communis, especially that belly of the muscle extending to the middle-finger, and the M. extensor pollicis longus, the extensor carpi radialis and ulnaris, the M. abductor pollicis longus, etc., of the right side, were paralyzed, while the affection of the left arm was limited to a feeling of weakness and trembling, in connection with a normal motor power in all the muscles. The electro-muscular contractility was lowered, in different degrees, in the several paralyzed muscles, most conspicuously in the M. extensor digitorum and extensor pollicis longus; the lateral movements of the hand were not impeded to an equal degree. The electro-muscular sensibility of the M. extensor digitorum communis and pollicis longus had suffered, though not to a corresponding extent. The application of an electric current of moderate force to the left arm gave rise to such quick, violent tensions, not only of the affected extensors, but also of the abductors and adductors of the hand, that the fingers were bowed over the hand. The irritation of the left extensor carpi radialis or ulnaris drew the hand to a position nearer the radius or the ulna than the patient could bring it by the simple force of will. The sensation accompanying the contraction was so intense that the patient was disinclined to a repetition of the experiment. The Mm. supinator, deltoideus, and triceps, both of the paralyzed and unparalyzed side, remained always constant and normal. The cure was completed in about six weeks.

Case 40.—Von S., a chamberlain, from Giessen, a healthy but somewhat sallow-looking man of fifty years, was attacked with a paralysis of the right hand, which had been coming on for three weeks, and which, on his first visit to me—March 12, 1857—was so far developed that the extension of the three middle fingers was absolutely impossible and the elevation of the wrist difficult. The thumb could be extended and abducted, and the arm was capable of pronation and supination; muscular atrophy was not exhibited. The electro-muscular contractility was depressed in the extensor digit. comm. and the extensor indicis propr., and, though to a less degree, in the extensor carpi rad. and uln.; in the other extensors and in the supinators it remained normal. Metacarpal intromescences were not exhibited. The patient had never had colics, but had frequently suffered from constipation. The only cause of the paralysis was the use, for the preceding twelve years, of snuff which had been packed and preserved in lead. A favorable prognosis, based upon the short duration of the patient's suffering, and the participation of but few muscles, was confirmed by the course of the cure.

CASE 41.—Miss Pauline L., apparently in her thirtieth year, formerly an actress, a woman of pale-yellow complexion, had suffered for many years with constipation, which, however, could be easily overcome by simple remedies. During a few months past she had frequently felt drawing pains in both shoulders and arms, accompanied, within the three preceding months, by a gradually-increasing paralysis of both hands, which finally rendered the elevation and extension of them impossible. The Geh. Rath Koner immediately perceived that the paralysis was one resulting from the poisonous effects of lead, and he ascribed its origin to the considerable proportion of lead found in the paint which the patient was accustomed every evening to apply to her neck. I saw the patient for the first time, March 17, 1856, and observed the following details: A prominence of the metacarpal bones of both hands; inability to elevate the wrist, especially of the right side; abduction, especially of the right thumb, impossible; the fingers, particularly the third and fourth, hanging relaxed and capable of only slight voluntary distention, though easily brought into contact; the supinators of both sides perfectly free in their action. The electro-muscular contractility was not entirely extinct in any muscle; the reaction was feeblest in the Mm. extensores carpi radiales, the abductor pollicis longus and extensor indicis of the right side, and in the extensor digit. comm. of the left side; the left extensor carpi radialis, both extensores carpi ulnares, the left abductor pollicis longus, and the extensors of the thumb had suffered less. The interossei ext. and the supinators exhibited throughout a normal electric condition.[1]

[1] [Two cases of lead paralysis, induced by the use of the cosmetic known as "Laird's Bloom of Youth," have recently come under my observation. One of these occurred in the person of a young lady whom I saw in consultation with my friend, Prof. Lewis A. Sayre; the other is that of a young married lady, whom I am now treating successfully with the direct and induced currents. In the latter case, all the extensors of both wrists and fingers and the interossei muscles were more or less affected. At the present date (March 24,

Often, for a long time after the paralyzed muscles have been restored to free, unrestricted activity, their electro-muscular contractility remains depressed. Thus, in the case of a house-painter who had been treated two years earlier for a paralysis arising from the poisonous action of lead, and who since then had not suffered a renewed attack, I found, in conjunction with an unimpaired motor power in the muscles formerly affected, a continued deficiency of irritability in the M. extensor digit. communis. This could not have been a symptom of an approaching attack of the same nature, for the patient during these two years had worked with white zinc in place of white lead. In the instance, also, of the patient whose case is described on page 181, and who since his recovery has abstained from the use of snuff, a depression of the electro-muscular contractility of the paralyzed muscles was exhibited for a long time.

Cases frequently occur of a paralysis of the extensors of the hand, accompanied with all the indications of a paralysis from poisoning by lead—as the integrity of the supinators, the prominence of the metacarpal bones, the slate-colored borders of the teeth, antecedent colics, and the peculiar electric condition of the muscles affected—and which, moreover, are cured by treatment with sulphur baths and faradization, but which, as regards their cause, remain wrapped in obscurity—an obscurity which all the efforts that have been put forth in the interest of practical medicine, with the view, namely, of preventing relapses, have not been able to clear up.

CASE 42.—Carl Hennig, forty years old, an operator in the machine-works at Borsig, in which, however, he was not

1869) the patient has been under treatment for about three months, and has almost entirely regained the use of the paralyzed muscles. In this case, the induced current at first failed to produce the slightest contraction of the paralyzed muscles. The direct current acted from the first. It is in such cases that the latter is especially necessary.—W. A. H.]

employed as a worker in lead, nor was brought in contact with the vapors of lead, had been attacked once or twice every year, for the last ten years, with colic, and, in the course of the last one or two years, had frequently experienced, especially while playing at cards, a cramp in the third and fourth fingers of either hand. From the end of November, 1866, he had been suffering with a paralysis of the extensors of both hands, which resisted the various remedies applied, among which were, in particular, hypodermic injections. Dr. Fraenkel, who at once recognized the case as a paralysis induced by the poisonous action of lead, having introduced the patient to me, I made, February 15, 1867, the following observations of the patient's condition: Hennig could neither elevate the wrist nor extend the fingers; but supination was on both sides unrestricted. The sensibility of the skin was dull, the forearm was flabby, the muscles of the hand lax. The electro-muscular contractility was much depressed in all the extensors of the fingers, especially the Mm. extensores digit. comm., and also in the right M. extensor carp. rad. and in the left M. extensor poll. long. The supinators of both sides reacted with normal power. The metacarpal bones of both hands were very prominent. The teeth were surrounded with a slate-colored border, more than a line broad. These symptoms indicated the necessity of a protracted treatment, and, in fact, in addition to the continuous employment of sulphur-baths, ninety applications of the electric current were necessary in order to render the patient again fit for work, which was not effected till the middle of June of the same year. The only cause which could be discovered in this case as possibly occasioning the disease, was the residence of the patient immediately over a type-foundry, a residence which lasted for two years, but was discontinued soon before the first attack of colic. Whether it is possible that the colics which were repeated every year since that time, as well as the subsequent paralyses, were induced by the residence of the patient ten years previously in an atmosphere impregnated with lead, I must leave undecided.

B. *Progressive Muscular Atrophy.*

Under the name of "Atrophie Musculaire Progressive" Aran[1] has described a disease, the characteristic sign of which consists in a disturbance in the nutrition of particular muscles or muscular groups, or of the entire muscular system, advancing at equal pace with a disturbance of the functional action of the affected parts. This form of disease was, however, not unknown to earlier writers; Charles Bell, Abercrombie, Romberg, and others had already described cases of this kind. Duchenne has sought to make the electric condition of the affected muscles available in the diagnosis and prognosis of the disease.

The affection generally begins with an emaciation of the M. interosseus primus of one hand, a feeling of fatigue and weakness in the arm; in frequent cases with pains in the back of the neck. The emaciation proceeds from the M. interosseus primus to the muscles of the hand and forearm, under certain circumstances to the muscles of the shoulder and the breast, the buttocks, or to the one or the other lower extremity; finally, it attacks the muscles of the tongue, the diaphragm, and the throat, and the patient, emaciated to a skeleton, sinks under bronchitis, or other pulmonary disease. Progressive muscular atrophy does not, however, always attack the upper extremities first; sometimes it begins with the muscles of the trunk, or of the nape, or other part of the neck, etc. The disease often develops only to a certain degree in the parts primarily affected, and then remains stationary for many years; thus, for example, it may be seated for a long time in the forearm, and suddenly, without apparently any method of development, leap to the muscles of the upper part of the arm, or those of the trunk, and de-

[1] Archives Gén. de Méd., 1850, p. 5, *et seq.*

stroy them. Of the muscles of the arm the deltoideus and the biceps suffer most frequently, the triceps least frequently.

To the gradually progressing emaciation correspond disturbances in the motor power of the muscles. The feeling of fatigue and weakness is followed by a certain clumsiness in the movements of the parts attacked, which gradually become less and less capable of action, till finally the patient is left utterly helpless. The peculiar muscular decay which characterizes this disease never follows some one nervous cord, but leaps, and with apparently regular advances, from the domain of one nerve to that of another, and is thus distinguished from the muscular decay caused by neuritis, with which it is often confounded, but which is confined strictly to the realm of the diseased nerve. In the majority of cases, fibrillous convulsions are added, which, at times, especially after unusual agitation or exertion, or when the muscles have been exposed to a draught, come on with increased force; these are frequently the first sign of a diseased condition on the part of muscles apparently perfectly sound. Throughout all these disturbances in muscular function, the sensibility of the skin and the muscles, under touch, pressure, or pricking, seems in most cases to remain normal, though in many anæsthesia is present; on the other hand, in the more advanced stage of the disease, the patients frequently complain of tearing pains, which at times have their seat in the joints, at times follow the path of certain nerves, at times are diffused. There also occasionally occur in the later stages certain swellings of the joints, such as have been described by Remak, Benedikt, and M. Rosenthal. In all cases, however, the temperature of the extremities attacked falls with the progress of the disease; the subjective sensation of chilliness is followed by excessive sensibility to the cold, and, finally, by a reduction of bodily heat objectively appreciable by the touch, and by thermometrical measurements. Feverish effects are always absent, unless occasioned by the addition of other acute diseases.

As regards the electric condition of the muscles affected, as exhibited under the induction current, the electro-muscular contractility remains in general undisturbed, so long as there is any normal muscular tissue left; the energy of movement, however, which is excited by muscular contraction, diminishes with the mass of the muscle; but not until the substance of the muscle is altogether gone, does the electro-muscular contractility become extinct. We often find various parts of the same muscle electrically irritable in different degrees. The electro-muscular sensibility decreases as the atrophy increases. In special cases, particularly in the outset of the disease, the sensibility of the nerves is heightened, and, in consequence of this, diplegic and centripetal reflex contractions occur whenever the intermittent current is applied, and with still more force upon application of the constant current. In the further course of the disease, irritability is still manifested near the central nervous paths, when in the more peripheric nervous branches and muscles it is extinct.

The electric condition of the muscles, as here described, corresponds to the pathological changes which we perceive in the muscles. By the side of perfectly sound muscles we find others which are in various stages of disease; and again, in the same muscle, we find, by the side of healthy fascicles, others which are included in the approaches of the disease. In this case microscopic examination exhibits, in the affected muscles, fibres, which are normal in texture and size; others, in which the transverse striæ are indistinct, broken, and here and there entirely gone, while the longitudinal striæ appear prominent; others, in which only longitudinal striæ are present, the transverse ones being no longer visible, and in which fat, in the form of round or oval cells or globules, is deposited; and lastly, bundles of fibres, which have relapsed into an amorphous mass. To the different stages of fatty degeneration correspond the various colors of the fibrous fascicles, namely, red, pale red, yellowish red, and yellow.

The changes in the muscles, which we have just described, are found, according to the common testimony of all authors, in all cases of true progressive muscular atrophy. Cruveilhier, however, in one case, reported in the "Arch. Gén. de Méd.," 1853, discovered, in addition to these changes in the muscles, a very considerable atrophy of the anterior nervous roots of the medulla spinalis, and on this account, regarding the affection of the nervous roots as primary, that of the muscles as secondary, felt justified in designating the disease a "paralyse." The result of this dissection was accepted as a finality, until Valentiner[1] published a second case, in which he discovered the same atrophy of the anterior nervous roots of the spinal cord, but, in addition, a very considerable number (about one hundred) of small, white, hard granules, from the size of a pin-head to that of a lentil, embedded in the tissue of the arachnoides of the medulla spinalis, and also a central softening of the lower cervical and upper dorsal portions of the medulla, together with an accumulation of granulated cells. Leubascher and Froniman[2] also found, in addition to a red softening of the anterior and lateral columns of the medulla oblongata, a transformation of the anterior and lateral columns of the medulla spinalis into a dark-white, formless substance, in which no whole nervous fibres could be distinguished, while in the nervous roots themselves no special attenuation of the anterior roots was perceptible.

Similar discoveries were made public at a later date by Lays, Reade, Touvenet, and others. On the other hand, Oppenheimer, Hasse, Friedberg, and Meryon, who, in numerous cases of progressive muscular atrophy of the most pronounced character, directed very careful examination upon these points, were unable to discover, either in the central organs or in the cerebral or spinal nervous centres, or in the peripheric branches, any departures from the normal condition; while Virchow and Friedreich found, associated with

[1] Prager Vierteljahrsschrift, 1855.   [2] Deutsche Klinik, 1857.

a soundness of the anterior roots, a gray degeneration of the posterior cords. Friedreich[1] thought he was able to show in the single case which he personally examined that "the diseased action going on in the muscles was carried forth by the nervous branches and roots distributed to those muscles, and thus finally excited in the posterior cords certain processes of degeneration.

After an unprejudiced examination of the facts adduced, it seems to be undoubtedly the case that the disease gradually advances from the muscles to the nerves and the spinal cord. In favor of this view are the following points: 1. In no one case which has fallen under dissection have the anatomical changes in the muscular fibres been absent. 2. The most skilful dissection and examination, of the bodies of persons who died of this disease, have developed no change in the anterior nervous roots or in any central organ. 3. The case reported by Friedreich, in which the progress of the disease was traced from the periphery to the centre. 4. The various stages in the diseased condition of the muscles, found sometimes side by side, in the several fascicles of the same muscle. 5. The electric condition of the muscles and nerves, as well under the intermittent as under the constant current—under the former, the preservation of electro-muscular contractility, so far as normal muscular substance remains—under the latter, the preservation of nervous irritability in the more central nervous paths, in connection with a contemporaneous loss of irritability in the peripheric nervous off-shoots and muscles ; while, if the progress of the disease was from the central nervous parts through the nerves to the muscles, a reversed relation would hold good.

On the other hand, the affection of the muscular substance itself seems to be the result of a disease of the sympathetic nerve. In favor of this view are, among others, the considerations adduced on page 252 ; but it cannot as yet,

[1] Ueber degenerative atrophie der spinalen Hinterstränge. Virchow's Archiv, Band xxi. und xxiv.

of course, be supported by any anatomical proof, unless we regard as such the isolated case, published by Schneevogt, in which was exhibited a fatty degeneration of the sympathetic nerve.[1]

While, however, in respect to the etiology of the disease, we know but little, certain it is that rheumatic affections, colds, long-continued and excessive exertion of particular muscles, and, above all, hereditary predisposition, exercise an important influence upon its origination. As regards the value of the last of these influences, Duchenne mentions an instance of four members of the same family suffering with this disease; Meryon gives a similar instance, and Oppenheimer instances a family in which three members suffered in like manner. Ordinarily this disease, like hæmophilia, is implanted only in the male issue. Friedberg describes a case in which both mother and daughter fell a sacrifice to it.

CASE 43.—Moses Jedwabnitzki, a teacher from Poland, 31 years old, was seized four years ago, after an obstinate intermitting fever, with trembling and weakness of the left arm, accompanied with an emaciation of the affected member. The emaciation, beginning at the shoulder, advanced rapidly over the upper arm, the forearm, and the hand, and at the same time the weakness increased to a degree of complete paralysis. For the past year and a half the shoulder and upper part of the right arm had also been growing emaciate, and, at a corresponding rate, paralytic. During the last three months, the left Mm. glutæi had been settling into a condition of atrophy. The temperature of the left arm was considerably depressed. The general health was undisturbed. Appetite and sleep good; the latter, however, sometimes interrupted by tearing pains in the loins and extremities. The pulse in both arms equally strong. Fecal and urinary discharges were regular and easy. The urine had a weak acid reaction; it was bright and clear. A more careful examination exhibited a com

[1] Nederlandsch Lancet, 1854.

plete atrophy of all the muscles of the left arm from the shoulder-blade, of which the fossae supra spinatae et infra spinatae formed cavities an inch deep, down to the hand, between the metacarpal bones of which, deep furrows were visible; the hand was bent to the forearm; opening of the fingers and extension of the forearm were impossible. The entire extremity could be thrown upward, and could be poised upon the acromion, but a slow elevation of it was impossible. On the right arm there was apparent a considerable atrophy of the M. deltoideus, and, though to a somewhat less degree, of the M. triceps and biceps; the forearm and hand were still tolerably muscular; accordingly, the entire arm could not be elevated, but the forearm could be adducted and abducted with some force, while the movements of the right hand were accomplished with freedom. The left leg displayed nothing abnormal except a noticeable emaciation of the M. glutaeus maximus. The muscles of the right leg, as well as those of the entire trunk and of the face, showed no variation from the natural condition. Fibrillous muscular contractions were observeable in various muscles of the trunk. When the degenerated muscles of the left arm were subjected to an electric current, no contractions arose, weak muscular twitchings were all that were perceptible; on the other hand, upon the irritation of the N. radialis, evident extensor movements followed. Upon the electric irritation of the muscles of the right arm, the contractions were more or less energetic, according to the more or less advanced stage of atrophy. The muscles of the right forearm, the right hand, both legs, etc., displayed a normal degree of electro-muscular contractility and sensibility. When, September 12, 1853, I again saw the patient, an interval of five months having intervened, which time he had spent partly in the Jewish Hospital of this place, partly at the baths of Gastein, he was complaining already of a feeling of weakness in the right leg; the emaciation of the right forearm had considerably progressed.

M. Rosenthal in his work, "Die Electrotherapie; ihre Begründung und Anwendung in der Medicin," Wien, 1865, reports on page 165 the following case, which we reproduce as embodying the characteristic traits of the hyperæsthetic form of this disease:

Katharina Gurda, twenty-four years of age, experienced in the spring of 1863, while at work in the field, a relaxation of the muscles of the left hand, in consequence of which, the objects grasped by it were apt to slip from their hold. Four or five weeks later, the fingers of this hand began gradually to bend inward; after several months, tearing pains broke out in the arm, a drawing cramp in the left shoulder, and frequent twitchings in the hand and fingers, which were never free from a disagreeable feeling of coldness. When Rosenthal undertook the treatment of the patient, who had been during three months subjected to faradization, her condition, now that her sufferings had lasted a year and a quarter, was as follows: The left hand, which had become blue as with cold, was utterly unfit for use, the thumb could neither be adducted nor brought into opposition, but lay in the hollow of the hand against the fingers, the phalanges of which were adducted; the elevation of the arm at the shoulder was restricted; the exterior angle of the shoulder-blade was sunken, the inferior raised and drawn toward the median line; upon the posterior side of the shoulder-blade fibrillous twitchings were perceptible. When the skin, in the neighborhood of the left interior angle of the shoulder-blade, was touched, energetic repulsive movements were aroused; when a pressure was brought to bear upon the left M. pectoralis, which was in a condition of tension, reflex extension of the arm followed; a pressure upon the dorsal vertebræ from the third to the fifth produced extension of the left arm and a sense of pain—all of which are signs of the hyperæsthesia of the nerves of the skin and muscles. The faradization of the thumb and the ball of the little finger, and the irritation of the Mm. interossei remained, without effect; the irritation of the extensor digit. comm. led at once to a cramping in the flexors; the application of both poles to the more central parts of the deltoideus effected, in quick succession, the extension of the hand, the extension of the arm, and the elevation of the latter to the head. In the left lower extremity, which, when the patient walked, showed a degree of weakness and dragged somewhat, there were also plain indications of cutaneous hyperæsthesia, for example, on the inner side of the upper part of the calf; there were also in this extremity evidences of increased reflex irritability, as shown by the faradization of the tibialis ant. or the extensor digit comm. (which caused flexion and extension of the ankle). The electric condition of the right lower extremity was normal. On the passage of a galvanic spinal-nerve current of fifteen elements through the left medianus, the arm turned outward so that the palm of the hand faced upward; on the galvanization of the left radialis, the arm trembled for a moment between flexion and extension, and at last was elevated and placed against the head. On the galvanic irritation of the right upper extremity, which was in a healthy, plump condition, similar indications of increased reflex irritability were observable; thus, for example, on the passage of a spinal-nerve-current through the right trapezius, centripetal reflex movements arose in the left arm, together with the extension of the fingers of the left hand and the elevation of the extended arm above the horizontal line.

The prognosis of progressive muscular atrophy is in general unfavorable and its cure uncertain. This is especially true of progressive muscular atrophy, properly so called, as described by Aran, and as distinguished from that form originating in neuritis. In the cases, then, that belong to this part of our subject, the prognosis is dependent upon various considerations: 1. The extent of the disease. If only one member of the body is attacked, and that to but a partial extent, and if the evil remains for a long time within these limits, the prognosis may be regarded as favorable. 2. The cause of the disease. If this lies in a sudden change of temperature, or a frequent straining of certain muscles, especially if these muscles are such as cannot be spared from future use, the prognosis is far more unfavorable than when an hereditary predisposition lies at the root of the disease. 3. The electric condition of the paralyzed muscles. A restoration of function can be looked for only in those muscles which still retain some sound muscular fibres, and in which, consequently, electro-muscular contractility is not yet fully extinct.

As regards the curative agents employed in cases of progressive muscular atrophy, electricity, especially in connection with prescribed gymnastic exercises, the use of iron, marsh baths, etc., has shown relatively the most favorable results. The electric treatment required consists either, as recommended by Duchenne, in the faradization of the muscles attacked—a course specially indicated where the irritation of the smaller muscles is demanded—or in the application of galvanic spinal-nerve and plexus-muscle currents—a mode which has this advantage over the former, that it brings the electricity to bear at once upon an entire group of muscles, the separate irritation of which, by faradization, would, where the affection is widely extended, be an impossibility—or, finally, in the galvanization of the sympathetic nerve, to which process Remak at last exclusively resorted, the diplegic contractions which are thus excited being, according to this author, peculiarly adapted to promote the nutritive restoration of muscles in a condition of atrophy.

Duchenne (page 535) communicates the following, in which the employment of faradization was crowned with the best results:

Bonnard, a mechanic, a large, strong man, twenty-five

years of age, who had previously enjoyed uniform good
health, observed for the first time in February, 1848—when,
in consequence of the political events of the day, he found
his regular work gone, and, in order to support his large
family, was compelled to struggle night and day amid priva-
tions of all kinds—a great degree of muscular weakness and
a certain inflexibility of the left arm, which could not be
accounted for by any precedent pain. This weakness, which
was continuous, was accompanied by a gradual emaciation
of the left arm, which from his youth he had been accustomed to use in preference to the right one; the emaciation
finally extended also to the trunk. Nevertheless, he continued at work without interruption till the year 1850, by
which time the left arm had become utterly incapable of
service, and in December of that year he applied to Duchenne for treatment. Duchenne found his condition as
follows: The thorax was emaciated to the skeleton; upon
its anterior side the skin seemed to lie immediately upon the
ribs, and was sunken in between them; upon its posterior
side, the shoulder-blades, when at rest, were at a great distance from the median line, and its spinal borders were
obliquely directed from below upward, and from within outward; the shoulders were even more depressed. The left
arm was about a third less in volume than the right, the
biceps having scarcely the thickness of the forefinger, the
triceps, however, though emaciated, still retaining a certain
development; in the forearm, the Mm. supinator longus and
radiales, in particular, were in a condition of atrophy. As
regards the electric condition of the muscles, the strongest
current excited only a few fibrillous contractions in the Mm.
pectorales, the two inferior divisions of the trapezius and
the latissimus dorsi, and then only when the exciters were
placed on those points where the muscular tissue was not
changed in its texture; the biceps contracted a little in its
superior part; the other muscles of the anterior side of the
upper arm could not be traced out. The triceps, when irri-

tated, extended the arm completely and energetically. All the muscles of the forearm were present, but the movements executed by the supinator longus and the radiales showed a little less energy in the left arm than in the right. The electro-muscular sensibility of the muscles in a condition of atrophy was considerably lowered, although the sensibility of the skin, even in those parts which covered the muscles that had wholly lost their vital power, was normal. The marked development of the muscles that retained their organic energy contrasted strongly with those whose vitality was suspended. Fibrillous contractions were also observable in most of the muscles which were apparently sound and were capable of movement. As regards the disturbance of motor power, briefly stated, the movement of the forearm was impossible, the extension of the hand laborious; Bonnard could not raise even the lightest hammer. General disturbances in the power of motion were not present, though, probably in consequence of an incipient atrophy of the diaphragm, the respiration for the last month had become difficult, so that the patient could scarcely walk a few steps without stopping to rest and to take breath. The faradization of the diaphragm, executed three or four times a week, quickly removed the difficulty of breathing, and rendered the patient able to take long walks and to go up-stairs without fatigue. The electric irritation of the muscles of the left arm, effected three times a week in sittings of eight to ten minutes, soon created an addition of strength and an increase in size, so that, after six months, Bonnard could again support his family by the labor of his hands. The frequent experiments which Duchenne undertook in the case of this patient, in the course of which he irritated in turn the various muscles of the trunk and extremities, also subdued the fibrillous contractions. The pectorales, the trapezii, and the latissimus dorsi, though they still remained much emaciated, did not by their weakness essentially hinder the patient in carrying on his work.

In my own practice, though many cases of this character were unsuccessful, a greater number were fortunate in their result; among the latter were included those, in particular, in which the disease was limited to the forearm and hand, or to the shoulder, arm and hand, of one side.

CASE 44.—Mr. S. had two years previously, while cutting ice—an occupation to which he was not accustomed—contracted a severe cold, in consequence of which, pains were excited in the nape of the neck, which gradually extended over the right shoulder, the upper arm, the forearm, and the hand, being particularly severe at the elbow, and at the basis of the metacarpal bone of the thumb. These pains were followed by weakness, emaciation, inability to use the arm, and a remarkable feeling of coldness. When, upon the request of Dr. Ichroider, I visited the patient (September 14, 1865), the right shoulder and the arm along its whole extent were emaciated, the elevation of the upper arm was difficult, and the extensor power of the arm limited. On every attempt to extend the hand, the three middle fingers fell forward; the index-finger could not be extended; the fingers could be separated to a distance of only a few lines, and could not be fully brought into contact. Together with these effects, there was an atrophy of the muscles of the shoulder, arm, and hand; the muscles of the ball of the thumb (with the exception of the adductor) and the interossei had suffered the most; fibrillous twitchings were exhibited over the greater part of the surface of the muscles attacked. Electro-muscular contractility was preserved in all the muscles, though the corresponding movements, especially those of the muscles of the hand, were less prompt. The application of the galvanic spinal-nerve and plexus-muscle currents, which was repeated 51 times, produced by the 20th November—at which time I was forced to interrupt the treatment, to make a journey—so considerable an improvement, that the upper arm could be fully raised, the hand extended, and the separated fingers brought into contact; the pains had ceased, the fibrillous twitchings were no longer apparent, the shoulder and arm were increased in size; on the other hand, the forefinger could not yet be extended, and the ring finger could be separated only a few lines from the middle finger; the interossei and the muscles of the thumb still showed an essential deficiency of assimilative power; and, finally, the temperature of the arm was still lowered.

When I saw the patient again (April 17, 1866), his improvement had come to a stand-still; his pains had gone and returned, and the feeling of coldness in the arm still remained. This condition of the patient compelled me to proceed to the galvanization of the sympathetic nerve; the application of this process, which was repeated twelve times, was crowned with such good results, that the patient considered further treatment superfluous, and determined to leave the rest of the cure to nature and cold embrocations of the arm. This hope did not deceive him; on visiting him, August 14, 1867, I found the entire arm well filled out, strong, and capable of every movement. All the muscles of the hand were developed in accordance with their various uses, though not to the same degree as those of the sound hand; the pains had not returned; the temperature was normal.

Whether the mode of practice here prescribed, including especially the galvanization of the sympathetic nerve, can sometimes also afford help in those cases of muscular atrophy in which the disease has attacked not only one or both of the upper extremities but also the lower ones, I dare not decide. At any rate, the experimental application of the process last named is to be recommended, because it may possibly have a central influence.

We must, in conclusion, mention still another form of paralysis, to which Duchenne[1] was the first to draw atten-

[1] Arch. Gén. de Méd., 1860. Sptbr.

tion, giving it the name of "paralysie musculaire progressive de la langue, du voile, du palais, et des lèvres," and which has also been made the subject of observation on the part of Chomel, Trousseau, Empis, Gerhardt, Schultz, and others. This disease—of which in nine years Duchenne had witnessed nineteen cases—attacks, without known cause, persons of forty to sixty years of age, seizing first upon the muscles of the tongue, then those of the soft palate, and at last those of the lips; in only a single case has this order been changed, the paralysis of the velum pendulum and the orbicularis oris preceding that of the tongue. The paralysis of the tongue is made known by a labored articulation and deglutition; the first consists in a difficult enunciation of the palatal and labial sounds, produced by the immovable position of the tongue in the cavity of the mouth; the second is caused by the difficulty of loosening from the walls of the mouth the saliva which is secreted in abundance, and which by its long retention becomes viscous and tenacious. When paralysis of the velum pendulum occurs, the tone of the voice changes, becoming nasal; the enunciation of the labial sounds, formerly natural, becomes indistinct, food and drink are regurgitated through the nose. The paralysis of the orbicularis oris prevents, at last, the contraction of the lips, and impairs the enunciation of *o* and *u*. Sometimes other muscles of the lips are embraced in the attack, as, for example, the levator lab. inf., the triangularis and quadratus menti, while the muscles of the face situated above these—the orbicularis palpebr., the zygomatici, the levator lab. sup. alæque nasi, the buccinatorii, etc.—always remain untouched. The disease is free from fever, digestion is not disturbed by it, but, in consequence of the difficult immission of food, which must necessarily be of a semi-fluid character, the strength of the patient gradually fails; or disturbed respiration and attacks of choking are followed by a hectic fever, which, in periods varying from half a year to three years, brings the sufferings of the patient to a fatal end, no means having yet been found to check the course of the disease, much less to effect its cure. The electric condition of the muscles of the tongue, the lips, and the soft palate, is uniformly normal.

In differential diagnosis, the disease is liable to be confounded with double facial paralysis—a fault into which I myself fell in the only case which I have yet had an opportunity of observing. In the latter malady, as in the former, the muscles of the lips are attacked, the velum pendulum is often affected, deglutition is difficult, and the speech indistinct and toneless; but, on the other hand, the preservation of the motor power of the tongue, the unchanged quality of the voice, the contemporaneous paralysis of the higher muscles of the face, and other indications, will, upon closer attention, present sure diagnostic criteria. In rare cases this disease may be associated with progressive muscular atrophy; it must, however, be distinguished from it, for, while in the latter the restriction of the motor power coincides in point of time with the degree of nutritive disturbance, in the former the paralysis always constitutes the first symptom.

Concerning the essential nature of this disease we know nothing positive. Duchenne's theory of its peripheric seat in certain muscles provided with the hypoglossus, the motor branch of the trigeminus (vagus), and with the facial nerve, is contradicted by the few dissections thus far made, especially by that reported by Gerhardt[1], who discovered in the pons varolii an unnaturally soft spot, violet brown in color, of the size of a pea, in which reddish-blue vascular lines and points could be seen with the naked eye, and also by that made by Schultz,[2] who discovered an atheromatose process on the basilar artery and osseous formations in the medulla oblongata. Schultz, in his interesting work, above

---

[1] Jena'sche Zeitung für Medicin und Naturwissenschaften. Band i., Heft ii., 1864.

[2] Berträge zu den Motilitäts-störungen der Zunge, in the Wiener Med. Wochenschrift, 1864. Nos. 38, 39.

mentioned, endeavors to explain the disease, even without the participation of the hypoglossus, as a bilateral partial paralysis of the facial nerve, for, according to him, the partial immobility of the tongue is occasioned exclusively by the deeper position of the hyoid bone, produced by the paralysis of the posterior belly of the digastricus and that branch of the facial nerve distributed to the stylo-hyoideus.

Duchenne publishes in his work[1] the following case, which he attended in company with Chomel, in the year 1852, and which first afforded him an opportunity of making out a complete synopsis of the symptoms of this disease:

The affection, induced by some unknown cause, began, about seven months before Chomel's examination of the case, with a difficulty of deglutition and of speech, which for the first two months was scarcely regarded. This difficulty gradually increased; deglutition became labored, and the saliva flowed from the mouth; the enunciation was rendered confused, and finally unintelligible. After a fruitless trial of various remedies, the patient was introduced to Chomel, who immediately perceived that the case was one of an affection of those muscles which are employed in articulation and deglutition, and called upon Duchenne to make an electric examination. The tongue was pressed down, and, as it were, fixed behind the lower row of teeth; its upper surface was somewhat furrowed; its power of motion was much restricted; the patient could neither raise the point, nor apply its upper surface to the palate; it could only be moved a little forward and laterally, the velum pendulum and the uvula exhibited no deformation, and contracted naturally when mechanically irritated. The voice was nasal, but of normal power, though the patient was obliged, in speaking, to make extraordinary efforts, which were undoubtedly necessitated by the immobility of the tongue. The patient could not whistle or blow out a light, except when he held his nose; and in like manner the articulation

[1] L. c., page 622.

of the labials "b" and "p" was less distinct when the nose was open than when it was closed. The mouth was always full of viscous saliva, which the patient could not spit out, having to remove it with a napkin. When he drank, he was obliged to pause at each swallow; a portion of the fluid, thus laboriously swallowed, was regurgitated through the nose. He could not appropriate solid food except when it had been cut up into small pieces and was previously moistened, and he had then to masticate it a long time. The tongue's sense of touch, as well as of taste, was not impaired; though the respiratory movements were regular, labored breathing was from time to time exhibited; for the last two months, weakness and emaciation had been added, although the assimilative and executive functions of the muscles of the limbs and trunk were still undisturbed. The electro-muscular contractility of the tongue and the muscles of the face, as well as those of the soft palate, had not suffered in the least. The employment for two weeks of the process of faradization had given volume to the tongue, and had rendered its surface smoother, and its movements as well as those of the lips easier, and the enunciation more distinct. This treatment, however, had had no influence upon the difficulty of deglutition and the excessive secretion of saliva; the introduction of a rheophore into the pharynx and the œsophagus had no effect upon these symptoms,[1] and accordingly the unfortunate patient went home, where, after a few months, he died by choking. Broth and milk were, during his last days, introduced into the œsophagus, without, however, appeasing the pangs of hunger.

[1] Schulz was able to check the superfluous secretion of saliva (which, as Claude Bernard has shown, is the result of a section of the facial nerve), by the galvanization of the facial nerve, and to excite a perfect act of deglutition by the irritation of the hypoglossus.

NINTH SECTION.

ELECTRICITY AS A CURATIVE AGENT.

In each of the three departments into which the art of healing is divided—medicine, surgery, and obstetrics—electricity has been employed with success.

In medicine especially it has proved of service in the cure of so many heterogeneous maladies, and has, according to the testimony of various authors, so frequently accomplished results of a wonderful, not to say incredible character, that a review of the vast amount of material dispersed through the various medical journals—in which the true is mingled with the false, intentional with unintentional deceptions, and so many superficial and unsatisfactory observations of cases prevail—would be a work of the severest labor; yet, in view of the many interesting reports of successful practice, published by scientific observers, such a review would greatly enrich the healing art. The diseases in which electricity has shown itself most efficacious are those that attack the nerves, and those that depend upon anomalous secretions and excretions.

In the chirurgical art, though electricity has been but a short time in this field of practice, it has achieved results not less satisfactory, and has won a permanent and important place, not only in consequence of the application of electrothermic processes in galvano-caustic operations, and of electro-chemical processes in the cure of varices and aneurisms, but also in consequence of the influence of the electric current, as scientifically established and practically confirmed, in the dispersion of exudations and tumors. Many other chemical operations, as the solution of calculi in the bladder, and the removal of poisonous metals from the system, are theoretically possible, as has been experimentally proven, but in practical medicine have been utilized in but few cases. But, on the other hand, the transportation of medicaments by means of the continuous current—an assumed operation which Klenke and Hassenstein have made so much of—has not been verified in practice; the investigations of Pelikan and Savelieff have, on the contrary, shown that even a transportation of iodine from one electrode to another, when due care and foresight are exercised against error, does not take place.[1]

In obstetrics, finally, the electric current has been applied by the English, to excite the activity of the parturient efforts, and to arrest metrorrhagia, and more recently by the French to overcome version and prolapsus of the womb; in Germany, little progress has as yet been made in the use of electricity in this branch of the healing art.

[1] A point, however, of great interest and diagnostic importance, is the use of the electric current in discovering the locality of a metallic body, which has been forcibly projected into the system. When Garibaldi was wounded by a rifle-ball in the ankle, it became necessary to decide whether the ball was still seated in the wounded spot. For this purpose, Nélaton fastened two metallic probes to the conducting wires of a single element, united with a multiplicator, and, without permitting them to touch, inserted them into the wound till they came in contact with some hard substance lying in their path; a marked deviation of the magnetic needle proved that a metallic connection of the probes was effected, and accordingly the ball was found and removed, and the wound perfectly healed.

CHAPTER I.

THE USE OF ELECTRICITY IN MEDICINE.

I. ELECTRICITY IN NERVOUS DISEASES.

A. *Hyperæsthesia—Neuralgia.*

In consequence of the uncertainty which has in general attended that treatment of neuralgia which aims at a removal of the cause—for, as Romberg remarks, in but few cases, and only where the disease is of brief standing, has this treatment been crowned with success—practitioners found themselves compelled to resort to other means. But neither the section of the suffering nerve, nor the internal employment of narcotics, nor the application of specific agents, as turpentine, arsenic, quinine, etc., has led to satisfactory results. The most numerous cures were still accomplished by the application to the external skin of revulsive agents, either in the form of mustard-plasters and irritating washes, or of vesicants and cauterants. The use of the burning-irons was particularly recommended by Jobert de Lamballe, and this mode of treatment, when united with the anæsthetic action of ether and chloroform, found a warm eulogist in Valleix.[1]

In more recent times, two other remedial agents have been brought into use, which are at once more easy of application, and more effective than those already named. These are electricity and hypodermic injections. But, while the latter, as A. Eulenburg says,[2] may be used with almost absolute certainty as palliatives, and in many cases as radical

---

[1] Guide du Médecin practicien. Paris, 1851. Tome iv., page 314.
[2] Die Hypodermatische Injection der Argnsmittel. Berlin, 1865. Page 71.

cures, yet electricity, on the other hand, affords, in by far the greatest number of cases of peripheric neuralgia, a satisfactory means of treatment.

The modes of application which have been employed are various: 1. Induction electricity in the form of the electric brush. 2. The induction current conducted by means of moist electrodes through the affected nerves. 3. The constant, or, according to Remak, stable current. 4. The perpetual galvanic current, as Hiffelsheim names it.

In regard to the first method, Duchenne applies the current to the skin in the neighborhood of the painful parts, first having dried the surface very thoroughly, and applied an absorbent powder. By this means the current is prevented penetrating to the deep-seated parts, and thus possibly increasing the pain.

In very chronic cases—especially in sciatic affections of long standing—where the strongest current, applied in the prescribed manner, does not produce an adequate degree of pain, Duchenne places an electric pencil upon the ear, or the ala of the nose. I have seen the intense irritation of the skin by means of the electric pencil, as recommended by Duchenne, successful in only those cases in which, in addition to neuralgia, a more or less extensive anæsthesia of the skin existed, and in which, consequently, the nerve which was deprived of the power of conducting the impression of the sense was nevertheless painfully affected—a condition which finds its explanation in the law of excentric manifestations.

Case 45.—Rothardt, a postman, fifty-four years old, being much exposed by his occupation to colds, and having suffered for a number of years with chronic catarrh, together with emphysema of the inferior lobe of the left lung, was attacked about the middle of the cold and wet January of 1854, without any direct cause that could be indicated, with a severe pain in the shoulder-blade, which extended afterward to the upper arm, then to the forearm, and finally to the hand, being especially severe in the third metacarpal space, and extending thence into the little finger, the ring-finger, and the ulnar side of the middle finger. The pain was boring and tearing, but not equally severe at every hour of the day; it was generally most violent in the morning hours, and in the course of the day subsided into a dull painful sensation, and at night ceased altogether. Every attempt to grasp any thing with the hand, immediately excited the pain, if not already present, and increased it when it was present, so that the patient was unfit for service. After he had for a long time employed sudorifics and exciting washes, and had thus subdued the violence of the pain in the shoulder, upper arm, and forearm, he came, January 31st, to me. Externally he presented no abnormal appearance, but a pressure upon the third metacarpal space was extraordinarily painful. The skin of the ulnar side of the hand, the little finger, the ring-finger, and half of the middle finger, was completely insensible (neuralgia et anæsthesia ulnaris). Upon a single application of the electric pencil, moved here and there over the anæsthetic parts of the skin, with force sufficient to excite a painful sensation, the patient immediately felt a marked alleviation of his sufferings, the stagnant feeling in the fingers was lessened, and, when portions of the skin, formerly insensible, were touched, a weak sensation was felt. On the next morning the pains were less severe and of briefer duration. At the end of the second sitting—February 1st—the sensibility of the skin on the inner and dorsal surfaces of the metacarpus was normal, and on the little finger improved; but it still remained about the same as before on the ring-finger and the ulnar side of the middle finger. On the following day, only an insignificant degree of pain remained, and Rothardt was already able to lift a chair. After the third sitting, the sensibility of the skin was perfectly normal, the stagnant feeling was gone, nor did any of the painful symptoms recur. On February 6th, the patient was again ready for service.

On the other hand, in numerous cases of neuralgia affecting the most dissimilar nerves—the ischiadicus, the plexus brachialis, the plexus cervicalis, the trigeminus, the Mm. intercostales, etc.—I have, with the happiest results, applied the electric pencil as a moxa, in the following manner:

I generally select, without, however, ascribing special importance to the points of application, either such places as lie as near as possible to the nerve on its egress from the central organ, or, with still greater preference, such as lie immediately over the nerve where it courses beneath the skin, and which are frequently discoverable by a special painfulness under the pressure of the finger (points douloureux). Thus, in the case of the sciatic nerve, I select the spot where it leaves the incisura ischiadica, or where it runs behind the trochanter major, or, if the pain extends still higher, at its point of egress from the for. intervertebralia. In neuralgia of the trigeminus, I operate upon the upper posterior part of the neck. Applying one pencil firmly to the point selected, I hold the other (just as Jobert does with the heating-irons) at a distance of about half a line from the skin and pretty near the first. This position is retained for a period varying from a few seconds to a minute, during which the sparks escape to the skin, with a distinct crackling sound; the fine hairs of the skin are raised, the skin becomes red; repeated applications on the same spot—where the skin is especially irritable, one only—will produce cauterization, and, in cases where the blood is in a bad condition, the livid mark of a bruise. The pain excited by this process is intensely severe; it may, however, be diminished or abbreviated at pleasure, according to the duration and severity of the neuralgia, its situation, the sensitiveness of the skin, etc. If it is requisite to operate upon only a small portion of the skin, as, for example, in the case of an intercostal neuralgia, instead of the pencil, a small, moist, pointed piece of sponge can be used to transmit the sparks. Sometimes, after a single application, the pain disappears and does not return; but generally it recurs again on the next day with abated intensity. Sometimes, soon after the application, a new attack comes on, which greatly exceeds in duration and severity those which have regularly occurred, but this is followed by a marked alleviation of the neuralgic pains. Frequently from one to three applications of the prescribed kind are sufficient to effect a cure, but generally six to eight are needed, and only in deep-rooted chronic cases of many years' standing, or when the patient is in a weak, decrepit condition, is a greater number of sittings (sometimes from forty to fifty) necessary to a complete cure. Among cases of peripheric neuralgia, those only seem to resist this mode of treatment which have their origin in some deeper organic affection, or in a mechanical cause, as a nervous tumor, a carious tooth, or in neuritis or periostitis.

The physiological action of the electric pencil, in cases of neuralgia, is probably the same as in all epispastica, namely, reflex. O. Neumann[1] has proved experimentally that weak electric irritations effect a decided acceleration in the flow of the blood combined with an evident contraction of the vessels, and a more energetic action of the heart; that, on the other hand, powerful irritations effect an evident retardation of the blood, combined with an expansion of the vessels, and a diminished action of the heart; and he consequently considers the change in the capacity of the vessels, and the activity of the heart, sufficient to explain the clinical effects of epispastica. The electric moxa, however, has an advantage over the epispastic preparations in common use, in the suddenness of the intense pain which it excites, and the facility with which this pain may be renewed at any moment, as required, in consequence of which the patient cannot accustom himself to it, and thus lose a part of its effect.

[1] Untersuchungen uber die physiologischen Wirkungen der Hautreizmittel. Prager Vierteljahrschrift. 1863. Page i.-xviii.

Case 46.—S., a school-councillor, a healthy man, about sixty-five years of age, had suffered for the last two years with a left sciatica, which for fourteen months had stubbornly resisted all remedies, but finally yielded under the employment of "vesicatoires volants," which were applied along the course of the nerve. On the 14th September, 1854, when he had been, for a few preceding days, suffering anew with sciatica of the same leg, I applied, at the request of his physician, the Geh. Rath. Eckard, an electric moxa, and, having repeated this treatment, on the 16th and 19th of September, dismissed the patient, completely and permanently cured.

Case 47.—B., a merchant, forty-four years old, formerly healthy, but recently rendered nervously excitable by harassing emotions, had suffered for six months with sciatica of the right side, which had been contracted in the beginning of October, 1857, as the result of a railroad accident that had befallen him on his way to Leipsic. The pain, which during his stay in Leipsic was endurable, gradually increased so much in violence that on his return to Berlin he was compelled to keep his bed for some time. Neither cupping nor embrocations were sufficient to remove the pains, which extended along the posterior side of the thigh, and from the knee down the inner side of the leg to the foot; they were increased by walking and every movement of the person, and were only quieted at night, when the body was in perfect repose; within the last fourteen days they had come on with renewed and intolerable severity. On the 21st of March, 1858, the first application of the electric pencil was made, the spot selected being one which was painful to the touch, situated behind the trochanter major; the pains disappeared at once, but recurred the next day, though with diminished severity. After the second sitting—March 23d—the pains decreased daily, and the patient was able to walk considerable distances without suffering, and only experienced a light drawing sensation in the spots formerly painful, making a third sitting necessary on March 27th.

CASE 48.—Mr. S. Rosenberg, thirty-five years of age, had been suffering for two months with a pain in the right shoulder, which passed over to the upper part of the arm, and followed the course of the ulna along the inner side of the arm down to the little finger, occasioning a partial paralysis of the hand, and hindering the patient in writing. By the application of uncleaned wool the pain was driven off, but, when at last this was removed, it returned with renewed violence, and for the last two weeks had undergone no alleviation day or night. The elevation of the arm was especially painful, and the feeling of numbness had extended into the fingers. An examination showed a neuralgia of the right supra scapularis, for the removal of which, the patient, at the suggestion of the sanitary councillor, Herzberg, applied to me, March 24, 1857. A pressure upon the N. supraspinatus, immediately above the collum scapulæ at the point where the nerve passes from the fossa supraspinata into the fossa infraspinata, excited an intense pain; the extension of the pain to the little finger and ring-finger, and the stagnant feeling which was associated with this pain, indicated the participation of the N. ulnaris. The electric pencil having been applied in the manner described, to the spot—lying above the spina scapulæ, which was so sensitive to pressure—the pain immediately disappeared and the patient slept well on the following night. The second application—March 26th—removed the feeling of heaviness and stagnation in the forearm and fingers.

CASE 49.—Gustavus Lehnhardt, a smith, twenty-three years old, apparently not very strong, was seized, probably in consequence of extraordinary exertion in his work, with a pain which extended from the furrow between the condyl. extern. and the olecranon of the right arm to the interior side of the elbow, and radiated, particularly when the arm was turned outward, to the forearm and to the little and ring-fingers. The pains, which, during the day and while the patient was at rest, were comparatively unimportant, increased in violence at night and with every movement of the arm, and at last compelled the patient to suspend his work. Fourteen days later, after a fruitless application of irritating lotions, he came to me, October 30, 1866, for treatment. I found a pressure upon the spot above indicated very painful to the patient (N. ulnaris dextra); there was no anæsthesia of the lower part of the inner side of the forearm. After a single powerful application of the electric pencil near the sensitive spot, the pain disappeared, leaving only a feeling of tension in the soft parts of the elbow, which, without further application of electricity, was fully removed in a few days by rubbing with warm oil.

CASE 50.—Mrs. A. F., thirty-five years old, a woman of small stature, graceful in form, and of a lively temperament, the mother of several children, had been suffering for the last seven years with a considerable degree of anæmia. On January 9, 1856, while present at an evening company, she caught a cold, which brought on a severe griping pain in the left ear and shoulder. Her domestic affairs having at the same time called forth unusual exertions, this and a perturbed emotional condition excited, about January 16th, a feverish state united with palpitation of the heart, labored breathing, and tearing pains in various parts of the body. A light antiphlogistic treatment, continued for fourteen days, removed all of these symptoms except the pains in the limbs, which harassed the patient more especially at night; these after a while concentrated in the left shoulder, extended thence into the left ear, and soon attacked the third branch of the trigeminus. On the 28th of January the pains, thus located, attacked her in a new and peculiar manner; the pain in the face came on like a flash, lasted from five to ten minutes, and then as quickly passed off. At first these attacks recurred after intervals of considerable length, afterward they visited her daily about ten o'clock in the evening, but always lasted but a few minutes; gradually they increased in frequency, intensity, and duration, being at last repeated five or six times a day, when they included also the other branches of the trigeminus, and robbed the patient of rest at night for whole weeks. Quinine, arsenic, a tonic diet, the removal as far as possible of all causes of excitement, a salve of veratrum—all were tried with none or at most but doubtful effect, and the patient consequently, upon the advice of Drs. Philipp and Friedländer, applied to me, May 3, 1856, for a trial of electric treatment. After the first sitting a marked exacerbation of the pains occurred; they raged for more than fourteen hours with the most fearful intensity; they then, however, underwent a marked subsidence, and after two applications repeated on the 5th and 9th, with weaker currents, the neuralgic symptoms completely and permanently disappeared.

CASE 51.—H., a building-inspector, a weakly, nervous young man, of pale-yellow complexion, had suffered for several weeks with an intense pain which, occasioned by some unknown cause, frequently attacked him, but always after mental exertion and emotional disturbance. Its principal seat was in the region of the interior angle of the left eye, but it often extended from this spot to the forehead and the left nasal cavity; it was fought, though unsuccessfully, with narcotics and metallic preparations. Whenever the pain came on, the lachrymal caruncle of the left eye, as well as the eyelids, particularly those parts near the interior angle of the eye, became red, and an excessive secretion of tears ensued. When the pain reached its height, which it regularly did in the morning hours, the lower jaw was convulsively turned upon the axis of the right proc. condyloideus, and the teeth of the left side ground together. The case thus presented was a neuralgia of the first branch of the trigeminus, including, secondarily, that branch of the motor portion of the trigeminus supplying the M. pterygoideus minor—a diagnosis with which the patient's physician, Dr. Housselle, agreed, and which was clearly indicated by the pain which a pressure upon the for. supraorbitale and the spina trochlearis produced. After the electric pencil had been applied —July 31 and August 2, 1860—in the region of the for. supraorbitale, a complete cessation of the pain followed, and, during an absence on my part of four weeks, only a few brief attacks of the pain recurred, brought on by the severe mental labor to which the patient's professional pursuits sometimes subjected him. Since then he has been in good health.

CASE 52.—Lieutenant von H., thirty-two years old, had been attacked four years previously, as the result of a cold, with a severe pain in the right shoulder, which continued for a long time, and greatly exhausted the patient. In the course of the subsequent years it had been frequently repeated, but often lasted only a short time, sometimes but a few days or hours, and was variable in its intensity, a dull pain being often interrupted by a severe shooting pain; it always, however, yielded to the use of Russian baths. Two months ago, he was again visited by his old foe, but on this occasion he ascribed its attacks to the circumstance of his having, when his head was heated, put on his helmet after it had lain all night on the moist earth. The customary remedy, Russian baths, had this time no effect; the pain increased daily, deprived the patient of his night's rest, and rendered him incapable of mental activity. During a period of eight to fourteen days it was seldom absent, although, while it preserved its general character, it was not at all times of the same intensity. On the 30th of October, 1858, on the advice of the brigade physician, Dr. Pesch, the patient came to me. He looked as if nervously affected; he described his pain as griping, shooting, intolerable, it went from the right posterior region of the neck above the os occipitale and extended thence behind the ear, on the right side of the head, to the crown, sometimes also to the right shoulder and down the right arm; the right processus transversus of the atlas, and the tuber parietale, were very sensitive under pressure. The case was accordingly a neuralgia occipitalis dextra. After the first sitting there was an immediate cessation of the suffering, and at night a quiet undisturbed sleep was enjoyed. A recurrence of the pain in a light form, generally toward evening, made a repetition of the treatment necessary on the 3d and again on the 5th of November. There then arose a furuncle on the spot which had been irritated, and the pains wholly ceased, nor have they since returned.

CASE 53.—Mrs. R., fifty-six years old, though subject to various nervous afflictions, had, however, remained tolerably healthy till she reached her climacteric year; since this time, however, she had been suffering with hæmorrhages, and had been so much troubled with piles that finally, in the winter of 1854, she was obliged to have an operation performed on them. This operation, which was otherwise successful, was followed by a violent pain that, proceeding from the loins, followed the right ischiadicus down to the foot. Gradually this pain passed off; but about a year later, just after the patient had been subjected to an unusual degree of emotion, sciatica of the right side again occurred, and, notwithstanding the employment of various antagonistic agents, increased daily in severity. The patient could not endure to stand or walk long at a time; she complained of a feeling of cold, stagnation, and deadness in the leg, especially in the lower part. The intensity of the pain robbed her of sleep, and accordingly when I visited the patient—February 7, 1856—I found her in a very exhausted condition. Forty applications of the electric pencil were in this case needed for a complete removal of the affection, but the amount of uric acid in the urine of the patient, as well as various swellings in the labia of the pudenda—which broke out five months after the completion of the cure, on her return from Marienbad—indicated very clearly a condition of dyscrasia.

The following case is one of more interest, because in it the employment of the mode of treatment which has been described was adequate to the permanent removal of a neuralgia of the left medianus, the Nn. thoracic. ant. and the N. thorac. post., evidently caused by a tuberculous process of the cervical vertebræ.

CASE 54.—Friedrich Muës, a compositor, thirty-five years old, who, up to the year 1850, had always been healthy, fell sick in August of that year with the cholera, which left, as a result, a diarrhœa that lasted till May, 1852. In the following year tuberculosis pulmonum had been gradually developed, and, since Christmas of 1853, severe pains, which could not be traced to any exciting cause, broke out on the left side of the neck adjoining the spine, extending from this place forward to the region of the left nipple, and posteriorly to the shoulder, compelling the patient, January 1854, to give up work. Cuppings, embrocations, and rest, had moderated the pain, so that Muës was able in two weeks to resume work, but, soon after, the pain had recurred with renewed violence, extending from the place described to the left upper arm, then to the forearm, and finally to the hand of the same side, including the index and middle fingers. The patient had at the same time experienced in these parts a feeling of stagnation and paralysis, as well as a constant painful itching which was excited to an extreme by the use of the fingers. The pain increased at night as well as whenever, by a recumbent position, the parts attacked were subjected to pressure. The remedies which had been applied had produced no effect; and Muës, on the 19th of May, 1854, upon the advice of his physician, applied to me for electric treatment. Pressure upon the four lower procc. transversi of the cervical vertebræ on the left side, as well as pressure on the medianus at the inner side of the upper arm, excited intense pain. The skin of the left index and middle fingers, especially at the points, was anæsthetic.

In this case the electric pencil was applied in the manner

described upon the sensitive proce. transversi; but also, in order to the reduction of the anæsthesia, the affected parts of the skin were stroked with the pencil for about five minutes. After only the first sitting, the patient experienced an essential improvement. After the sixth sitting—June 5th—the anæsthesia at the points of the fingers was removed, pressure upon the proce. transversi was not so keenly felt; the patient could grasp different objects without pain, and his nightly rest was undisturbed. After the twelfth sitting —June 18th—the patient was dismissed cured. I saw him again two years later, a short time before his death, which was caused, toward the end of 1856, by pulmonary consumption.

An abscess was formed on the left side adjoining the upper dorsal vertebræ, caused probably by a carious process of the lower dorsal vertebræ. Since the electric treatment, the neuralgic pains had not returned.

The electric pencil, applied in the manner described, often produces still another favorable effect. In consequence of the intense cutaneous irritation which it causes, it excites, by a reflex action, venous bleedings within the cavity of the pelvis (the pressure, thus induced, probably occasioning the phenomena exhibited by the sciatic nerve), or else, in cases where there exists an impetiginous tendency, it excites, by direct action, exanthematic developments, such as boils, impetiginoid eczema, etc., with the appearance of which the neuralgic symptoms pass off. I adopted this mode of treatment in the case of an officer who, four years before he came under my care, had suffered a slight hæmorrhage, and who now was affected with a double sciatica, which, after the hæmorrhoidal bleeding which followed the third electric sitting, immediately and permanently disappeared.

CASE 55.—The post-revisor, R., fifty-seven years old,

from his youth had been subjected to rheumatic attacks, which always held on for a long time, frequently for years; thus for many years he suffered with an exudation in the tendon achilles, and also for a long time with a rheumatic inflammation of the eyes, which almost utterly destroyed the sight of the left eye; finally, with a swelling of the wrist. In April, 1857, he was attacked with sciatica of the left side, which, notwithstanding the employment of cuppings, purgatives, and narcotics, increased in severity, rendering a sitting or recumbent posture excessively painful. Standing and walking were impossible; in the night, especially, the patient suffered fearfully. Having, at the request of Dr. Koerte, visited the patient—May 3, 1857—I found him with his legs drawn up in a cramped manner upon the abdomen, as every other position increased his tortures to an extreme degree. Pressure upon the ischiadicus behind the trochanter was very painful. On the first application of the electric pencil, the pains immediately subsided, and the patient passed a quiet night. The third sitting—May 7th—completed the cure. There then broke out a severe itching eruption, of an eczematous character, which especially affected the left leg, and continued for months with greater or less intensity. The patient is still much subject to cutaneous eruptions. Since the treatment, the pains have not returned.

Sometimes the desired result is attained by the milder treatment previously mentioned, and which consists in transmitting through the affected nerve, by means of moist electrodes, an induced current of moderate strength, lasting from five to ten minutes. The mode of application depends upon the capacity of the current to reduce directly the irritability of the nerves. In consequence of the slight pain which this operation causes, it is well, in the case of very irritable patients, to give it the first trial, though in certainty of result it stands far behind the method already described.

CASE 56.—Carl Maass, thirty-four years of age, a journeyman baker, short and thick-set in form, previously healthy, had for the last few years been frequently subject to rheumatism, and, about three months before the treatment of his case, had been suddenly seized with an attack of lumbago, to which was soon afterward added a continuous pain in the posterior and lateral portions of the right thigh, extending to the knee. The pains were particularly intense in stormy weather, very severe at night; and whenever, after sitting a long time, the patient stood up, they became so intense, that he was often obliged to support himself with both hands before he was able to take a step. Cuppings, vesicants, and Russian baths, were employed with none or at least but transitory effect. The patient had consequently found himself compelled to give up his employment, which was one requiring a standing posture. On the 19th of April, 1861, he applied to me for treatment. He complained of a constant, penetrating pain, near the tuberosity of the ischium adjoining the point of egress of the N. ischiadicus, which from evening to midnight was especially severe, but did not trouble him during the morning hours; it was greatly intensified by pressure. The skin over the suffering parts was, when pinched, very sensitive; but, on the other hand, the pressure of the femur on the cotyloid cavity produced no pain; the appetite was good, evacuations regular, pulse normal. One of the conductors, having been applied in combination with the apparatus of Stöhrer, to the point of egress of the sciatic nerve, the other behind the capitulum fibulæ, a current of about ten minutes' duration was transmitted. The patient was at once able to walk with more ease; he still went up-stairs laboriously, but, by treading carefully, he could go down without pain. The pains continued till past midnight, and recurred again late in the following evening, though with much less intensity than before, and toward midnight passed off. After the third application of induction-electricity, made in a similar manner, and for the same length of time, the sciatica disappeared, and the patient returned from Spandau to Berlin—a distance of about two miles—on foot, so as to assure himself of the perfect success of the cure.

Becquerel[1] reports the following cure of a case of neuralgia supraorbitalis:

A servant-maid, nineteen years of age, was seized about the end of August, 1856, with a neuralgia supraorbitalis duplex, which came on daily about eleven o'clock, and kept increasing in intensity till two at night; up to four of the afternoon it was sufficiently endurable to permit the patient to discharge her regular duties, but from five to two at night, it was so intense that the forehead and eyelids suffered severe convulsive twitchings, and the patient screamed with the pain. At two o'clock the pain began to subside, and at five ceased altogether, permitting the patient to sleep till eleven, when the attack renewed its former course. Quinine, opium, and morphine, were employed endermatically and otherwise till the end of October, without assuaging the violence of the attacks or lessening their duration. Becquerel at this time brought electric treatment to the patient's help, and for three successive days—always at one o'clock—applied an intermittent induction current of moderate strength, and of ten to fifteen minutes' duration, to the temporal and supraorbital region. On each occasion the attack ceased, and the patient remained free from pain till six o'clock. Becquerel then applied the treatment twice a day—at one and at six—and in ten days a complete and permanent cure was effected.

The following case is especially interesting, in which, probably in consequence of a periostitis of the metacarpal bone of the left thumb, a neuralgia of the left radial nerve

---

[1] Traité des applications de l'électricité à la Thérapeutique. Paris, 1857. Page 270.

ensued, which, progressing gradually, soon affected not only the arm and leg of the same side, but also proceeded to the right arm, and which was entirely cured after sixteen applications of a mild induced current across the primarily-affected bone.

CASE 57.—Miss Marie S., a nervous girl seventeen years of age, while jumping out of a cab on November 23, 1862, injured, either through the forcible opening of the door, or in consequence of her falling upon her left arm, the ball of the thumb of her left hand, which soon became tender and painful. Neither arnica lotions, nor compression by means of a bandage for fourteen days, alleviated the pain, till finally the application of leeches and warm poultices relieved the patient sufficiently to enable her toward New Year's to walk without carrying the arm in a sling. After a few days, however, perhaps in consequence of a cold, the pain reappeared stronger than before. Now, not only the thumb began to swell, but also the whole hand; warm poultices and the repeated application of leeches failed to give any relief, the hand grew thicker and stiffer; the pain now attacked the index and middle finger, and thence extended along the arm, shoulder, and back, into the left leg; and then the right arm also became painful, while the right hand likewise was affected at certain times with violent pains.

Upon the advice of Dr. Kloatsch, the patient consulted me for the first time on January 22, 1863. As a pressure upon the metacarpal bone of the thumb was felt very much by the patient, an induced and slightly painful current was directed through it by means of wet conductors. After the third application the motion of the left hand became easier, the swelling and the pain diminished, especially the pain felt in the right arm, and that in the left leg ceased entirely. The next thirteen applications, in which the same method was employed, sufficed to render the arm free from pain by the end of the month of February, and also to fit the hand for every kind of manual labor.

The third method, the treatment of neuralgia by means of the continuous current, is employed in such a manner that the positive pole is applied as nearly as possible to the centre (upon the nervous ramification or the nervous root in neuralgia of the trigeminus, at the cervical vertebra near the mastoid process), while the negative pole is placed upon the several painful points in the course of the respective nerves, or, in case such cannot be found, in the vicinity of the peripheral terminations of the nerves, and the current is allowed to act in this manner usually for the period of from two to five minutes. Concerning the strength of the current, from 6 to 10 elements are mostly sufficient where the trigeminus is affected, while a neuralgia of the brachial nerves or of the great sacro-sciatic nerve requires from 20 to 40 elements, in order to obtain a deflection of the galvanometer-needle of 5° up to 20°, which is mostly sufficient. The feeling of tension in the muscles which often accompanies a neuralgia, and especially sciatica, is usually soon relieved through a few interruptions by means of the metallic current-changer. Usually the pain is already, after the first application, alleviated, if the employment of the current is to be successful at all. Yet but a few cases are benefited in three to five applications; usually, the treatment must be continued for five or six weeks, in order to remove all morbid symptoms, and it must be borne in mind that, as soon as the symptoms are considerably diminished, the last residues, the removal of which requires the longest time, disappear gradually by themselves under the employment of the proper treatment. According to my opinion, the electric moxa cures the affection quicker than the continuous current; the latter, however, is much less painful, and on that account to be preferred in the treatment of irritable patients; the latter is also especially indicated in those not rare cases in which a swelling of the neurilemma (neuritis), or a periostitis, is the cause of the disease. I prefer to employ, in the last mentioned cases, the *polar method*, by applying the positive conductor to the inflamed, the negative pole, however, to any remote and less tender spot, in order to avoid every irritation of the nerve through the negative electrode. The same method, namely, the application of the positive pole to the irritated place, with the simultaneous application of the negative electrode to a more remote point, is to be employed in such cases of tic douloureux, etc., where Remak found the starting-point of the pain in one of the cervical ganglia of the sympathetic nerve, and which he cured through this method. We shall communicate his observations which are published in the Berlin Klin. Wochenschrift of 1864, page 229. The manner of action of the continuous current in neuralgia is explained partially through the irritation of the skin, partially through the diminished excitability in consequence of the long-lasting influence; in those cases, finally, in which the neuralgia is caused by hyperæmia and swelling of the neurilemma or by an irritation of the sympathetic ganglia, through the removal of the existing anatomical changes.[1]

CASE 58.—Mrs. D., aged fifty-four years, midwife, after having assisted for several days in succession in some difficult confinements, experienced a violent pain beginning between the fifth and seventh dorsal vertebræ, and extending thence to the right and anterior parts in the course of the corresponding ribs. The pain, which prevented a complete inspiration, rendered the erect position of the body difficult, and only ceased in the night when the patient kept perfectly quiet. It had already lasted for three weeks, during which period neither cups applied to the back, nor embrocations of chloroform, gave any relief when she desired my aid for the removal of an intercostal neuralgia. After the first application, lasting in all from five to six minutes, in which I applied the small conductor connected with the copper pole, successively to the central places of exit of the fifth, sixth, and seventh intercostal nerves, and kept in the same man-

[1] Remak's Catalytic Effects.

ner the zinc pole at the corresponding intercostal spaces near the sternum, a decided mitigation of the pain immediately ensued, and the treatment terminated successfully after the third application, on the 7th of February.

CASE 59. — Our revered colleague, Privy-Councillor Wilm, aged forty-one years, was taken sick at the end of September, 1865, in consequence of a severe cold, with the usual symptoms of an occipital neuralgia. The pains occupied the entire occiput, and thence radiated toward the temporal region. The attacks happened at irregular periods, beginning frequently in the evening, lasting during a part of the night, and preventing the patient from sleeping. As reflex symptoms, spasms appeared in the muscles of the face, neck, and arm. The points of Valleix, tender upon pressure, were proved especially plainly in this case. After the usual remedies, such as the iodide of potass, quinine, flying vesicatories and warm baths, were administered in vain during the months of October and November, the continuous current was employed at the beginning of December. Fifteen applications sufficed entirely to remove the disease, which had weakened very much the strength of the patient, in consequence of its intensity, long durability, and the want of sleep produced by it for weeks. In this case, the polar method was used, so that the positive pole was placed upon the painful points, and the negative pole upon the lateral cervical region. The first application was followed by a quiet and refreshing sleep, while the spasms were considerably diminished.

Remak reports, in his Galvano-Therapeutics (page 442), the following case:

Ferdinand R., a farmer, after having contracted a cold, was, in the beginning of the year 1855, attacked with sciatica which defied all known remedies, and finally, in the month of August, 1856, compelled the physicians to recommend to him a trip to Töplitz. As the pain became unbearable on the way to Berlin, the patient applied to Dr. Remak for advice. The paroxysms were strongest mornings and evenings, and also while the patient was sitting, so that he was obliged to take his dinner partially while standing. He limped while walking, as he stepped on his toes on account of a secondary contraction of the flexor muscles of the thigh. Pressure upon the trunk of the sacro-sciatic nerve caused violent pain. From the 25th to the 29th of August, and therefore for five consecutive days, electric currents, generated in a battery containing from 25 to 30 Daniell's elements, were passed along the course of the nerves down to the external angle for 4 to 5 minutes each time, which relieved the patient so much that he gave up the journey and returned to his home.

Case 60.—Miss C. B., from Rostock, aged twenty years, contracted a sciatica of the right side, in consequence of over-exertion in climbing mountains during the catamenia, which did not yield, in spite of the employment of every imaginable remedy. Every attempt to walk caused pains in the hip, which, after continued walking, extended to the knee, and thence soon after to the external ankle. After standing for a long time, a feeling of weight and numbness ensued in the right leg, which, while lying on her back, was frequently followed by spontaneous pain. The catamenia were regular. At the examination made on the 12th of April, 1866, no tender points could be found along the course of the nerve, only a pressure upon the parts next to the second and third sacral vertebræ was painful, and produced, when long continued, a slight pain, corresponding to the course of the nerve down to the knee. To this spot the copper-pole was fixed, while the zinc-pole was attached to some place in the vicinity of the spine. The patient improved perceptibly after a few applications, yet, not until after forty-nine applications did recovery take place, which, however, was so complete, that, as I was afterward informed, she could gradually make the greatest journeys without any difficulty.

The following is an instructive case of neuralgia of the cervico-brachial plexus, in consequence of neuritis, copied from M. Rosenthal's Electro-Therapeutics:

Th. Schreiber, an old servant, twenty-seven years old, perceived in November, 1862, after having washed in cold water, a sharp pain in the right hand, which, however, did not prevent her performing her accustomed kitchen-work until the end of January, 1863, at which time the pain, becoming more frequent and violent, and spreading from the neck over the arm, together with spasms of the flexor muscles of the fingers, rendered her right hand entirely unfit for every kind of work. Pressure upon the spinous processes produced pain of the cervical vertebræ from the sixth upward, while a swelling of the right half of the neck could be plainly perceived. Pressure in the supraclavicular region upon the brachial plexus of the same side also caused violent pain. Besides one painful point in the lower third of the deltoid muscle, there was also a large number of *points douloureux* along the median, radial, and ulnar nerve, from the shoulder down to the ball of the thumb. The patient designated several of these points as the seat of severe pain. After each paroxysm, a violent reflex spasm of the flexors of the carpus and fingers set in, and the spasmodically closed hand could not be opened even with the use of force. After six to eight hours, gradually first the outer and then the inner fingers relaxed. In this case there was, undoubtedly, an inflammatory swelling of the soft parts of the right half of the neck, caused by the long-continued irritation of cold, which also probably attacked the neurilemma of the brachial plexus. As large doses of quinine, veratrine ointment, and morphine injections, had not prevented a return of the painful paroxysms and spasms, as warm baths had quieted the cramps but for a few hours, and as faradization of the antagonistic muscles repeated eight times had caused a transient and painful stretching of the fingers, without, however, producing any lasting result, Rosenthal proceeded to employ the continuous current, by leading stable plexus-nerve-currents of eight and afterward of twenty of Daniell's elements through the affected extremity. On the morning after the third session, the patient was, for the first time in two months, able to use her right hand in combing her hair. Of the painful points, one situated on the radial nerve between the supinator longus and the brachialis anticus, two, placed in the median and ulnar nerves about an inch above the wrist-joint, resisted longest the influence of galvanization. After fourteen applications, the neuralgia was removed from all points. The spasms of the flexor muscles did not appear during the galvanic treatment, so that, at the beginning of April, she was enabled to reënter upon the discharge of her usual duties.

After she had enjoyed perfect health till the middle of November, the same symptoms reappeared, in consequence of the same cause; namely, her washing again for several hours with cold water. The examination made at the end of November showed the symptoms to be exactly the same as in the first attack, except that the spasms were more severe, and usually existed for more than twenty-four hours. The methodical use of the tepid and steam bath, as well as the employment of the continuous current, produced no change for the better during the first fourteen days. Then the inflammatory symptoms disappeared, the paroxysms assumed a milder form, and the patient felt easier after each application, although twenty applications were necessary to remove all the painful points.

CASE 61.—Mrs. A., twenty-eight years of age, a healthy, strong blonde, had already in March, 1866, while nursing her third child, experienced frequently a feeling of weight and numbness in the thumb and first three fingers of the left hand. Having, in the month of June of the same year, lost two children with the cholera, the morbid sensation increased in violence, and was soon followed by a disturbance of the motor power, so that the hand when semiflexed could not be opened without great pain. Especially in the morning, the hand was closed spasmodically, no relaxation ensuing until some time in the course of the day. The patient in the mean time having again been delivered, and also nursing the child herself, the evil increased every day in spite of all remedies (narcotic embrocations, baths, etc.), until the 13th of August, 1867, when the patient was advised by Dr. Wolff to seek my aid. The hand was half shut; every attempt to open it caused the most violent pain. Besides the sensation of numbness, the patient experienced a feeling as if scalded, especially in the middle fingers, while anæsthesia predominated more in the thumb and index-finger. The arm was thicker above the wrist-joint, and the median nerve perceptibly swollen to the extent of three-quarters of an inch, which proved beyond doubt a neuritis of the median nerve. The conductor connected with the positive pole being applied to this spot, and the other connected with the negative pole placed upon the anæsthetic fingers, a stable current of twenty elements was passed for about five minutes. Having been obliged, on account of a journey, to interrupt the treatment after ten applications (August 23d), the pain had been diminished very much when trying to straighten the hand, which now at times opened spontaneously. The swelling of the arm and the pain produced by pressure upon the median nerve were less; the thumb was entirely and the ring-finger tolerably free from pain.

I saw the patient again on the 10th of November. She had continued to improve; the tenderness of the median nerve, especially across the wrist-joint, and the swelling existing there before, had entirely disappeared upon the use of the iod. of pot. ointment. As, however, the spasm of the hand, although less severe, still continued, and the abnormal sensations in the index and middle finger also existed, I tried to find a second point douloureux; which I soon discovered in the shape of a tender swelling of about half an inch, at the junction of the upper and middle third of the humerus. For this swelling the same treatment was employed, with apparently so good results, that the patient, after fourteen applications, considered herself fully cured on December 5th, and she discontinued the treatment against my wish, as the swelling was not yet entirely removed. She put herself again under my care. The abnormal sensations had not returned, but the hand, and especially the index-finger, was spasmodically closed every morning until 10 A. M. A few more applications sufficed to relieve her entirely.

The following case of tic douloureux cured by means of the continuous current is reported by Remak:

A woman aged thirty-six years, of healthy exterior, who was married ten years since, but without children, observed for the last twelve years that the right half of her face was very sensible while washing it, and that spasms followed upon her face being touched. She thus continued for six years, when she felt, while walking on the street one day in the summer of 1856, as if she had been struck with a club on the right side of her head. Upon looking round, she was astonished to find nobody near her. Since this occurrence, a very violent pain set in, which usually originated at the frontal bone, shooting back into the interior of the head, affecting the lower and upper margin of the orbital cavity, the right half of the tongue, the maxillary bones and teeth, affecting all the parts supplied by the trigeminal nerve at once, or attacking them consecutively, for the last six years, so that she was but for a few intervals free from pain so as to be able to sleep. On the last time the pain had increased to such a degree, that she had hardly any rest even for a few minutes. The slightest touch on the right cheek, for instance, with a handkerchief, or a movement of the mouth while eating or speaking, produced a violent paroxysm of pain. After a few applications, Remak discovered that the spasm and pain ceased for many seconds as soon as he pressed the finger upon the second transverse process of the corresponding right side, but the pain reappeared as soon as the finger relaxed or did not press upon one exactly-defined spot, against which Remak directed the treatment with considerable success from the 5th of March until April, when he was taken sick himself.

In the month of June, the patient again appeared at his office, complaining of unbearable pain, and again the same treatment was followed by a daily increasing improvement. Remak also, in July, discovered that from the same spot were produced *diplegic contractions* in all the muscles of the right arm and hand, and that, consequently, the medulla spinalis cervicalis of the right side existed in a state of increased excitability: one more reason for persevering in the same kind of treatment. After this had been done energetically for several weeks, the paroxysms of pain and spasm—ceasing entirely after each application—decreased day by day in strength and duration until they nearly disappeared in the beginning of August. Remak saw the patient again in August, 1862, and in May, 1864. She was, and remained cured.

4. THE CONSTANT GALVANIC CURRENT OF A CHAIN (for instance, of a Pulvermacher's or Marie Davy's, etc.) is employed by Hiffelsheim[1] not only at stated times, but also daily and nightly for weeks and months (unless particular reasons cause a temporary interruption), in such a manner, that the chain, moistened with vinegar, is applied according to the seat of the pain, to the forehead, chest, hip, etc.

We copy the following observations from the "Annales de l'Électricité," pages 279 and 281 :

Mrs. F., aged fifty years, suffered, twelve years ago, from a sciatica of the right side, lasting for six months. Fourteen

[1] Annales de l'Éctricité médicale, 1860–'61. Allg. Wiener, Med. Zeitung. 1865, No. 8–19.

days ago, an attack ensued which, beginning at the hip, gradually extended to the heel, and increased so much in violence, that she was prevented from walking or standing, while turning in bed became very painful. Hiffelsheim began the treatment on the 27th of July, 1867, by moistening a chain, consisting of 40 elements, with equal parts of vinegar and water, and then placing it spirally around the thigh. On the next morning, the patient declared she had slept better, the pain in the thigh had diminished, in consequence of which she could turn easier in bed. On August 1st, pain existed only in the region of the calf; the patient slept well and sat up in bed. On August 2d she was able to walk. On the 5th, after a storm, she felt pain near the malleolus, which, however, disappeared the following day. On the 18th the patient was discharged cured.

L., twenty-two years of age, a lady's maid, delicate and nervous, was received into the Charité on the 18th of August, while suffering from typhus. Four weeks afterward, having hardly become convalescent, she was taken with a very violent neuralgia of the trigeminus, which extended over the head and face. The head was so tender that she could neither raise it, nor shut the eyes. Chewing and speaking were equally impeded. After four days, the neuralgia was complicated with-drawing pain in the ears and teeth. On the 25th of September she came under the treatment of Dr. Hiffelsheim, who found the following symptoms: the highest degree of insomnolence, no appetite, fever at 5 P. M. Pressure upon the points of exit of all the nerves supplying the head and face was equally painful. A chain of 24 elements, dipped into an equal mixture of vinegar and water, was led from the right temporal region, across the cheek to the chin, a moistened compress having been placed beneath it. The patient slept for an hour during the night. On the next day, little change had taken place, but in the morning of the 27th the pain became tolerable; the pain, however, jumped from one place to another, now from the right to the left side, now from the temporal to the frontal region. For these symptoms, H. applied the chain to the several painful regions for twelve hours in succession. On the 30th the patient had one more violent attack in the teeth. On the 2d of October a general improvement took place. The violent paroxysms and the perforating pain at the bottom of the orbital cavities had ceased. On the 3d of October she considered herself cured, the chain was removed, and the patient was dismissed after the administration of tonics for a few days, for the purpose of strengthening her general health.

The long duration of the treatment usually required by this method, as well as the metastasis of the pain from one nerve to another, indicates, with regard to the discussed methods, the use of the *constant galvanic current only in such cases where neuralgic pains affect nervous individuals simultaneously in many nerves, or where the pain frequently changes its place.*

B. Anæsthesia.

In ANÆSTHESIA OF PERIPHERAL ORIGIN happening to the nerves of the skin in consequence of over-irritation or depression (influence of a very cold temperature), or in consequence of primary spasms of the arteries,[1] or on account of rheumatic influence, or by means of a long-continued pressure, etc., as well as in anæsthesia following hysteria, where it is caused by a changed nutrition of the peripheral nerves; finally, in anæsthesia of the nerves of special sense, which is produced by similar causes, also, by inactivity or want of exercise, a cure may be expected through the electric current, as the reproduction of the nerves of special and general sense is heightened through the increased supply of blood. In anæsthesia caused by a lesion, or section of the nerve, electricity cannot give any relief, unless

[1] See Nothnagel, Deutsches Archiv für klinische Medicin. Band ii., Heft II., page 175, *et seq.*

a union of the injured nerve-ends has taken place by a reproduction of the nervous fibres—a fact the microscopic proof of which occurrence, Steinrück first,[1] and afterward Brown-Séquard, have furnished.

As soon as the nerve-fibres have united, the irritability of the respective nerves returns; the power of motion, however, is still absent, the restitution of which is accomplished by locally stimulating means, and especially by the employment of the electric current. No time can be determined during which a regeneration of the power of sensation after peripheral lesions is possible. It varies from four weeks to three or four years, and never takes place in those cases in which the cicatrix consists exclusively of fibro-cellular tissue followed by no restoration of the nerve-fibres.

In anæsthesia of central origin, however, the peripheral employment of the current is of no use until after the removal of the central cause, which, as will be shown in the chapter on paralysis, is frequently accomplished through the central employment of the current.

It is important to distinguish between cutaneous and muscular anæsthesia (anæsthesia cutanea et muscularis), both of which may occur simultaneously, or one after the other. In the former, the patient is insensible to touch or pain, and is unable to keep the lightest substance in his hands; neither can he determine the probable weight of a body—in the latter case, however, the patient suffering from muscular anæsthesia feels the touch or pain, but the grasp of his hand is powerless; he cannot hold even the slightest body unless he fixes it with his eyes, while those suffering exclusively from cutaneous anæsthesia may weigh the gravity of a body with the affected hand, but are insensible to the superficial or deep touch, and unable to determine the temperature of the substance in contact with the skin. On the other hand, it is necessary to distinguish between anæsthesia (insensibility against an impression caused

[1] See his Dissertatio inauguralis de nervorum generatione. Berol, 1838.

by the special sense against external contact), and analgesia (insensibility against pain), a difference caused probably by a diminished sensibility of the superficial layers of the skin, while the deeper ones may retain the normal amount, or *vice versa*.—In order to form a correct opinion of the degree of diminished sensibility, it is of the greatest importance to know the normal amount of sensibility, which has been ascertained most carefully by E. H. Weber,[1] with regard to the sense of touch and the power of perceiving warmth. He found that the clearness and keenness of the sense of touch varied considerably in various parts of the skin: thus two points of the compass, applied to the tip of the tongue, could be distinguished as two separate impressions at the distance of $\frac{1}{2}'''$, while the palmar surface of the last phalanx of a finger required a distance of $1'''$, the skin over the back and anterior part of the thigh, a distance of $30'''$. In the face, the acuteness of sensation is the less, the farther the part is from the mouth and the median line. The chin and external surface of the lips are provided with a remarkably fine sensitiveness. Concerning the *perception of taste*, the experiments of A. Klaatsch and A. Stich[2] prove that only a small portion of about $2'''$, extending around the tongue at its margin as well as its root and posterior third, and finally a part of the soft palate transmit the taste.

We refer, with regard to the cure of anæsthesia generally, to pages 141, 154, and 165; the following points, however, are to be borne in mind: 1. Where the deeper layers of the skin, or the muscles, are in a state of anæsthesia, the skin is moistened before the brush is applied. 2. With the gradual return of sensibility, the strength of the exciting current is also gradually diminished. 3. Where anæsthesia exists along with other disturbances of nervous function, whether

---

[1] De pulsu, resorptione, auditu et tactu. Annotationes anatomicæ et physiologicæ. Lipsiæ, 1834.

[2] Ueber die Geschmacks-Vermittelung, Virchow's Archiv, Band xiv., Heft iii., page 225, *et seq*.

hyperæsthesia or motor paralysis, the anæsthesia is first to be treated, the removal of which (see Case 45, and Duchenne's case, page 205) is frequently followed by a spontaneous disappearance of all the other symptoms of abnormal irritation, or depression of nerve-power. 4. In anæsthesia existing in consequence of a lesion or section of nerves, the treatment by electricity is never begun sooner than four weeks after the accident, as this is the shortest period during which the entirely severed nerves will be reunited. 5. Generally in anæsthesia following a peripheral cause, the intermittent current will give a more favorable result—if it is desired to employ the constant current, it is best applied in such a manner that the negative conductor is placed upon the anæsthetic portion of the skin, and the positive upon the respective nervous trunk; which being done, the latter is, with a slow kind of stroking motion, moved to the former. 6. Anæsthesia from neuritis usually disappears without any local treatment, through the galvanization of the nerves.

CASE 62.—Albert Mohricke, machinist, thirty-eight years of age, found at the beginning of May, while awaking during the night, that his right arm, which had been hanging over the back of a chair on his bed, was paralyzed from the shoulder down to the hand, motionless, benumbed, and painful. The paralysis appeared the same night, soon after the arm had been placed in a proper position, but he noticed the following morning that the ulnar side of his forearm and hand was anæsthetic to such a degree that neither the prick of a needle, nor a red-hot coal falling upon it, produced the slightest pain, and that the involuntary motion of the last three fingers was made but imperfectly.

After the long-continued and useless employment of an irritating liniment, the patient was placed under my care by Dr. Carl Hoffmann, for the purpose of being treated by electricity. On examining the patient on the 19th of June, I found the ulnar side of the forearm absolutely insensible to the prick of a needle; the same state existed on the dorsal, palmar, and lateral surfaces of the little and ring-fingers, and the ulnar side of the index finger. Mohricke complained of a sensation of cold, numbness, and weight in the paralyzed parts; the temperature of the hand was perceptibly reduced, the paralyzed muscles of the hand, especially the interosseous muscles, began to be atrophied. We had evidently to do with an anæsthesia of the principal trunks of the ulnar nerve, and, as a consequence, with a paralysis and atrophy of the interosseous, abductor, and opponens digiti, and accordingly we faradized the anæsthetic portions of the skin and the atrophied muscles. The result was satisfactory throughout. The patient had already, after the fifth employment of the apparatus, a clear, although still benumbed feeling, on touching the formerly anæsthetic portions of skin. At the same time, the temperature increased, while the motion of the fingers also became easier. In this case it was interesting to observe the return of sensibility progress from the peripheral borders toward the centre. Thus the points of the fingers and the middle of the forearm had already recovered their sensibility, while those portions of the skin situated over the inferior part of the ulna and metacarpal bone of the little finger were still void of sensibility. After twelve applications, the anæsthesia, together with all its consecutive symptoms, was entirely removed.

Case 63.—Mrs. Charlotte Schulz, aged forty-three years, always healthy, and with normal catamenia, contracted while washing, in the month of November, 1850, a severe cold. Neuralgic pains affected the neck and right arm, which were followed afterward by complete paralysis of these parts. The patient, after having used various internal and external remedies, came, in the month of May, to Professor Romberg's clinic. At that time, the arm had again become movable, but she now complained of a feeling of numbness and insensibility in the right cheek. A closer examination, by the introduction of needles, showed the insensibility to exist in the skin over the temporal region, the upper eyelid, the frontal region, in the tongue, in the floor of the mouth, in the gums, the lower lip, in the skin covering the right half of the face, as well as in the skin of the posterior portion of the head and neck, while the mucous membrane of the nose on the same side was sensible to a certain although diminished degree. This consequently proved to be a complete anæsthesia of the first and third branch of the trigeminus, and also of the occipital and subcutaneous nerves of the posterior branches of the first four cervical nerves, together with an incomplete anæsthesia of the second branch of the trigeminus. Headache was not present, but frequently a painful burning sensation was felt in the right eye and in the mouth. The seat of the disease, therefore, had to be sought for in the common place of origin of the upper cervical nerves, and of the trigeminus at the superior cervical portion of the spinal marrow. Cups were applied to the neck, followed by iodine ointment, iod. of pot. was administered internally, and warm baths afterward ordered.

This treatment was continued till August 2d, when the anæsthesia of the right side of the face had disappeared, a feeling of cold remaining. The patient also complained of a constant bitter taste in the right half of the tongue, of a feeling of burning in the tip of the tongue and in the membranes of the right eye, and also a feeling as if water escaped continually from the dry eye. The power of vision was also diminished in the affected eye, so that, the left being closed, every thing appeared as if covered by a veil. The anæsthesia of the cervical nerves still remained. After the electric brush had been applied three times, the anæsthesia of the cervical nerves was entirely removed, the veil before the right eye and the bitter taste also disappeared, while only a sensation of weight in the formerly insensible places, and the burning in the eye and tip of the tongue, remained. These abnormal sensations disappeared after the sixth application, and the patient was dismissed, cured, on August 13th.

We are indebted to the kindness of Dr. Klaatsch, for

the following case from the clinic of Privy-Councillor Romberg:

In June, 1856, the Widow Ringe, aged fifty-three years, applied for aid at Romberg's clinic. Her complaints were manifold, without being exactly defined. She said that for some time her general health had become weaker, she was unable to work or walk long, her hands and feet soon getting tired. She had a feeling of lameness all over her body, while her taste had become weak and indistinct. She also maintained that she had suffered for several years from violent neuralgic pains in the head, frequently changing their seat, and causing the sensation of serpentine movements. On inquiring about her appetite, she declared that she always was hungry, and never felt satisfied, however much she ate. She thought her complaint was caused by the frequent colds and drenchings which she could not avoid in her occupation as a laundress. The temperature influenced her health greatly, stormy weather always increasing her pain. Otherwise all the functions were normal, menstruation having ceased three years ago. She had been confined nine times, and had never been seriously ill. As far as could be ascertained, she had no hysterical symptoms.

A careful investigation of the patient led to the discovery of a considerable decrease of sensation. The feeling of pain had disappeared all over the skin, and in all the mucous membranes accessible to examination, so that deep prickings with a pin produced not the slightest pain, either on the surface of the body or in the oral and nasal cavities. Chemically irritating substances were equally indifferent to her. Although the patient, when smelling caustic ammonia, or acetic acid, noticed something sharp going up her nose, yet she felt no pain, and could bear acrid vapors for any length of time. The eyes became red and watery, but active: subjective symptoms failed. The mucous membrane of the larynx and lungs was equally insensible, the inspiration of ammonia vapors causing no cough. A high temperature aroused the general sensation. The patient having put her fingers into hot water, kept them there quietly for three seconds, after which time she took them suddenly out, remarking that the water was "very hot." She put her fingers into water at a temperature of 60° R., without finding it too warm.

The feeling of touch had not suffered in the same degree as the general sensation, although softly touching and stroking the skin and mucous membranes was not perceived by the patient, who also was unable to distinguish by the touch whether a substance had a smooth or rough surface, yet a stronger pressure with a dull object, or pricking the skin with a needle, was not only felt by her, but she could also pretty certainly designate the place thus touched. She could also distinguish two impressions made upon two different places of the skin, and tell whether she had been touched on one or two places. The distance necessary for the two points of the compass to be perceived as two separate impressions, was greater than the one ascertained as normal in the healthy skin by E. H. Weber. It amounted to one-third on the right and to one inch on the left side of the face, on the forehead to one inch on the right and left side; on the last phalanx of the index-finger, one inch; on the extensor side of the forearm in the transverse diameter, two inches; on the longitudinal diameter, three inches; on the flexor side of the forearm, two inches; on the neck four; on the lower part of the thigh, two and a half inches. The sense of smell was entirely extinct; she could smell neither ethereal oils nor assafœtida. The taste still continued in a low degree. A strongly concentrated solution of extract of quassia having been spread extensively over her tongue, she pronounced it, after a long period, as "somewhat bitter." The muscular feeling had not suffered. She nearly correctly ascertained the weight of substances held in her hand. The patient was also able to distinguish smaller substances from greater ones by touching them with her hand, even if they did not differ very materially in size. She could quickly and surely place the finger or toes upon any given point.—Her affection consequently was an extensive anæsthesia of the skin, and an analgesia, also a complete anæsthesia of the olfactory nerve, and of the gastric portion of the par vagus, and finally a paralysis of the glossopharyngeal nerve.

The treatment was begun with the use of Russian vaporbaths, which, however, did not have the slightest influence upon the anæsthesia. Then the electric brush was employed. In applying this, the patient felt nothing in the beginning; after a minute she perceived a burning sensation, which increased to a violent pain. After the brush had acted for a short period, the places touched by it became sensible to the prick of a needle. The electric brush was applied to limited parts of the neck and face. After four applications, the patient was again carefully examined with regard to her sensibility, when it appeared that not only the electrified spots, but also her whole body, had become almost entirely normal. She perceived everywhere the prick of a needle as painful, and was able to distinguish smooth from rough surfaces by touching them. The distance at which the two points of the compass had to be applied, in order to produce two separate impressions, was only a little farther than those ascertained by Weber as being normal. Now she could no more bear the inhalation of ammoniacal vapors, but turned her head away as soon as they were held under her nose. The feeling of excessive and insatiable hunger was gone; the painful sensations, winding serpentlike from one limb to another, had also disappeared. She now was again enabled to work with her hands, which she could not do before, not so much on account of the want of muscular power, as in consequence of the absence of sensibility.

CASE 64.—Carl M., aged nine years, of a rather scrofulous diathesis, a lively and smart boy, showed suddenly, in

May, 1862, signs of difficult hearing, which frightened his relatives, the more as already several members of the family suffered from a similar difficulty. Dr. Ehrhard, being of the opinion that the evil was a rheumatic affection, as the examination of the ear showed no disease, ordered corrosive sublimate and baths of potash. After eight days, the little patient could hear even a low conversation, musical sounds, rappings, etc.; however, he heard but very little. Iodide of potassium was now substituted, and the potash-baths continued. Now this peculiar symptom appeared, that the baths had no action on the skin, while in the first week they produced a copious diaphoresis; yet, the perception of spoken words improved, while other sounds were absolutely unheard. The vibrating tuning-fork, held against the skin, produced no sensation; its application to the thorax caused the surprising discovery that there was an anæsthesia, not only of the whole face, but also of the whole body, especially of the upper portion. As the continued administration of the above-mentioned remedies brought about no change, on the 14th of July, upon the advice of Privy-Councillor Romberg, my aid was sought with regard to the application of electricity. One application of the electric brush to the face, forearms, and hands, sufficed to remove the anæsthesia in its whole extent, and with it also to relieve the difficulty of hearing. The increased temperature of the skin following this operation, and the free perspiration now ensuing each time after the use of a potash-bath, caused in a short time a complete restoration of the sense of hearing, so that the patient could perceive both words and sounds as well as ever.

Duchenne has, in a large number of cases of so-called nervous deafness (where during life no organic changes could be proved), happening sometimes in hysterical persons, also after measles, scarlatina, and typhus, obtained an improvement, or even a cure, through the employment of the intermittent current. For this purpose, after having introduced a wire, isolated up to the point, into the meatus auditorius externus, filled half with tepid water, and applying the second conductor to the mastoid process, he allowed a weak current to act for a few minutes. The sensation of taste, felt in the tongue during the operation, which he considers a sign of the integrity of the chorda tympani, and the noise originating in the inner part of the ear after each intermission, which, according to Duchenne, is caused by the vibration of the tympanum, the ossicula auditoria, and the membrane of the fenestra ovalis, are valued by him as prognostically favorable symptoms. He also was so fortunate as to relieve, by the method, a few cases of deaf-mutism considerably, and to cure almost entirely one (page 1015), a short history of which follows:

A boy, eight years of age, deaf and dumb from birth, of whom at least the presence of the sense of hearing could never be ascertained to any extent, was, in 1856, put under Duchenne's care for relief from this affection. On inquiring into the history, Duchenne found that the boy heard neither loud shouting nor the striking of a loud alarm-clock even if made close to his ears, neither did he perceive the sound of a tuning-fork held against the cranial bones. He, therefore, began the treatment with but slight hopes. After the first application, the boy seemed to hear the sound of the tuning-fork on the left side, while the right side remained insensible; on the following day a hand-organ, playing in the yard, excited him greatly. After the seventh application, he heard vowels pronounced close to his left ear, and repeated them distinctly, although with difficulty. The distinction between the *e* and *i* was especially troublesome. After the twelfth application, he heard with both ears not only the tuning-fork and the striking of the alarm-clock, but also its ticking, and that too at a distance of several centimetres. At the same time the whole nature of the boy changed; having been wild and unmanageable, he now became more quiet and docile. After the twentieth application, in which the patient learned to pronounce the words "papa," "mamma," "bon bon," the treatment was suspended. In April, 1857, the patient was again placed under Duchenne's treatment; the results gained before were not only preserved, but he had also made further advancement. The boy, having been a member of a singing-class, tried to repeat the musical sounds, he knew and pronounced all the letters of the alphabet, began to spell, asked for bread, water, etc.; his voice had no more the guttural sound peculiar to persons deaf and dumb from birth; he turned his head in the direction whence his name was called, etc. A new course of treatment, comprising thirty sessions, was now begun, during which such favorable progress was made that a governess was engaged for the boy's education, who was required to make herself understood only through the sense of hearing. After a year (May, 1858), the boy read fluently and wrote a plain hand; his pronunciation was distinct, although a little hasty; on entering, he greeted Duchenne with the words, "Bon jour, Monsieur le Docteur Duchenne de Boulogne;" on leaving, he said, "Adieu." He asked for every thing he wanted, inquired the appellation of things unknown to him, and retained the newly-learned words very readily. Although the last thirty applications still improved his hearing, it was not to such a remarkable extent as the former applications.

B. Schulz[1] first directed attention toward the fact that some cases of impotence are characterized by a diminished electro-cutaneous sensibility of one (mostly the left) half of the glans and prepuce, and that in these cases the impotence disappears with the removal of the anæsthesia through the continued employment of the electric brush.[2]

[1] See *Heilung der Impotenz mittelst Electricität* in the Wiener Med. Wochenschrift, 1854 and 1861.
[2] Besides those cases of impotence connected with anæsthesia, the induction current is also used with advantage in such cases where atony of the bulbo-

He uses the following method: A brush, connected with one conductor of the induction apparatus, is placed upon the several anæsthetic points for from one to two minutes, while the other conductor is either applied by the patient himself upon any portion of the body or is introduced into the rectum, isolated up to the point. Schulz communicates the following case pertaining to this category:

Mr. S., forty-three years of age, married, a man occupied with governmental duties and scientific pursuits, of a slender, yet healthy constitution, complained of nothing else but a hæmorrhoidal affection, and a frequently-returning sciatica. From his early youth given to serious studies, he could not devote sufficient time to satisfying the sexual instinct; he did not, however, neglect altogether its peremptory calls. About two years ago, after having indulged more than usually this desire, he noticed a decrease of the strength of the erections to such an extent as to render cohabitation impossible. Abstinence, practised for more than a year, causing

cavernosus and ischio-cavernosus muscles causes insufficient erections and, consequently, impotence, or where the latter depends upon a relaxation of the seminal vesicles and of the ejaculatory duct. In the latter case, Duchenne, after introducing one excitator up to the verumontanum and applying the other to the perinæum, allows a current of medium strength to act for several minutes. I have also obtained splendid results with the electric brush in those cases of impotence arising so frequently from hypochondriasis.

The constant current, however, is indicated in those cases in which a hyperæsthesia of the respective portions of the skin is combined with excessively frequent pollutions, or where the ejaculations happen prematurely. In such cases a constant current of from fifteen to twenty of Daniell's elements is passed through the spinal column from its middle portion to the os sacrum for three to four minutes; then the positive pole is placed upon the perinæum, and the negative pole upon the glans, or, gradually progressing, upon the dorsum in such a manner that the whole time of the application amounts to about eight minutes. I shall here relate the case of a young Rabbi who, probably in consequence of former self-abuse, suffered from pollutions occurring repeatedly every night, which diminished his physical and moral power to such an extent as to render him unfit for the further administration of his office. A treatment of five to six weeks sufficed to reduce the number of pollutions to one, or, at the highest, two per week, and to allow him to reënter upon his official duties. I saw him two years after, a happy husband, and father of one child.

no change, the patient applied to Dr. Schulz for medical aid, who discovered, besides the symptoms of anæsthesia, considerable varicosities of the testes and anus. After using the brush for four months, the patient was cured, the erections again became strong, and cohabitation satisfactory, the above-mentioned varicosities disappearing at the same time.

We must, finally, mention a peculiar form of anæsthesia which first has been thoroughly examined by Nothnagel (*l. c.*) under the name of "vaso-motor neuroses." According to his opinion, they are caused by a spasm of the arteries and a diminished supply of arterial blood in consequence. Such cases are cured by the employment of the induced current in the shape of the electric brush, as well as by the stable constant current. Nothnagel reports the following case:

H. S., a servant-woman, thirty-seven years of age, had suffered for ten years from a frequently-recurring sensation of numbness of both hands and forearms, preventing her from working. Six months ago, pains supervened without any known cause, which increased very much in violence during the last five weeks. On her reception, patient complains of a feeling of stiffness and formication in both hands, with pain in her hands and forearms. The formication and the numbness disappear almost entirely after hard work, but return as soon as the hands are at rest, often increasing, especially in the night, to an intolerable degree. The first and second fingers of either hand are most affected, those of the right hand more than those of the left. When this affection is at its height, these fingers are white, and not, like the others, red. This paleness is the most conspicuous in the morning soon after rising, lasting sometimes for an hour, sometimes for a shorter period. Inspection and palpation of the affected parts show nothing abnormal in the interval. Sensibility to the prick of a needle and electro-cutaneous sensibility, also perception of temperature, are somewhat blunted, in both hands and forearms, but more so on the right than on the left side. Temperature on the right 35.5°, on the left 36.3°. The constant current was so used that the positive pole of a battery, consisting of 10 to 20 elements, was placed upon the brachial plexus of either side, and the negative pole upon the neck, thus allowing the current to pass through steadily for from three to eight minutes. After sixteen applications the patient was cured.

On page 189, Nothnagel communicates a case differing from the one just mentioned, in the seat and extent of the affection, for here disturbances of coördination were present in consequence of the diminished sensibility of the hands and feet, as is characteristic of gray degeneration of the posterior roots. All motions were perfect, as soon as the eyes compensated the want of the sense of touch. Electrocutaneous flagellation, foot-baths with mustard, scrubbing of the skin, etc., produced a complete cure.

C. Spasms.

Romberg[1] designates enhanced excitability and increased irritation of the motor nerves as the common character of spasms—muscular contractions of an either frequently-changing or a continued type—clonic or tonic spasms as the expression of this irritation. Only the tonic spasms appear to be continuous; actually, they are composed of an infinitely large number of contractions rapidly following each other. Transient contractions are convulsions; if they occur in a still weaker degree, trembling ensues; permanently remaining contractions are denominated contractions.

All central or peripheral irritations of motor nerves, either directly or by reflex action, may cause spasms. Their

[1] On Nervous Diseases, 3d edition, vol. ii., page 335.

occurrence is facilitated through the circumstance that the irritation may be transmitted from one cerebral half to the other, that it is conveyed in the spinal marrow, not only in the longitudinal, but also in the transverse direction by means of the ganglionic cells of the gray substance; finally, because general spasms can be produced from every point of the spinal marrow, as is proved by Weber's experiments with the rotation-apparatus. The occurrence of spasms is also favored by an abnormal irritability of the nerves and spinal marrow, existing, congenital or acquired, in many individuals, and depending almost always upon anæmia. The spinal marrow may be the source, or it may transmit spasm, either as the organ conveying irritations of sensible origin (irritations of motor origin almost always terminate in paralysis), or in consequence of the increase of its independent motor activity, as in chorea, or finally by its manifold connections with the sympathetic system.

All those spasms are decidedly unsuitable for electric treatment which are caused by a deep disturbance of nutrition of the brain and spinal marrow, or their bony coverings (meningitis, encephalitis, myelitis, tumors, etc.); or by plethora, or congestions toward the central organs; also those reflex spasms caused by dislocations or other diseases of the uterus or ovaries, etc.; or finally the contractions resulting from cerebral hemiplegias and maintained by cerebral irritation.

The employment of the electric current, however, is indicated in the removal of those spasms developed gradually in consequence of a continued local irritation (spasmus facialis after photophobia, vocal spasm after pertussis), or in those caused by over-exertion of single muscles, or by neuritis (several forms of writer's paralysis), also in those forms of trembling which accompany poisoning by lead or mercury, or which appear locally as symptoms of nervous irritability. Contractions which affect healthy muscles in consequence of a paralysis of their antagonists, or which suddenly appear through rheumatic influences or through over-exertion, or those resulting from the reflex action of painfully-affected articulations; finally some kinds of spasms depending upon an affection of the sympathetic system (spasmus facialis from irritation of the cervical ganglia of the sympathetic), etc., are benefited by the electric treatment.—I have also seen good results obtained from the employment of electricity in a number of cases of chorea after the acute stage had been passed.

The electric current exerts here a sanative influence, inasmuch as its use in spasms, depending upon asthenia, anæmia, or nervous irritability, increases the supply of blood to the weakened muscles, thereby improving their nutrition, and thus rendering them not only fit for their normal functions, but also giving them a greater power of resistance against external influence. For these purposes both the interrupted and constant current may be employed. Those contractions, resulting from a paralyzed condition of the antagonistic muscles, naturally require an exciting current, either the intermittent or the constant stable one, to be directed toward the paralyzed muscles, while those muscles affected and contracted by rheumatism will be more suitably relaxed with a constant and stable current of medium strength, or by single shocks.

Equally favorable results were also obtained from these electric shocks in chorea, by applying large conductors to the cervical and lumbar portions of the spinal column, probably on account of their directly reducing the irritability of the spinal marrow. It is often difficult, in reflex spasms, which so frequently come under medical treatment, to discover and attack the real starting-point of the affection, yet the success of the treatment depends entirely upon it. Sometimes it is possible to find regions or points tender by being touched or pressed upon, against which then, by way of trial, the treatment must be especially directed, by applying to them the positive pole of the battery, while the negative pole is placed upon any other remote spot. The ganglia of the great sympathetic appear, in some cases, to be especially such tender points, the influence of which system upon the voluntary muscles can hardly be doubted, since late researches have successfully proved the intermixture of vasomotor nerve-tubules with motor and sensitive nerve-fibres in a considerable number of motor and mixed nerves. Remak, especially, having, in an interesting treatise on "spasm of the facial muscles,"[1] pointed out the cervical ganglia of the sympathetic system as the frequent starting-points of this affection, succeeded in curing it through the galvanic treatment. No successful result can be obtained from the employment of electricity in paralysis agitans, by reason of the anatomical changes found in the brain and spinal marrow after death; yet, if the case be recent, and trembling restricted to one extremity, the use of the spinal marrow-root current in such manner as to apply the copper-pole to the spinal marrow, and drawing the zinc-pole slowly along the corresponding nervous roots on its side, the trembling may be diminished, and the functional power of the extremity increased.

In irritable individuals it is especially necessary to begin the treatment with very weak currents and to continue them for a short period, with intermissions of from one to two days, otherwise the local spasms may become general, or even turn into the most frightful convulsions. On the whole, it will be more suitable, in such cases, to precede the use of electricity by the employment of remedies causing a strong derivation upon the intestinal canal, or having a directly sedative influence upon the nervous system. For these purposes, metallic preparations, arsenic, and narcotics, may be used, the latter especially in the shape of hypodermic injections of morphine and atropine.

CASE 65.—Thekla von K., a strong, healthy girl of thirteen years, very much developed physically, but who had

[1] Berliner Klin. Wochenschrift, 1864. Nos. 21-23.

not yet menstruated, was, about two years ago, in July, 1849, attacked with pertussis. In spite of the different means employed, the paroxysms increased in violence and frequency, until they occurred every ten or fifteen minutes, lasting from two to three minutes, and finally resulting in hoarseness, and afterward in complete aphonia. This state lasted till January 24, 1850, when the patient again, for the first time, uttered a sound. In the next four weeks the patient improved so much that, at the end of February, she was, the still-continuing hoarseness excepted, perfectly well.

Toward the end of September, 1850, a slight pulmonary catarrh set in, which gradually increased, and was accompanied by convulsive attacks of coughing, followed by hoarseness and finally by aphonia. Leeches were applied to the throat, cups, etc., to the neck, ointments of veratrine, iodine, and narcotics, rubbed into the laryngeal region, nitrate of silver, musk, dissolving and quieting remedies were administered without producing the slightest change in the symptoms, with the exception of a transient improvement following the use of the musk. Even the appearance of the menses after the employment of pills, consisting of aloes, galbanum, and iron, had no influence whatever upon the course of the disease. Then, in the month of May, 1851, the patient came to Berlin for the purpose of consulting Dr. Romberg. She was affected with a complete spasm of the glottis, recurring every quarter or half an hour, and lasting up to twenty minutes. Single, convulsively-expelled coughing-sounds were interrupted by a deep, sonorous, trumpet-like noise accompanying the inspiration. This noise, apparently rising from the lesser bronchial tubes of the larynx, introduced, as it were, the spasm, and predominated also during the attack, yielding only toward the end to the more or less connected coughing-sounds. At the same time the face was deeply reddened, the muscles of the face and neck spasmodically distorted, the hands and feet moved convulsively, and the pulse became accelerated. These paroxysms were most frequent in the morning, diminished somewhat in intensity in the afternoon, and ceased entirely at night. The aphonia, however, still continued the same without any intermission, so that the patient could not produce even the slightest sound. Otherwise all the functions of the patient were normally performed, and her appearance was not such as to indicate disease. Romberg first caused a solution of nitrate of silver to be pencilled repeatedly over the mucous membrane of the larynx, while the carbonate of copper with belladonna was given internally in increasing doses. As, in spite of the continued employment of these means, the paroxysms diminished but little in violence, frequency, and duration, he finally ordered the induced electricity to be applied to the suffering organ.

When I first saw the patient, July 18, 1851, the attacks occurred about every half hour, lasting for fifteen minutes, and accompanied by the above-mentioned symptoms. This was undoubtedly an affection of the inferior laryngeal nerve. After sixteen applications of the induced current, made in sixteen consecutive days, each lasting for half an hour, an interval of two to three hours ensued between the paroxysms, the duration of which was now shortened from two to five minutes; both the trumpet-like sound and the spasmodic action of the muscles of the face and neck also became weaker. From the 4th of August two applications were made daily, in consequence of which, the number of paroxysms decreased so much that, on the 10th, they recurred but twice, each having a duration of about four minutes, and from that day till the 16th of August, when the patient left for her home, she remained perfectly free from spasms. According to letters received afterward, she continued to do well; the aphonia, which on her departure had improved so much as to enable her to utter a few feeble sounds with a hoarse tone, did not disappear until after a year—without, however, the further use of any medicine.

CASE 66.—Miss T., an apparently healthy and robust

girl, sixteen years old, with a regular but feeble catamenia, put herself, upon the advice of Dr. Nagel, under my care on the 26th of January, 1863. The disease having had a mild beginning, had now existed for one year and three months. It had, however, increased so much during the last months, that it occurred every few minutes while she was awake, unless her attention was very much engaged; only in the afternoon a slight interval of fifteen minutes ensued. It was accompanied by a noisy, inspiratory murmur, which could be heard in every part of the house, and was followed by a short expiration, accompanied by a peculiar odor of the food. I need not mention that, besides the iron, every narcotic and nervine had been used. There was in this case, beyond doubt, an affection of the pneumogastric nerve, as singultus appeared as little during the electric irritation of the phrenic nerve as in diaphragmatic pleurisy. On this account, both the induced and the stable constant currents were directed against the vagus on either side. As the former seemed to have more effect, I used the induced current exclusively after the twentieth application (May 9th), yet thirty-one more applications were necessary in order to relieve the patient entirely. A slight relapse occurring after some time, was quickly removed by means of a simple dietetic regimen.

Hiffelsheim[1] cured the following case of pharyngeal spasm by means of the continued current:

A man, twenty-six years old, who had used arsenic for acne rosacea, was attacked with a difficulty in swallowing, and he finally, in consequence of a spasm, found it impossible to swallow any thing at all. As soon as the food arrived at the pharynx, it was rejected through the mouth, while liquids returned through the nose. After Hiffelsheim had first applied both electrodes of a large chain of Pulvermacher on either side of the neck on a level with the pneumogastric, he applied, on the second day, the current of

[1] De la Dysphagie, etc. Annales de l'Électricité. Janvier, 1861.

fourteen small elements of Daniell for fifteen or twenty minutes. After three applications the patient could swallow finely-cut meat; and was cured after the fifth application. In order to prevent a relapse, he was subsequently galvanized four times more.

Popper[1] reports the following case:

An apparently healthy girl suffered from a continual distention of the stomach through gases, tenderness upon pressure, constricting pain in the stomach, especially after eating, eructation, and vomiting. No remedy gave any relief. Popper placed both poles of an induction-apparatus near each other upon the gastric region before eating, and allowed the current to pass through it for five minutes. After the first application, the vomiting diminished, and after the twelfth application the patient was cured. Still the treatment was continued for some time.

In very desperate cases of nervous vomiting of pregnancy, Bricheteau met with success in three cases by the following method : He placed both electrodes of a weak current, at the beginning, in the middle, and toward the end of each meal, for several minutes upon the epigastrium.

Unfortunately, the employment of electricity is not successful in many cases where it is apparently indicated : thus I treated, without any success whatever, a girl twenty-five years of age, a patient of Professor Henoch, who suffered from singultus; also a patient of Dr. Steinrueck, a girl of the same age, suffering from a spasmodic cough (the so-called sheep's cough), where, however, there were no special symptoms warranting the assumption of its being caused by reflex action. The same negative result was naturally obtained in a case of spasm of the diaphragm attacking an apparently very healthy girl daily from five to eight times, inasmuch as the first illness of the patient could be deduced from a fall down-stairs happening a year and a

---

[1] Heilung des Erbrechens durch Electricität. Oestr. Zeitschr. fuer pract. Heilkunde, 1864. Page 43.

half ago, followed immediately by dysmenorrhœa (caused, as the examination showed, by a retroversio uteri), and, a few months afterward, by the first diaphragmatic spasm in consequence of violent mental excitement. In this case, the galvanic treatment, undertaken only upon the urgent desire of the parents, had naturally no success, but the local treatment of the displaced uterus seemed to have a favorable influence upon both dysmenorrhœa and spasms.

CASE 67.—Paul Staeger, aged eleven years, weak and scrofulous, was, without any known cause, taken about four months ago with a trembling in the right arm, which, although it disappeared after some time by observing perfect rest, yet temporarily returned after any mental or physical exertion. Since October, 1857, the mother noticed a remarkable increase, which attained its height between the 19th and 22d of October, so that the little patient was unable to keep the arm quiet for one moment, the hand flying all over the paper at every attempt to write. Upon the advice of Dr. Bartel, the patient was placed under my care. After having faradized the muscles of the arm and hand on the 22d, 23d, and 25th of October, the movements ceased entirely, and the boy was able to write again. The cure was permanent.

CASE 68.—Hermann Beermann, aged fourteen years, for two years suffered from a gradually-increasing trembling of the right arm. He was sent to me on the 30th of September by Professor Traube, when I treated him with the constant current by allowing a stable current to ascend from the radial nerve to the brachial plexus, afterward irritating the extensor muscles of the arm and hand with weak labile currents. The patient improved in a marked manner from the third application (October 3d), so that he was able to keep the arm extended for half a minute without trembling. After the tenth application (October 13th), he could, by exerting himself, write for a quarter of an hour without trembling. I finished the treatment with the nineteenth application, as the trembling had ceased for eight days, not only in a state of rest, but also in writing.

E. Fliess,[1] having investigated the sedative action of the constant galvanic current on the impulse of the heart in twenty-four cases, of which, in nineteen, no organic lesion could be proved, while five had a structural disease, found a diminution of the symptoms in all, while he obtained a perfect cure of a large number of those belonging to the first category after from five to six applications. Fliess used for this purpose mild currents, causing a moderate, rarely a strong burning, by applying them to either vagus daily, or every other day, for from one to two minutes; the descending current proved to be more efficacious than the ascending. The patient felt relieved and relatively better a short time after the opening of the circuit, and the improvement lasted for a longer or shorter period of the same day, after the first application. After several, and sometimes after many applications, this feeling of comfort became permanent, even in cases of organic disease of the heart. Later, a perceptible decrease ensued in the intensity and frequency of the impulse, and of the sounds of the heart.

The same physician reports the following case, which, in the course of the galvanic treatment, was repeatedly subjected to a careful examination by Dr. Ph. Munk, lecturer on medical diagnosis.

Carl Berg, twenty-six years of age, a shoemaker by trade, relates that having had two years ago an attack of

[1] Observations on the Influence of the Constant Galvanic Current upon the Morbidly-increased and Augmented Impulse of the Heart. Berl. Klin. Wochenschr., 1865. No. 26.

inflammatory articular rheumatism, he suffers since that time from palpitation of the heart and shortness of breath increasing in violence after every mental or physical exertion. He is prevented from lying on the left side by this palpitation becoming so violent as to shake the whole body. Diagnosis of Dr. Munk: Insufficiency of the mitral valve and constriction of the left auriculo-ventricular opening, dilatation without considerable hypertrophy of the right ventricle (for the second sound of the pulmonary artery is but little increased). Radial pulse 80, small, regular. After the first application (December 11th), the patient professed to feel more quiet, yet this was not permanent even after the second application (December 15th); the difficulty of breathing, however, was less. After the seventh application, the dyspnœa had disappeared, the violent palpitation ensued only after great exertions, such as fast walking, mounting stairs, etc. The pulse continued unchanged in frequency. After a few more applications, the patient was enabled to lie on his left side without any difficulty. On February 2d, after twenty-eight applications, Dr. Munk affirmed that there existed a compensating hypertrophy of the right ventricle, with an increase of the second pulmonary sound, which probably accounted for the greater ease of the patient. Neither could the *frémissement catoire* be felt any longer. The further treatment improved the health and appearance of the patient so much that, on March 4, 1861, he was dismissed, after the forty-third application, the impulse of the beat not being too strong, with a frequency of 80. On April 7th and May 21st of the same year, the patient called again, informing me that his health was tolerable.

CASE 69.—Wilhelm May, twenty-one years of age, a fusileer of the eighth regiment, enjoyed always good and robust health, until he was, in November, 1850, received into the special hospital of the fourth army corps on account of a rheumatic inflammation of both eyes, predominating, however, in the right. The disease continued for five months with frequent exacerbations and remissions, without producing any local change or leaving any other residue, except an extraordinary photophobia, causing a spasmodic closure of the eyes whenever exposed to a sun-ray, while the patient could open them always in the dark. The morbid irritability of the orbicularis palpebrarum affected also, during the month of March, several other muscles in the vicinity, viz., the corrugator supercilii of either side, the zygomaticus major and platysma of the right side, so much, that these muscles were affected with spasms after each attempt to open the eyes. Toward the end of the month the disease had not only gradually increased, but also attacked the more distant muscles of the right side, viz., the sternocleidomastoideus, the scaleni, and the longus colli, so that now the head with its twitching muscles was continually rotated in a semicircle from the right to the left, which motion was only interrupted during sleep. The pendulum-like, rotatory motions of the head proceeded evidently from the spasmodic convulsions of the orbicularis palpebrarum which at first only happened when the patient tried to open the eyes, but afterward became spontaneous. In addition to which, involuntary motions of other muscles followed in consequence of the nervous irritability of the patient, caused by the length of the affection, and the long-continued antiphlogistic treatment. On the 3d of June, I began for the first time to treat this patient by electricity. I faradized every single affected muscle, and had the pleasure to remove the convulsions of the facial muscles after the second, and the spasmodic motions of the cervical muscles after the fifth application of one-quarter of an hour's duration.

The so-called wryneck (torticollis), depending upon a clonic spasm of the sternocleidomastoideus, usually with the coöperation of the rotatory muscles of the occipital region, is mostly of a crossed origin. It is developed either in consequence of an asthenia (paralysis, atrophy) of the antagonists, from a tendency of the healthy muscles to keep the head in its normal position, in which case it is cured by the induced current being directed to the antagonists (see Case 70), or it is caused, according to Remak, by a myelitis lateralis of the opposite side, within the region of the lateral columns of the cord, from which the roots of the accessory nerve take their origin, and then it is treated successfully by removing the myelitis through the constant current (see Remak's case).

CASE 70.—Mr. von R., a high official, of a weakly constitution, had been suffering from his youth from a hyperæsthesia of the nerves, which caused him so much mental anxiety, that at times he became tired of life. He married in 1846, being then thirty-six years of age. In the next year his general health improved, yet the slightest deviation from his accustomed way of living caused intolerable pain in the head and back, which only yielded to absolute rest. At this time also a hæmorrhoidal affection began to show itself. In 1855, the patient noticed that his right hand made, while he was writing, involuntary motions, and in 1856 his head also followed these movements. In the mean time, profuse hæmorrhoidal hæmorrhages had taken place, increasing his weakness day by day, and depressing him mentally and physically. The use of the Franzen bath and a subsequent cold-water treatment alleviated these symptoms, but it was not till the year 1859 that his strength increased to any noticeable extent; he now became more self-confident, and all his functions were more normally performed. From this time, however, an increasing weakness of the right side, difficulty of writing, and a numbness of the last three fingers of the right hand, became apparent. Finally, he noticed a considerable inclination of the head to the right side, so that he was unable to keep it in its normal position, unless he powerfully exerted the left sternocleidomastoid muscle while at rest, or by pressing the cane against the right side of the chin while walking. When the patient, upon the advice of Dr. Wolff, applied to me on May 6, 1860, I found the left scaleni muscles remarkably relaxed, withered, and emaciated, their electro-muscular contractility and sensibility being very much reduced; the reaction of the other cervical muscles was normal. After the eighth faradization of the left scaleni, the patient was enabled (May 18th) to hold the head for a few moments in its normal position. Sixteenth application (June 7th), patient can now hold the head straight when walking, without the support of the cane, neither does the head follow the motions of the hand when he writes slowly. On July 23d I finished the treatment with the thirty-fifth application, in order to allow the patient to use the marsh baths in Franzensbad. The left scaleni muscles had increased considerably in volume; when the patient sits still, his head is nearly straight, his walk is free and easy, neither is he now troubled by the rotatory movements while writing. I had repeatedly occasion to see the patient afterward; the spasm had not returned in 1865, when he died of phthisis pulmonum.

Remak reports the following case in the Med. Central-Zeitung, 1862, page 182:

Lindner was, in November, 1860, taken with torticollis, after having been exposed to cold, and after having, the day before, leaned one-quarter of an hour over a chair with his neck twisted. Being unable to work, the patient was received into the Charité. Here spasm in the right accessory and, corresponding with it, in the right sternocleidomastoid muscle having been diagnosticated, the right side was, for four weeks, treated with antispasmodics and electricity, without, however, accomplishing any thing. Remak, to whom the patient now applied, found, in the trigonum cervicale of the opposite (left) side, knotty, painful swellings (about the nature of which, whether belonging to the lymphatic glands or to the nerves, he was doubtful), and applied to these spots leeches, unguent. hydr., etc., and the constant current. The patient improving, but not yet being cured, went, after four weeks, to the clinic, where the hot iron, unfortunately without any result, was used on the right side.

On April 18, 1861, Lindner again applied to Remak, being then in a worse condition than before. He was now perfectly unable to hold his head still, which he could do at least for a few minutes before. There were, besides, insensibility of the left side of the pharynx, and a limited anæsthetic spot in the fossa cervicalis. The constant current was again applied to the left side, and a perfect cure obtained after a two months' treatment, from the middle of April to the middle of May, and from the middle of June to the middle of July. On the 6th of December there remained only a small hardened place in the right sternocleidomastoid muscle as the residue of the reflex spasm which did not again return.

Remak maintains that, although, according to his experience, there is no part of the central nervous system or of the sympathetic nerve from which a lateral or double chorea cannot originate, in general, the most severe cases have a compound origin. Thus he ascertained, in a case of chorea magna, the spasms of which were so violent that the patient, a girl ten years of age, could only be kept on the bed by exerting great force, that the real starting-point of the convulsions, which had begun in the left half of the body, was situated within the region of the right side of the cervical portion of the spinal marrow, and of the cervical portion of the sympathetic nerve. On the right side there were also symptoms of neuritis, and a knot the size of an almond in the tibial nerve. Remak[1] adds, that in severe cases of chorea at least, in the earlier stages, the neuritis disappears by itself during the central treatment with the constant current,

[1] Med. Central-Zeitung, 1863, page 158.

while, on the contrary, the peripheral, although quieting temporarily, acts rather injuriously than otherwise.

I have treated a series of attacks of chorea (chorea minor), affecting three girls at the ages of from seven to ten, and one of sixteen years, with shocks of a battery consisting of about thirty elements (twenty-four to thirty in one application), and observed after each application an improvement followed by recovery, so that I cannot but urge a further examination of this method, which failed me but once in a recent case where the symptoms increased rapidly. The number of applications necessary for a complete recovery varies between five and twenty-four, but the first application always produced an evident improvement.

Case 71.—Miss P., an anæmic girl of sixteen years of age, a patient of Dr. Friedheim, suffered for about six weeks from an insecurity of the movements of both halves of her body, but more so of the right side, which, hardly perceived in the beginning, increased from week to week. The patient was unable to sit on a chair without moving her whole body or her arms and legs. On attempting to grasp anything, she dropped it, having no control over her hands; she could neither write nor play on the piano; while walking, her legs performed rotatory movements; while her arm and shoulder were raised anteriorly, posteriorly, or laterally.

The patient was placed under my care on January 27, 1865. After the fifth application (February 11th), an improvement was noticed; after the fourteenth application, her hand was sufficiently steady to write a few lines tolerably, and to play on the piano. At the end of March (after twenty-four applications), the patient had fully recovered.

Benedikt thinks he has met with no ill success in more than twenty cases of chorea minor, through galvanization of the spinal column in such a manner as to let a barely perceptible current ascend for from one to one and a half minutes; moreover, he found the worst cases improve the most, as here, after a few applications, the chorea-like movements were reduced to a minimum.—I have not been as successful by this method; its employment failing in several cases caused me to rely upon the above-mentioned method. Benedikt quotes, among others, the following case:

Fanny Wascher, aged eleven years, on being received for treatment (December 10, 1862), had suffered for six weeks from a violent chorea minor in the muscles of the extremities, trunk, head, and face. The patient was moving continually, and was unable to make any fine movements, not even the buttoning of her dress. On an examination with the descending spinal marrow-nerve and nerve muscle currents, the sensible and motor excitability were found to be heightened to an enormous degree, especially at the opening of the current. After the first sitting, in which fourteen elements were employed in the described manner, such a calm immediately ensued, that she was enabled to button her dress without any difficulty. After the fourth (December 13th), the patient could knit, in which state she remained till the 22d of December. On December 27th, another examination was made, when her excitability was found to be very much diminished. On December 30th, the morbid movements became so rare that it was necessary to observe her for several minutes in order to notice any spasm of the extremities. On January 8th she was galvanized for the last time, and was discharged from the hospital on January 19th cured.

Writer's paralysis, for the alleviation of which, probably, the aid of electricity is most frequently sought, offers, on the whole, no favorable prognosis. First, because those afflicted with this disease are usually able only for a short time and at a sacrifice to give up their occupation, which originates and maintains the affection; second, because the affection is met with in a variety of forms, the anatomical and physiological explication of which is exceedingly difficult, yet necessary for a rational treatment. We must especially distinguish between three kinds. In the first, the disease consists of a reflex spasm depending upon an irritation of the nerves of the hand and wrist; the second is caused by a paresis of the extensor muscles; while the third proceeds from a neuritis. The spasm naturally assumes another type in the last case, according to the seat of the disease, whether the radial, median, ulnar, or other nerve is spasmodically affected. With regard to the treatment, I was so happy as to cure a case of the first category, with a coexisting anæsthesia of the skin of both thumbs and index-fingers, with the induced current, and the use of the brush (see Case 72); that form which depends upon an asthenia of the extensor muscles is best removed through their faradization, while the neuritis is cured by the use of the constant current (see Case 74).

CASE 72.—Mr. Joachinii, a secretary, aged forty-one years, was, at the end of the year 1851, probably in consequence of over-exertion in writing, affected with spasms in the thumb and index-finger of the right hand, compelling him to leave off writing for several months, but permitting him to resume his occupation after that period. Soon, however, he perceived other morbid symptoms in his right hand, viz.: pain in the inner side of the ends of the fingers, and in the joints of the thumb and index-finger, which followed every attempt to write. Neither Töplitz, which the patient visited in 1854 and 1855, nor the long-continued employment of the constant current, had any perceptible influence upon it. Yet Joachinii was enabled, although with great pain, to continue his occupation as secretary till May, 1859, when the upper joint of the thumb became so much affected as to make it impossible for him to hold the pen in the usual position, compelling him to grasp the pen alternately between the index and middle, or the middle and ring-finger, or to fasten it, by means of an ingenious device, to a thimble. The hypodermic use of morphine caused violent burning and constricting pain from the place of injection, along the thumb, which finally obliged the patient to resort to his left hand for the purpose of writing. After four weeks, the left-hand writing also was made impossible on account of the violent pain arising in the joints of the left thumb and index-finger. The unhappy patient was now unable to dress without help, or cut his food, and he was finally compelled to give up his occupation altogether. After the third visit to Töplitz, from June till August, 1860, had hardly improved his condition, the despairing patient came, upon the advice of Dr. Wolff, to my office.

The examination proved that it was impossible for the patient to extend fully the thumb and index-fingers (especially of the left side), a condition which was undoubtedly caused by a hyperæsthesia of the nerves supplying the joints of the fingers, which made the patient anxiously avoid even the slightest extension; anæsthesia of the skin of both thumbs and index-fingers was also discovered. In accordance with the result obtained by the examination, the electric brush was applied to the anæsthetic portions of the skin. After the first application, Joachinii was able to write for a quarter of an hour with the pen held in the normal position. After the fourth application (October 15th), he wrote an account of his affection, extending to five pages. After thirty-three applications (toward the end of December), he was able to extend tolerably well the thumb and index-finger, while he could also hold lighter substances with his left hand. Still, as the pain fluctuated frequently, caused partially by his continued use of the pen, partially by unknown influences, it was necessary to use the brush twenty times more, till the 23d of March, in order to remove entirely the neuralgia with the anæsthesia. The extensor muscles of the fingers were also faradized during the last applications.

I saw the patient again on the 7th of May. He was now able to attend to his customary duties as a secretary; the pain, however, caused by the morphine injections, had not yet fully disappeared, his right thumb was, to use his own expression, painfully enclosed by a tight-fitting net.

Case 73.—Mr. Richard Fabricius, twenty-seven years of age, continually engaged as a clerk for six years, always enjoyed good health until eight or nine months ago, when, after having written for a long period unusually much, frequently eight to ten hours, he experienced, while writing, a stinging, contracting sensation in the wrist-joint, which thence extended into the fingers, especially into the thumb and index-finger. The thumb was then spasmodically bent in the last joint, approaching the palmar surface of the hand, and drawn tightly to the index-finger. The pain in the wrist-joint began whenever the patient tried to write; after having written for a quarter of an hour, spasm of the fingers followed, obliging him to stop if he had necessarily to continue writing; nevertheless, the pain in the wrist and spasm in the fingers not only increased, but the pain also extended along the extensor carpi ulnaris to the forearm, making any further writing impossible. After the evil had, for seven months, increased in intensity, the patient was advised by Dr. Wegscheider to put himself under my treatment.

This affection apparently consisted of a spasm of the flexor longus pollicis and the adductor-pollicis, the former causing the flexion of the last joint of the thumb, the latter, besides the adduction, assisted by the muscles situated on the inner side of the ball of the thumb, producing also the opposition of the thumb, that is, its moving into the palmar surface and its approaching the little finger. The examination made with regard to the electric action, showed a deficient contraction of the abductor pollicis brevis, and of the extensores pollicis, longus, and brevis, the extensor muscles of the other fingers acting normally. The continued faradization of these muscles, made, at the beginning, twice a week, allowed the patient, who, although with intervals, continued to write, to attend to his clerical duties for fourteen hours in succession, so that, after this, I electrified him but once a week, terminating the treatment at the beginning of August.

CASE 74.—Privy-Secretary H., a patient of Dr. Simonsohn, forty-eight years of age, a strong and healthy man, came under my professional care, February 12, 1865, having suffered for a year from writer's paralysis, which showed the following symptoms: the thumb and index-finger stiffly embraced the pen; the wrist was drawn spasmodically to the forearm and rotated outward, so that he was unable to write a few words without interruption, the pen falling out of his hand unless he stopped writing. If compelled to continue, a pain ensued in the arm along the radial nerve going up to the shoulder; the local examination proved the existence of a painful swelling at least half an inch long, in the radial nerve immediately over the elbow-joint. The constant current having been applied sixty-five times to this place, the evil was removed, and the patient declared, a year after the termination of the treatment, that since that time he had no difficulty in pursuing his occupation.

Remak[1] has, in a series of lectures, delivered before the Medical Society of Berlin, on "spasm of the facial muscles," mentioned several cases cured by him by means of the constant current. These cases were either such as proceeded from a periostitis and were cured by the local treatment of the affected part, or they followed a neuritis cervico-brachialis, when they were cured by removing the knotty swellings situated in that region, or they were finally those in which the cervical ganglia of the sympathetic nerve of the same or of the opposite side acted a prominent part, through the galvanization of which, by placing the positive electrode upon the region of the ganglion, the spasm was quieted.

[1] See Berliner Klinische Wochenschrift, 1864. Nos. 21-23.

The following is the synopsis of a case belonging to the last-mentioned category:[1]

The patient, a baker by profession, thirty years old, was, about three years ago, affected with a spasm of the right orbicularis palpebrarum. Thence the spasm extended, within a year, to the other facial and especially the zygomatic muscles. After another year, the orbicularis of the left side was also attacked, and, finally, after a few months, all the muscles of the left side, the right side, however, being mainly affected. The spasms varied in their character; the majority of the facial muscles of the right side were subject to an almost continuous twitching; besides this, greater attacks of violent tonic spasms, beginning in the right orbicular muscle, affected the other facial muscles, occurring seven times an hour, and oftener. He could produce these spasms at will, by closing the right eye, as is usually the case in such mimic facial spasms. This act was inevitably followed by spasms, usually of a tonic nature at first, more strongly marked on the right than on the left side, lasting for minutes, and longer. The spasms then assumed a clonic character; brisk twitchings of all the facial muscles followed each other quickly in succession, terminating in slight, trembling motions, or convulsions of the respective muscles. The history of the case gave no explanation of the origin, neither could Prof. von Graefe discover any points, painful under pressure, which, in such cases, indicate neurotomy. Then Remak noticed such a painful point on the right side of the cervical portion of the vertebral column, in the vicinity and on the anterior surface of the fifth cervical transverse process (where the ganglion cervicale medium is usually found). Pressure upon this point did not stop the spasmodic attacks, but the introduction of the positive electrode of an intense galvanic current suspended them. After the current had been employed at intervals for three weeks, the spasms were, on the 1st of February, reduced to such an extent as to enable

[1] *L. c.*, page 207.

the patient to resume his work, and to continue it for three months without interruption. Having been no more galvanized during this period, he had but very few slight attacks of tonic spasms, occurring about once in a week or a month. Now, a tonic contraction of all the muscles of the right side of the face ensues only when he voluntarily shuts his eyes firmly; otherwise he feels so well that he has no desire to undergo another course of treatment for the purpose of removing these last residues.

Remak mentions, on this occasion, cases, in which facial spasms have been followed by EPILEPTIC CONVULSIONS, and in which he also obtained favorable results through the galvanic treatment of the cervical portion of the sympathetic nerve. He is of the opinion that, in such cases, indirect catalytic actions take place—that is, such actions proceed from the nerves to the blood-vessels supplied by them—by causing a dilatation of the vessels and a resorption of exudations, etc., by means of exciting a current of liquids in the interior of the tissue. He is, hence, inclined to ascribe quite a peculiar importance to the vertebral branch of the first thoracic ganglion, as this branch supplies the vertebral artery, and thus may possibly exercise a catalytic influence upon the base of the brain.

In consequence of rheumatic affections, be it either a simple muscular rheumatism or a rheumatic exudation into the muscular substance itself, there happen frequently distortions, especially of the muscles of the neck and shoulder. In the first case, the pain primarily causes the patient to give to the respective parts an abnormal position, which afterward becomes customary, and finally habitual, in consequence of the disturbances of nutrition developed in the inactive muscles. These disturbances of nutrition, being perfectly analogous to those cases in which muscles are, for a long period, kept in a state of inactivity, in consequence of a firm, long-continued bandage, or in consequence of a former apoplectic attack, are frequently removed, in a surprisingly short time, by the employment of the constant current, as well as by cutaneous and muscular faradization. Those RHEUMATIC DISTORTIONS, too, depending upon an exudation into the muscular tissue itself, may also be cured by directing an uninterrupted current upon the lengthened muscles simultaneously with the cutaneous faradization of the portion of skin over the distortion, thereby increasing their contractile power sufficiently for the extension of the shortened muscles. Passing a stable current through the diseased muscle may also accomplish a cure.

Erdmann reports[1] the following case belonging to this category:

Mr. W., a straw-hat manufacturer, had contracted a rheumatism, compelling him to turn the head strongly to the right side, anteriorly and downward. In the beginning he was still able to place the head in the right position, although only with pain, and only when aided by the hand; later he failed in this, and he thus remained, in spite of the use of vapor-baths, cataplasms, embrocations, and depletions. Four months after the beginning of the affection, the patient applied to Dr. Erdmann, who found a perfect torticollis rheumatica. The chin almost touched the right clavicle, while the left sternocleidomastoideus could be felt very taut under the skin. The patient was able, with the aid of the hand, to move the head somewhat backward, but not to the left side. Passive motions caused him an extraordinary pain. The electro-muscular contractility and sensibility of the sternocleidomastoideus were somewhat diminished. After the first employment of electro-cutaneous irritation of the neck, the motion of the head became immediately more free, and remained thus for several hours. On the following day Erdmann faradized, at the same time, the splenius capitis of the

[1] L. c., page 209.

left side and the upper third of the sternocleidomastoideus, when the head became straight, and even inclined to the left. The motions now remained easier, and, after the tenth application, the patient was perfectly cured.

M. Rosenthal cured, with the constant current, the following case:[1]

Therese Kummer, having been sent to the city on an errand, returned, after a few hours, drenched from a sudden violent rain, and with a distortion of the right trapezius, her head inclining to the right and behind, her chin turned to the left. The clavicular portion felt hard, and became painful whenever the patient tried to raise the head. The passing of a constant current through the affected muscle caused immediately a freer motion of the head. The next morning a second galvanization was made, which removed the abnormal position of the head entirely, and allowed the patient to resume her usual work.

D. *Paralyses.*

In the treatment of paralysis, the electric current has, from the oldest times, been extensively and successfully employed; indeed, it is, on account of its inlying qualities, to be used in preference to all other means.

1. *Electricity is a stimulus.* Accordingly, it causes, like all other organic or inorganic, chemical or mechanical irritations, when applied to motor nerves, a contraction of those muscles supplied by the irritated nerves. This happens as long as the nerve is still irritable, without regard to its being connected with or separate from the brain and spinal marrow. Applied directly to a muscle, electricity suspends contractions; if directed to sensitive nerves, or their extensions, sensation is produced as long as the communication with the brain and spinal marrow is intact. It is, finally, the only known agent which excites all the nerves of special sense,

[1] *L. c.*, page 105.

while through any other means only one can be excited. Thus the vibrating air affects the auditory, volatile substances the olfactory nerve, soluble substances, the sense of taste, etc. The constant and the intermittent current, however, differ in several points from each other with regard to their action on the nerves and muscles, for sometimes, in deeper disturbances of nutrition, the galvanic irritability is preserved, while the faradic is extinguished, and only through the irritation of the cutaneous nerves, by means of the secondary interrupted current, may single convulsions be produced as a consequence of reflex action. This difference probably depends upon the fact that, of the agents causing, according to Von Bezold and Fick, the irritation, namely, the fluctuation of intensity of the current and the duration of the uninterrupted current, the latter, under certain circumstances, becomes of greater importance than the former.

2. *The electric current increases the supply of blood to the irritated part of the body.* If an uninterrupted current is passed through the thigh of a frog, so as to cause tetanus, without irritating the other limb, the blood-vessels of the skin in the galvanized part are not only strongly dilated and filled with blood, but the muscles are also engorged, so as to cause the bright-red blood to pour out of every cut, while the flesh of the non-electrified thigh presents the usual pale, bloodless appearance.

3. *The electric current augments the temperature and increases the volume of the irritated part.* With regard to this, we have mentioned the observations of Matteucci and Ziemssen on the increase of temperature and augmentation of volume.

4. *The electric current enhances the contractile energy of the vascular walls.* We refer to the experiments of Weber made on the mesenteric arteries of the frog, already quoted. J. S. Schultze[1] has proved that the narrowing of the lumen

[1] De arteriarum notione, structura, constitutione chemico et vita. 1850. Page 52.

caused by the induced current takes place also in the larger arteries.

5. *The electric current counteracts the secondary changes occurring in inactive nerves and muscles.* John Reid[1] made a section of the nerves of the lower extremities of some frogs through the spinal canal, so as to destroy entirely their nervous connection with the spinal marrow. He then galvanized daily the muscles of one of the paralyzed legs, while those of the other leg were not touched. After the lapse of two months, the former had lost neither in firmness nor circumference, contracting, upon the galvanic stimulus, in a corresponding degree, while in the latter the volume was diminished about one-half, and they were relaxed and withered.

6. *The electric current is capable of restoring to nerves and muscles their lost functional power.* Nerves and muscles possess, like every other tissue, an activity corresponding to their degree of development. The electric current being capable of improving the nutrition of the muscular substance through contraction of the muscles—which, on their part, causes a fuller supply of arterial blood to their tissue, and with it an increase of the endosmotic power of the fibres—the endosmotic quality of the muscular fibres being also in a certain proportion to their power of action, the electric current is capable of increasing the diminished and of restoring the lost functional power. Whether the electric stimulus may cause a regeneration of muscular fibres in muscles atrophied to the highest degree, or whether, probably in such case, as asserted by Zenker,[2] a new formation of muscular fibres takes place, is exceedingly doubtful. Still, if the latter be the case, the electric current will be useful, by restoring the disturbed relations of nutrition in the new formation of muscular elements.

[1] On the Relation between Muscular Contractility and the Nervous System. Edinburgh, 1841. Pages 9-11.
[2] Ueber Veränderung der Willkürlichen Muskeln in Typhus Abdominalis. 1864.

7. *The electric current is capable of developing a supplementary function in muscular fibres not yet paralyzed.* L. Hepp[1] has proved that, in hypertrophies of muscles, the increase in thickness of the primitive muscular fibres is alone sufficient to explain the augmentation of bulk; that, likewise, the differences in the size of the same muscle, caused by age and exercise, depend solely upon the different thickness of the primitive muscular fibres. Thus the electric irritation causes also an increase of thickness and, at the same time, an increased capability of function in the normal muscular fibres.

8. *We are enabled, through the electric current, as shown by Erb,[2] to act directly on the brain and spinal marrow.* Moreover, the galvanization of the sympathetic nerve and its ganglia appears to us to have pointed out a method by which to cure, indirectly, cases of paralysis originating in the brain and spinal marrow. We have noticed a similar treatment for the removal of spasm.

9. *Even if the direct electrolysis has but little influence upon the process of resorption which we expect for the removal of certain paralytic processes, still the capability of the current, to effect a transmission of liquids from one electrode to the other, seems the more to be of greater importance in these procedures.*

If we now turn to the several forms of paralysis, those of cerebral origin will, undoubtedly, in accordance with the pathogenesis, hold out the least prospect of being cured by the electric current; yet, its employment is here also useful by removing or diminishing those frequently only secondary symptoms, such as the feeling of cold, the anæsthesia and atrophy, the contractions of the flexor muscles, etc., thereby reducing, as it were, their actual amount and extent. In

[1] Beitrag zur Lehre von der Hypertrophie der Muskeln in Henle and Pfeuffer's Zeitschrift für rationelle Medicin. Neue Folge. Band iv., Heft ii., page 257.
[2] Deutsches Archiv für klinische Medicin. Bd. iii., page 240, et seq.

apoplectic paralysis especially, its use becomes more prominent, as it acts often in a twofold manner: First, the cerebral portion around the apoplectic focus, rendered incapable of performing its usual functions on account of the hyperæmia, serous infiltration, etc., is again made active through the direct passage of the current, thus preventing the anatomical changes proceeding gradually from the extravasation through the cervical spinal marrow to the nerves and muscles; and second, these secondary symptoms themselves are afterward, although but imperfectly, removed. The following are the methods usually employed in these cases: 1. *The treatment through the head*, in which Remak galvanizes the sympathetic nerve, or places one pole on the cervical portion of the vertebral column, while the other pole is applied to the frontal half opposite the seat of the disease. 2. *The galvanization of the paralyzed muscles.* 3. *Their faradization.*

Concerning the first method, Remak, believing that every cerebral hemiplegia is to be considered a traumatic inflammation of the brain-substance caused by the extravasation, advises its employment immediately after the use of local depletions (from temporal and occipital regions), resorbing ointments, and blisters. Through these means he professes to have obtained a complete recovery even in hypersthenic hemiplegias which, according to his experience, would, at a later period, have become incurable. Yet this method has not yet been adopted by any one, so far as I know. At a later period, however, when the treatment is conducted more with regard to the removal of secondary symptoms, I have met with favorable results by galvanizing the sympathetic nerve with or without the appearance of diplegic contractions. I was not so fortunate as Remak and Benedikt to obtain a temporary or permanent solution of the contractions.

The peripheral treatment consists in the employment of the galvanic spinal marrow-nerve and spinal marrow-muscle currents, or in faradization, which latter course enables the practitioner to remove slight contractions of the extensor muscles as well as to restore the functional power to the affected parts. The removal of the contractions is also facilitated by faradizing the respective flexors with but rarely interrupted currents. It is naturally understood that but weak currents (eight to twelve elements) are to be employed for only a few minutes, if it is desired to begin the galvanization of the brain early. The same care must also be taken at a later period in this method as well as in peripheral galvanization and faradization, as long as tonic contractions indicate an irritated state of the brain. It is in such cases usually best to institute a few applications by way of trial, and to desist from any further electric treatment, unless a visible progress is caused by it, for then nothing can be expected by persevering; while on the other hand even a perceptible progress does not warrant in any way any exalted hopes for the final result. An isolated paralysis of single muscles of the eye, often appearing as first and only symptoms of a limited apoplectic focus, allows mostly a favorable prognosis with regard to its removal through the local employment of the constant and interrupted current, but it is frequently the precursor of new and more dangerous apoplectic attacks.

CASE 75.—Max Bunzel, eight years of age, was, in 1865, taken sick with an encephalitis accompanied by unconsciousness and violent spasms, and followed by a total paralysis of the left side of the body. In May, 1866, the little patient began again to walk, and the nutrition of the left leg also improved. When I saw the boy (January 23, 1867), for the first time, the arm was still perfectly useless, cold, and drawn to the thorax; elbow and hand were flexed, and could not be straightened nor removed farther than an inch from the trunk. A passive extension of the arm and hand, as well as a passive raising of the arm, was easily made. The deltoid muscle, and the extensors supplied by the radial nerve, were partially paralyzed, the ulnar nerve was entirely so. The electro-muscular contractility was intact in all; even in those partially very atrophied muscles (for instance, the interossei muscles); the sensibility was not disturbed. The farndization of the paralyzed muscles caused, after thirteen applications (February 27th), such an improvement, that the patient was enabled to raise the arm on a level with his shoulder, to stretch the hand, and to abduct the fingers somewhat. After twenty-seven applications (end of April), the deltoid as well as the triceps muscle acted normally, the fingers could be adducted and abducted, several of the fingers could also be extended, so that, at the end of June, the treatment terminated to our great satisfaction, after forty-two applications, and after the muscular tissue of the forearm and hand had become more developed.

CASE 76.—Mr. A. F., secretary, went to Dr. Graefe's clinic on account of double vision, which he first noticed several weeks ago while leaving his office for his home, and which had affected him ever since. The objective symptoms seemed to show nothing abnormal in his eyes; the examination of diplopia furnished at that time no exact localization, neither was it evident that a paretic affection had occurred simultaneously to several nervous trunks, especially of the left eye. The suspicion of the cause of the disease being central was confirmed by this circumstance as well as by its sudden origin, and a feeling of dulness in the head, of which, among other symptoms, the patient complained continually. He was treated for four and a half months with iodide of pot., Stahl's pills, the repeated application of the ferrum candens along the spine, etc., and, at the end of May, placed under my care for the purpose of an electric treatment. The symptoms of the patient were, according to Dr. v. Graefe, the following: the position of the axis of vision of the left eye showed under no circumstances any noticeable degree in the deviation of the angle from the normal position, so that, from the external appearance of the

patient, no conclusions could have been made concerning his
affection, if it had not been manifested by the characteristic
(corresponding to an existing paresis of the obliquus superior
muscle) position of the head (turning of the head round its
transverse axis anteriorly, and, at the same time, round its
vertical axis to the healthy, in this case, the right side). It
was only during the diagonal movement inward and downward—the direction in which the wanting function of the
superior oblique manifests itself most remarkably, on account of its moving the eyeball the strongest upward—that
it became evident that the left eye was not moved perfectly
inward and upward (corresponding to the function of the
trochlearis to the outward and downward), so that under
said circumstances a convergent squint with a deviation in
height ensued. The diagnosis could be completed from the
symptoms of diplopia, after analyzing which, it appeared
that the patient suffered, in addition to the above-mentioned
paralysis of the obliquus superior muscle, from a slight paretic affection of the rectus internus. The paresis had already changed in such a manner as to produce a slight contraction of the obliquus inferior, that is, the affection had
already begun to pass into the concomitant squinting of the
oblique muscles. This double vision annoyed the patient
very much, and he found it especially difficult, while examined, to ascertain the dimensions of height. In order to
obviate this, he was ordered prismatic glasses (130) with the
basis downward. He recognized, with great joy, the favorable results derived therefrom, but was still unable to read
or write by using both eyes at the same time.

After having, for four weeks, electrified the patient by
placing one conductor upon the frontal bone, while the
other was applied to those points of the closed eyes from
which the superior oblique and internal rectus muscles could
be easiest reached by the current, the examination made in
Graefe's clinic gave the following result: the paretic affection of the suffering muscles had considerably receded, dou-

ble vision could only be provoked by arranging the axis of vision for objects so situated that the two muscles must exert themselves mostly in a downward and right oblique manner. Symptoms depending upon a slight degree of contraction of the inferior oblique muscle still existed. From July, 1856, the patient was enabled to resume his occupation as secretary. The subsequent period furnished the sad proof of the patient suffering, indeed, from a cerebral affection. After the lapse of six months, during which he became entirely unable to work, repeated attacks of dizziness and loss of consciousness ensued, followed by partial deafness, and weakness in the lower extremities, so that, in the spring of 1859, he was obliged to resign. A paralysis of the muscles of the eye did not again appear.

Benedikt publishes the following case in the Medic.-chirurg. Rundschau, 1864, case 47:

Joseph Steiner, sixty-nine years of age, a merchant by profession, had, on the 24th of August of last year, at the grave of his wife, suffered from a hemiplegic attack, accompanied by loss of consciousness and speech, but not of the memory of words. On being received, May 7, 1863, the right lower extremity had returned to its normal condition, the articulation of vowels and single consonants was possible, the right facial nerve was paralyzed; the tongue was not perceptibly inclined, and was moved convulsively; the mental functions were normal. All the muscles of the forearm and hand, the muscles of the ball of the thumb excepted, were paralyzed; the flexor muscles of the phalanges and wrist-joint, as well as the pronator muscles, were contracted. Flexion and extension of the elbow-joint were normal; he raised the arm only as high as the ear, and moved the hand with difficulty to the shoulder of the opposite side. The electro-muscular contractility was considerably reduced in the paralyzed muscles, with the exception of the supinators; the same state existed in the otherwise unaffected triceps muscle. Galvanic treatment of the left cerebral hemisphere from the occipital to the frontal region caused immediately a passive flexion of the phalanges and the wrist-joint. May 13th (eighth application): patient could extend well the metacarpo-phalangeal, and somewhat the phalangeal joints. June 4th: slight supination. The patient was dismissed, as he did not seem to make any further progress.

Case 77.—Mrs. D., aged thirty-five years, widow, healthy, and with normal menstruation, never pregnant, although married for five years, suddenly, in the middle of December, 1864, lost the power of speech without any apparent cause; it returned, however, after a few minutes. This attack recurred on January 7, 1865, while the patient was sitting on the sofa conversing with somebody. She did not, however, this time, regain the power of speech, but was, in the following night, affected by loss of consciousness and complete paralysis of the whole right side of her body, in spite of a venesection made at the urgent request of her relatives. At the request of Dr. Steinmeck, I saw the patient, on the 1st of March, 1865. She was lying in bed, unable to turn from one side to the other; her right arm was still entirely paralyzed, the hand spasmodically closed so that the contraction of the flexors could only be overcome with difficulty, the leg could be drawn toward the body to some degree, the face was somewhat distorted, sensibility reduced, loss of speech complete, pain in the left frontal region. The electro-muscular contractility was normal. The faradization of the paralyzed muscles was accompanied by such an apparent improvement after each application, that the patient was enabled, on April 4th (after thirteen applications), to come to my office and walk up-stairs. The arm could be raised to an angle of 60°, the sensibility had increased, only the headache and loss of speech still existed, the latter making the patient especially unhappy. The galvanization of the brain from the left frontal region to the cervical portion of the spinal column removed this evil for a short time, but was of no material influence upon the other symptoms of paralysis

On the whole, the improvement, being at first so rapid, progressed now very slowly in spite of the employment of the plexus-nerve and nerve-muscle currents alternately with faradization, so that the patient, having terminated the treatment after fifty applications (August 10th), was able to raise the arm at about a right angle. The motions of the fingers were somewhat difficult, the sense of touch was undecided, and she could speak but few words. At this time (March, 1867), the patient drags the foot behind her while walking, she is able to knit and make embroidery, although the sense of touch is not normal; she still speaks very indistinctly. Her headache disappeared after a visit to Homburg.

CASE 78.—Mr. H. St., merchant, twenty-six years of age, suffered for many years from palpitation of the heart, depending upon hypertrophy, especially of the left ventricle, without valvular disease. He became, on the 5th of May, dizzy after great mental emotion, and fell down, without, however, losing consciousness. After being carried to his home, he became unconscious, and fell into convulsions, followed by a complete sensor and motor paralysis of the whole left side of his body as well as of the bladder. In the Catholic Hospital, where the patient spent four months, he improved so far as to be able to walk a considerable distance, although he still dragged the left foot. He was able to raise the arm to an angle of 40°, and also to move the fingers a little; the paralysis of the bladder had disappeared with the exception of a frequently ensuing desire to pass water. When the patient, upon the advice of Dr. Ulrich, consulted me on April 1, 1867, about two years after the attack, he could raise, with some difficulty, the left arm to an angle of 70°. He was emaciated and cold, the sensibility reduced, and even annihilated on the outer and inner surface of the hand, and especially in the fingers, being unable to feel a touch, while the prick of a needle was perceived but slightly; there existed also easily overcome contractions of the pectoralis minor and biceps muscles, while the flexor digit. comm. was still more contracted. An attempt to extend the hand failed on account of the uselessness of the interosseous muscles. Patient was lame, and complained of dulness in the head, troubling him at certain times. The treatment, applied two to three times weekly, consisted in the faradization of the sympathetic by placing the positive pole upon the portion of the neck corresponding to the left superior cervical ganglion, and the negative pole on the right side at a level with the fifth or sixth cervical vertebra. The result, accompanied by simultaneous diplegic reflex convulsive motions, was very satisfactory, for the patient could, at the end of April, after twelve applications, raise and extend his arm perfectly; the temperature had also improved greatly, the sensibility was increased and the foot dragged less. After each application his head also became freer. After fifteen additional applications, in which descending currents were employed together with the irritation of the sympathetic nerve, the movability of the hand improved so far as to enable him to extend it, July 28th, perfectly, while the fingers could also be adducted and abducted. When I terminated the treatment, on August 12th, after thirty-eight applications, the patient could execute all the movements of the fingers, and seize and hold small things, although he was still obliged to use his eyes for that purpose. The temperature of the arm was nearly normal, the nutrition was improved considerably, and he could again pursue his business without difficulty. He was, however, unable to distinguish any thing by merely touching it.

Remak succeeded, by means of galvanizing the sympathetic nerve, in curing a case of complicated paralysis of several muscular nerves of the eye, of the nerves of the face, of the hypoglossus in conjunction with the nerves of respiration—in short, a case of extensive paralysis, the starting of which had to be looked for in the posterior fossa of the skull. We copy this case from the "Berliner klin. Wochenschrift," 1864:

A farmer, aged sixty-nine years, always healthy, was exposed to a cold while engaged in heavy outdoor work in November, 1863, which suddenly terminated in double vision. This affection gradually increased, a falling down of the eyelids with an œdematous swelling, especially on the left side, ensued, followed by difficult motion of the face, impossibility of moving mouth and tongue in the normal manner, and finally, a catarrh with impeded expectoration. In the course of several months, the ptosis had assumed such a degree, that the patient, being unable to work, went to Berlin for the purpose of applying to Professor v. Graefe, who, after the fruitless administration of the iodide of potash, sent him, on April 24, 1864, to Remak.

Upon an examination, the following symptoms were noticed: The palpebral fissure did not measure more than one and a half lines; the pupil of the right eye was perfectly invisible, the eyeball being turned upward and outward in consequence of a paralysis of the internal rectus muscle, while the left pupil was also but little visible. The muscles of the eyeballs were in an unsymmetrical paralyzed condition; of the two sides of the face, the left was more paralyzed than the right, and the cheeks more than the frontal portion. The motion of the tongue was impeded and its pointing impossible; all paralyzed muscles could be excited by the electric current.[1] Another series of paralytic symptoms affected the respiratory muscles. The thorax did not expand during inspiration, neither could the patient cough. With

---

[1] The extinct electro-muscular contractility of the paralyzed muscles induced me to ascribe the cause of the paralytic symptoms to a diffuse exudation in the posterior fossa of the skull, and not to a disturbance in the circulation of the blood depending on the vaso-motor nerves, which point Remak left undecided.

regard to the general symptoms, it was found that the impulse of the apex of the heart was weak, the sounds of the heart dull, pulse seventy to eighty, and the face was of a corpse-like pallor, especially around the mouth and the point of the nose.

Remak galvanized the sympathetic nerve, and noticed, after a few applications, a decided improvement. After fourteen days the patient was out of danger; the respiratory motions, especially, became easier, and the muscles of the face, tongue, and eyes, also improved in a corresponding manner. Remak presented the patient to the Medical Society of Berlin after a treatment of four weeks, having been obliged to allow him to leave for his home on account of urgent business, although he had not yet fully recovered. At that time the right eyeball was still a little turned upward, and double vision also ensued to a slight extent whenever he looked to the left side; the motion of the eyelids, however, was perfect, he being able to open and close them rapidly and without difficulty. The facial paralysis had not entirely disappeared, but the patient was now able to perform normally the act of inspiration, expiration, expectoration, and of laughing. The electric excitability of the facial muscles had returned *ad integrum ;* the color of his face was healthy and fresh.

The spinal paralyses are to be divided, as Benedikt correctly remarks, into two classes with regard to their therapeutics: 1. Those in which the disturbance of motion is caused by a diminished power of the respective muscles—spinal paralysis proper. 2. Those in which the isolated muscular motions may be performed more or less normally, but where the power in coördinated movements is disturbed—tabetic paralysis.

Cases of spinal paralysis proper do not become amenable

to the electric treatment until the acute stage is passed, when we are called upon to remove the secondary disturbances, resulting from the lesion, as in traumatic injuries, or in paralytic affections caused by partial myelitis or myelomeningitis, meningitis spinalis, or by an effusion of blood into the membranes of the spinal marrow, etc. In all these cases, faradization of the paralyzed muscles, or galvanization by means of descending labile spinal marrow-nerve or nerve-muscle currents, may be employed with equal advantage. In choosing either method, especially in infantile spinal paralysis, of which we have treated above, I am led by the sensations of the little patients themselves, to whom, frequently the burning, caused by using the constant current, is far more disagreeable than the sensation experienced by using faradization by means of slowly interrupted currents. In cases of this kind, which always require great perseverance on the part of the physician and the relatives of the patient, in order to succeed, I frequently suspend the treatment for a long period (during which, baths, embrocations, frictions, and proper mechanical contrivances are used), in such a manner as to subject the children once or twice a year to an electric treatment, lasting each time for about four weeks, which method I cannot too urgently recommend for adoption. If, in spinal paralysis, there is still a state of irritation existing, recognized by a pain, occurring on a certain place of the spinal column, either spontaneous or in consequence of pressure, galvanization of the spinal column, by means of stable currents, is to be employed so as to apply the + pole to the irritated spot, while the — pole is placed upon any other somewhat remote point; here a peripheral treatment by means of galvanic or faradic currents would only do harm.

CASE 79.—The letter-carrier, Anton Schœffer, forty years of age, having always enjoyed good health, experienced, from the middle of April, 1858, a frequent desire to urinate without any known cause, happening at first every half an hour, afterward oftener, which was soon followed by an involuntary passage of urine. These symptoms, however, only appeared while he was walking, being absent while lying in bed. In addition to this, he was attacked, in the beginning of May, by violent pain in the back and both legs, especially in the right calf, a feeling of numbness in the whole lower portion of the body, involuntary defecation, and, finally, cutaneous and muscular anæsthesia to such an extent that he was unable to perceive either the touch or the introduction of needles, especially in the nates and posterior side of the thigh. In spite of local depletion in the sacral region, the employment of the tartar-emetic ointment, and the internal use of the iodide of potassium, the evil continued increasing till, at the end of May, the patient was entirely unable to walk. During the months of June and July the patient improved gradually, so that he was able to walk greater distances, although with difficulty and great exertion, at the time he consulted me, August 12th. The other symptoms, however, still continued, such as a frequent desire to urinate, followed by the involuntary emission of urine, unless attended to immediately, neuralgic pains in the legs, especially in the course of the sacro-sciatic nerve, intestinal tenesmus, a feeling of numbness and heaviness in the legs, and anæsthesia of the bladder, nates, thigh, and leg. After twelve electric applications (September 8th), in which the electric moxa was first applied behind the trochanters, and the electric brush to the anæsthetic parts of the skin and muscles, pain and anæsthesia of the skin and muscles had disappeared almost entirely, the walking also getting easier and freer. The difficulty about the bladder and intestines still continuing, I was induced, from the 1st of October (application twenty), to pass the current into these organs also. The anæsthesia of the bladder was so great, that the patient did not perceive the first introduction of the most intense and rapidly-striking current of Du Bois's apparatus. Thirty-second application (November 1st): the anæsthesia of the bladder has diminished, the urine passing with the proper force, the patient also being able to hold it back for a longer period than before, except that, when he is obliged to walk more than usual, an exceedingly violent tenesmus of the rectum and bladder ensues. Defecation does not occur any longer spontaneously, still there is a tendency to diarrhœa, which, however, is easily removed by the administration of an opiate. For this reason the patient was unable to resume his arduous duties before the forty-third application, on December 1st, when the electric current was passed several times simultaneously into the rectum and bladder. He is now (1868) perfectly well.

CASE 80.—Lieutenant W. L., of the first regiment of infantry, was, after a fatiguing brigade-drill, taken sick with a rheumatic fever on August 6, 1854, which lasted for eight weeks, followed by a general relaxation, especially a great weakness of his legs. A journey of ninety miles to his country-seat, made at the beginning of October for the benefit of his health, caused a trembling of the arms, followed by thoracic spasms, stitches in the cardiac region, palpitation, and other symptoms of nervous excitement. Although these symptoms disappeared after a few days of rest, they reappeared more strongly after a trip of sixteen miles, the motion of the wagon causing the patient great inconvenience. He was attacked by spasmodic pains in the head, heart, thorax, and legs, at times so violent as to make him yell; the points of his fingers and the heels were exceedingly sensible. In the spring of 1855 these nervous symptoms disappeared, allowing him to go to Berlin at a slow rate of travelling; still there were symptoms of spinal irritation developed. The careful touch of the spinal column, especially of the fourth, seventh, and eleventh dorsal vertebræ, reproduced all the nervous symptoms. His pulse was intermittent, the extremities cold, and the patient greatly excited. This state of his health caused his physicians, Drs. Vehsemeyer and Lauer, to recommend a longer sojourn at the baths of Landeck. Here his strength increased and the nervous symptoms diminished; the sensibility of the spinal column disappeared, but in the same ratio the uselessness of the legs increased, so that the patient, after having spent eight weeks at the bath, returned with a complete paralysis of both legs. After the continued use of irritating ointments, etc., the patient was placed under my care at the end of November, 1855. Both legs were completely paralyzed, they could be adducted simultaneously, but not one without the other, while abduction was entirely impossible, extension of the leg could not be made, extension and flexion of the toes of both feet only to a limited extent. The patient could move forward only by jumping and supported by two crutches, as it was impossible to separate the legs from each other. The electro-muscular contractility was considerably reduced in the crural, vastus internus, and externus, in the rectus and glutæus muscles, there being not much difference between either extremity, while anæsthesia of the skin existed more strongly on the right side. The muscles of the back reacted on the right less than on the left side; the adductor muscles were contracted. The state of the bowels was nearly regular; a frequent desire to pass water annoyed the patient a great deal. Reflex motions, ensuing often spontaneously and always upon an irritation of the skin, induced me to desist at first from the employment of the brush, in spite of the simultaneous existence of anæsthesia and paralysis, and to use only mild induction currents twice a week, lasting in the beginning from ten to fifteen minutes. After the sixteenth application (January 18, 1868) the patient was able to stand without the aid of crutches, and to walk with crutches, by putting one foot before the other. From the twenty-fifth sitting (February 10th) I faradized the anæsthetic portions of the skin, thus restoring its normal sensibility in a short time. In the thirtieth application (May 3d) the patient could walk round the table by leaning the arms against it; the tenesmus of the bladder had also disappeared.

On the 21st he was able to walk up and down his room with two canes instead of the crutches heretofore used. On the 25th of June (thirty-ninth application), he promenaded, with the aid of one cane, in the garden for a quarter of an hour. In July he left for a watering-place on the North Sea, whence he returned perfectly well after a sojourn of four weeks.

CASE 81.—Captain G., thirty-eight years of age, was, six years ago, often exposed to the influence of cold, while on special duty in the cannon-foundery of Spandau. Since that time he noticed a certain restlessness in both legs, to which, however, he paid no attention until a peculiar feeling of cold and insensibility spread over the whole left side of his body which appeared to be divided into two halves. These anomalies of sensation gradually disappeared, instead of which he was affected with a continually increasing weakness and unsteadiness in the left thigh, reflex movements in both legs, a considerable emaciation of the left nates and thigh, and a feeling of pressure in the dorsal region. For these symptoms he was ordered a cold-water treatment, Russian baths, iod. of pot., and, in the spring of 1863, electricity; which latter agent improved him so much that, after a visit to Marienbad, he was able to ride on horseback without difficulty, and even walk with a slight dragging of the leg. He continued improving slowly in this state—interrupted only temporarily by gastric derangement or by slight excesses in the use of alcoholic liquors, when his limbs became perfectly immovable—until October, 1867, at which time he fell out of a carriage, and was unable to rise again without the help of other persons. Since that time, the lameness and unsteadiness of the leg increased greatly; he could not walk unless he kept the knee-joint perfectly extended. Walking down-stairs also caused him great inconvenience. There were, likewise, strong reflex motions of the legs, with a progressing and very decided emaciation of the left thigh. When I saw the patient, January 13, 1868, the examination showed, besides the above-mentioned symptoms, only a pain on pressing the dorsal region without any derangement of sensibility and coördination. This case being a circumscribed myelitis, I applied the + pole upon the painful spot of the spinal column, and the — pole upon the region of the left crural plexus. By this method I shortly obtained a very favorable result, for after the ninth application (January 27th) the nutrition of the leg had improved a great deal, the lameness was very much reduced, ascending a staircase became again possible, greater distances could be walked on foot without difficulty, and the reflex movement ensued less freqnently. This improvement continued without interruption until the departure of the patient, February 12th.

Hitzig reports in Virchow's Archiv., 1867, vol. xl., the following case of traumatic myelo-meningitis spinalis, which he cured through the use of the constant current:

Sergeant Hermann Rothbart, aged thirty-five years, of a strong physique and well-developed muscles, was, in March, 1865, thrown off his horse, falling upon the lower portion of the back. Although, since, he always suffered from pain in that region, he performed his duties until May, when he was taken sick with pleurisy, rendering him unfit for duty till the month of July. From this time the pain in the back gradually increased, in addition to which, he suffered from excentric pain in the extremities and great sensitiveness of the skin. The patient experienced frequently, especially in the lying position, a feeling of formication and numbness of the feet; besides these symptoms, he always felt as if there were cushions under his feet. Involuntary, fibrillar, partial and local muscular spasms supervened, the motor power was more and more diminished, without, however, an actual paralysis existing, with the exception of a temporary diplopia. Finally, the patient suffered three to four times weekly from pollutions, without being impotent in the beginning. The insecurity of locomotion increased daily, he was unable to walk or stand in the dark or with his eyes closed, while in daytime or with open eyes he could only move in a bent position, dizziness and increased pain in the back ensuing whenever he tried to assume an erect position. His sleep being disturbed and appetite wanting, he became very much emaciated. After the useless employment of nitr. of silver, iodine, etc., the patient applied to Dr. Hitzig, on the 8th of January, 1866. He stooped, and was unable to raise himself without tottering; on closing his eyes he groped about him, fearing to fall. There was no paralysis, the pupils reacted normally; a slight touch of the skin, except on the face, with a pin's head, was almost entirely unperceived. Touching the skin, the extremities, and the trunk, caused violent reflex spasm in the limbs and trunk. The vertebral column, especially about the intervertebral spaces, was very sensitive. The patient was treated with stabile descending currents. After the eighth application, January 16th, sleep lasting for seven hours, almost no spontaneous pain, a feeling of ease in the legs. Gastric derangement required the proper remedies, but did not necessitate an interruption of the electric treatment; on the contrary, the treatment of the sympathetic nerve exercised a favorable influence upon the general health. In addition to this, the two crural nerves were also treated, after January 28th, in the same manner, with such a good result, that the patient was able, on the 8th of February, to stand with closed eyes for fifteen minutes, the feeling of cushions on the lower surface of his feet having, in the mean time, almost entirely disappeared. The experimental employment, however, of labile currents on the 9th and 10th of February, rendered him decidedly worse, which, however, was soon obviated through the galvanization of the sympathetic. This latter method of treating the large, nervous trunks with descending currents, and the spinal marrow by applying the positive pole over the painful vertebræ, improved the patient to such an extent that, on the 22d of February, after the treatment had been continued for six weeks, none of the above-described nervous symptoms remained, except a moderate pain on pressing several intervertebral spaces. The patient walked greater distances, sometimes even for hours in succession, in consequence of which, he was discharged, on the 20th of March, and soon after appointed a messenger for the laity court. A relapse, ensuing on November 10th, was nearly removed at the end of December, without preventing him from the discharge of his duties, when great exertion and a heavy cold, in the first days of January, produced the same state of disease as in the beginning, with a far stronger expression of the nervous symptoms (convulsive movements in the left thigh and leg). A greater psychical depression and a considerable gastric derangement also appeared, necessitating another two months' treatment analogous to the above-described, until he received the appointment of letter-carrier to the same court, on the 1st of March of the same year. In the course of the treatment, Dr. Hitzig repeatedly availed himself of the occasion to examine the patient's sense of touch in the legs and feet. He has added some drawings representing the gradually progressing improvement up to the nearly normal state.

With regard to tabetic paralysis—a name still to be retained for the present, inasmuch as the gray degeneration of the posterior columns forms at best the final result of the morbid process, the ataxia being neither peculiar to this species of disease, nor existing in all cases of this category—its prognosis is by no means as bad as it used to be considered. In the first place, affections of the spinal marrow sometimes occur, having all the characteristic symptoms of tabes, which are perfectly cured in the beginning by absolute rest in the supine position and a corresponding dietetic regimen. In the second, the use of the nitrate of silver and of electricity in the more advanced stages of the disease has been accompanied by results sufficiently favorable to warrant us in pronouncing them cures. Of these two remedies, the nitrate of silver has but little fulfilled the expectation entertained about its employment, although it has an unmistakable influence upon the removal of a possibly existing paralysis of the bladder, and of a coexisting gastric and intestinal catarrh, to which, perhaps, may be added an improved security of the gait by its reducing the reflex excitability of the spinal marrow. Still, the case lately published by Eulenburg[1] encourages new experiments with this remedy. The use of electricity, however, has produced a larger number of improved, and even cured cases. To the latter category those cases especially belong, in which the patients complain spontaneously of pain at a certain point of the spinal marrow, or where a careful examination reveals a spot particularly sensitive to pressure. This spot, the probable seat of a primary or secondary meningitis, must especially be taken into consideration, as treatment with the constant current renders it sometimes possible to remove the characteristic symptoms of the disease. The following is the method to be employed: The positive electrode of a pretty powerful battery (thirty to forty elements) is placed upon the tender spot, and there kept for from three to five minutes, while the negative pole is applied to the back near the spinal column.

I am indebted to the kindness of Dr. Drissen for the following cases, treated by himself and belonging to this category:

CASE 82.—Mr. S. O., aged fifty-two years, had suffered for six years from neuralgic pains, of an eccentric type, in the legs. A fire breaking out two years ago, he jumped out of bed in the night in order to assist in extinguishing it. He received a severe cold; ataxia followed, which increased to such a degree that he was at last unable to walk. After some time a slight improvement took place, giving the patient an opportunity to go to Berlin. When he first presented himself, his gait was insecure, he fell as soon as he

[1] Verhandlungen der Berl. med. Gesellschaft, vol. ii., 1867.

closed his eyes, and was hardly able to keep on his legs, supported by a cane. The right leg was worse than the left, and, consequently, the anæsthesia of the sole of the right foot also greater. The upper extremities were not affected.

As the first lumbar vertebra was found to be sensitive on pressing it, the treatment was directed exclusively to this vertebra, to which the positive pole was applied, while the negative pole was placed alternately upon the right and left hip. After the fifth application, the tottering, while the eyes were closed, was hardly perceptible; the numbness of the soles of the feet had disappeared, and the patient was able to walk greater distances without being tired and without even using a cane. I was prevented from observing the patient any longer, as he declared himself cured, leaving Berlin after the sixth application.

CASE 83.—J. W., aged thirteen and a half years, presented the following symptoms, gradually developed in the course of a year: He was hardly able to walk a few steps without getting immediately tired; the left leg especially was strongly thrown forward while walking, and the whole gait offered the picture of a patient suffering from tabes. He was unable to place the right leg upon a chair, and the left leg only by holding on to something. Patient complained of an indistinct sensation under the soles of the feet, although objectively no considerable derangement of sensibility could be proved. He tottered strongly whenever he closed his eyes. The third dorsal vertebra being painful on pressure, the positive electrode was attached to it, while the negative was placed upon the region of the hip. After the first application the patient was immediately able to place the right leg upon a chair; the improvement, however, disappeared at the first time of the treatment after a few minutes. This treatment continued, with frequent interruptions, for seven months, when J. was able to walk for hours in succession, and to run without any great fatigue. Since that time his body has been developed normally, and now he is a robust boy. After the lapse of a year, there exists, as the only morbid symptom, a slight tottering while the eyes are closed.

CASE 84.—The merchant P. K., thirty years old, suffered for several years from frequent pollutions and nightly erections, a slight fatigue while walking, and a feeling of tension in the inner surface of the thighs; in addition to which, lately, a feeling of being bruised between the shoulder-blades, pressure upon the chest, and lancinating pains in the lower extremities supervened. In this case the positive pole was placed upon the fifth vertebra, it being tender on pressure, and the negative upon the hip-joint. By this method the patient, who felt better if not too often galvanized, was treated for six weeks, until the perfect removal of his complaint, twelve applications having in all been made. In about a year the former symptoms reappeared, after he had repeatedly performed the sexual act with great excitement. He recovered, after having been galvanized three times in the same manner.

In a majority of cases of this kind, however, no such painful spots can be found, probably because the cells of the central nerves are primarily affected, while the spinal meninges remain intact. These offer, with regard to the result of the treatment, a far more unfavorable result. Remak, trying to ascertain their local seat, has, in accordance with the different symptoms, constructed a tabes lumbo-sacralis, lumbo-dorsalis, dorsalis inferior and superior, cervicalis, basalis, and cerebellaris,[1] a division of some practical importance, inasmuch as he bases his method of treatment upon applying every time the positive conductor to that place which he believes to be the local seat of the disease. How far this division is defensible on anatomical grounds the results of *post-mortem* examinations must decide; but it cannot be denied by those witnessing his presenting some patients to the Berliner Med. Society,[2] on July 13, 1864, that he obtained by

---

[1] See Allgem. med. Central Zeitung, 1862, p. 869, et seq.
[2] See Berliner klinisch Wochenschrift, 1864, p. 893.

this method very favorable results. We shall briefly give the most pregnant symptoms upon which his division is based, by comprising the first four species under the name of tabes dorsalis proper, as they possess less characteristic symptoms distinguishing them from each other. Their characteristics are—insecurity of gait, constant affection of bladder, rectum, and the genital organs; no other disease of the eyes except, perhaps, a dilatation of the pupils; pain, if at all present, never as violent as in the other kinds. Tabes cervicalis is not only distinguished by the small size and immovability of both pupils, but mainly by exceedingly violent attacks of excentric neuralgia of the arms and legs; the paraplegic symptoms may for many years remain of a low grade. Tabes basalis generally begins with derangement of the eyes—double vision or squinting. There are, in addition, also, amblyopia and atrophy of the retina, while pain is mostly absent. Tabes cerebellaris makes itself known by the highest degree of uncertainty of gait and a receding of all other symptoms. Pain never occurs.

If the catalytic action of the current in this method of application takes an important position, we must seek another explanation for the method, which consists in passing a weak current, generated from ten or, at the highest, twenty elements, through the neck to the lumbar region, and which also has been accompanied by good results. Here, unless we take it for granted—what has, however, not yet been proved by any fact—that it is possible to revive, by means of the current, the functionless fibres and ganglion-cells of the spinal marrow, the unmistakably favorable influence of the current can only be accounted for by assuming that it renders the diseased and inactive elements, which are still capable of performing their functions, fit for activity. This is similar to those cases of congenital facial paralysis observed by me, in which a single or double faradization rendered the buccinator muscle supplied by the motor portion of the trigeminal nerve capable of permanently performing its function, although they did not come under medical treatment until after ten and even nineteen years.[1] Weak currents are here especially indicated, because most of the patients affected with disease of the spinal marrow suffer from great nervous irritability, and consequently their nervous system is easily exhausted.

Dr. Seeligmueller[2] has published the following case of this kind:

Thielemann, a mason, aged forty-two years, had had an apoplectic attack, first five years and then two years ago. After the first attack his four extremities were variously paralyzed to a high degree, and he did not recover till half a year afterward. The paralytic state brought about by the second attack still remained to the same degree and extent when he was received into the institution. Concerning the motor disturbances, he appears on the street as if he were drunk; his left leg and right arm are especially weak. Every attempt to stand with closed eyes is followed by an attack of dizziness. He is unable to mount a chair without help. The following are the symptoms of deranged sensibility: Pain in the sacral and lumbar region; deafness, and formication in the hands and feet; impossibility of feeling small, thin substances, like coins or needles, or to take them off the table; and, finally, a sensation as if his chest were compressed by a strap. The anæsthetic zone extends from the level of the spinal scapulæ up to the vertex and laterally to the side-whiskers. In this zone the prick of a needle is well localized, but sensation is dull, the same as in the fingers and toes. He denies any excess in venery. Has had seven children, the last ten years ago. Is impotent, having no erections. The urine does not come out with the proper jet, and sometimes escapes involuntarily.

The patient was treated daily, for ten minutes, with a

[1] See Cases 31 and 32.
[2] See Correspondenzblatt der Vereins der Aerzte der Regierungsbezirks Merseburg, 1861, No. 7.

current of ten elements descending the spinal marrow, by placing the positive pole above the anæsthetic dorsal zone, and the negative pole on the upper lumbar region. After the first application, the result was wonderful. The pain in the back ceased, sensibility in the thumb and index-finger of both hands improved a great deal; he walked more securely, and crossed the street, for the first time, without a cane. After the second application he was able to turn the head in every direction without getting dizzy, as before, whenever he looked behind while walking. About an hour after the second application he perceived a higher sensibility in both middle fingers. After the third application the feeling in both hands, the little fingers excepted, was very good; he also felt the floor better, and the left leg was stronger. He said that, since the third application, he constantly felt, for a short time after each application, an increased tickling, first in the more paralyzed foot, then in the left arm, then in the right arm, then in the right foot, and finally in every extremity alike. After the fifth application, the walk of the patient had visibly improved. He was now able to walk upon the pavement for a whole afternoon at a time; furthermore, he perceived plainly the slightest touch in the anæsthetic zone; his sleep, formerly very restless and short, had now become long and deep. During the seventh application the current was felt in the little finger of the right hand. As he now complained only of a painful stiffness of the neck, six elements were passed through it, in addition to the ten applied to the vertebral column. In this manner, also, the patient's last complaint was removed almost entirely after seven additional applications, so that he could be considered cured after fourteen applications.

Dr. Seeligmueller saw the patient again a year and a half after the treatment. The results obtained by it were substantially the same. He had been able to work continually, and nothing remained of his former disease except a slight dragging of the left foot.

Few such pronounced cases are on record up to the present time. More frequently the progress made after the first applications is astonishing, but soon arrives at its limits, which cannot be overstepped, probably on account of the existing anatomical changes. Frequently we must remain satisfied with having improved one or the other symptom, and often even this is not attained. Sometimes it is advantageous to add a peripheral to the central treatment, partially by employing the spinal marrow-nerve current, partially by direct galvanization of the sensitive nerves, which, if indicated—that is, after removal of the irritation of the spinal marrow—are not without influence upon the security of gait. In each case the experiment must decide on their suitableness.

I have myself met with as much success, through faradization of the anæsthetic skin by means of the electric brush, as could be obtained by galvanization.[1] On one hand, probably the direct influence on the sensible nerves, on the other hand, the reflex action produced by the brush from the sensible upon the motor nerves, has contributed to the attained result. It is, of course, understood that the latter method is made use of by way of experiment only in such cases where there are not only no symptoms of inflammatory irritation of the spinal marrow, but where, also, there exists even no increased irritability in decrepit, old individuals.

CASE 85.—Professor Z., born in 1803, although not a strong child, still always enjoyed good health. While a young man, he was very much devoted to his studies, leading necessarily a most sedentary but in every respect temperate life. In 1844 he noticed for the first time, especially after an unusual mental exertion, a decided relaxation of his limbs, with a violent headache, against which neither Kissingen nor Franzensbad gave any relief. His complaints even increased since that time, especially in 1846, he fre-

[1] See Case 95.

quently fainting in consequence of the headache. A sojourn of six weeks in Homburg, a journey through France and Belgium, and finally the sea-baths of Ostend, relieved the headache entirely, without its ever returning again. In the year of 1848, however, which caused him many mental emotions and excitements, an abdominal derangement began, increasing gradually in violence. Diarrhœa followed constipation, blood and mucus passed from the rectum, and finally he was affected with prolapsus ani. The Marienbader Kreutzbrunnen and the subsequent use of sea-baths did not produce the slightest change. In addition to this, there supervened, in 1851, violent pain in the back, extending to the chest, or the hips and thighs, or the hands, in which latter case writing became very inconvenient to him. This state continuing about the same till 1857, with the exception of a few exacerbations caused by too much mental exertion or by the changes of temperature, he became much worse in the summer of the same year. The use of his hands and feet failed him nearly entirely; while walking, on the 11th of August, he suddenly lost all power of sensation; abdominal and vesical derangement also ensued. I saw the patient for the first time October 2, 1857. He was then fifty-four years old, anæmic, emaciated, and cachectic. An attempt to stand, or walk a few steps, his eyes closed, produced such tottering that he seemed to fall every moment; at the same time there began a continual vibrating motion of the orbicularis palpebrarum. Changes in the pupil were not observed. The patient complained of a sensation of constriction originating from the lumbar vertebræ, of a neuralgic pain along the course of both saphenous and ulnar nerves, of a feeling of heaviness in his hands, stiffness in his feet, and especially a perfect insensibility in the left great toe; also a frequent desire to pass water, with a scanty evacuation, especially in the daytime, while in the night the urine often escaped involuntarily, it being thick, alkaline, and containing sediment. The bowels acted slowly, usually requiring injections of cold water. The anus was prolapsed, the nates relaxed and emaciated. Concerning the electric condition of the muscles, the electro-muscular contractility and sensibility were reduced to a very moderate degree; the skin, however, was anæsthetic in the lower ulnar regions, in the soles of the feet, and in the toes. The feet were constantly cold, the skin dry, appetite pretty fair, sleep frequently interrupted by pain. Thinking that there was but little chance for improving a case apparently so far advanced, I deemed it sufficient to allow the electric pencil to act in a plainly perceptible degree upon the legs and feet, and upon the anæsthetic portions of the arms. The result was surprising. The patient was able, after the third application, to stand easier, and to walk through the room without assistance, the pain also diminishing. Sixth application (October 20th): the improvement continued, passing the urine became easier, the patient felt stronger and more courageous, the feet warmer. Ninth application (October 30th): patient can write easier; pain reappeared, being, however, but slight and of short duration; the gait was easier, the tottering less. Thereafter the muscles of the leg, quadriceps femoris, and the glutæi muscles, were stimulated by mild currents. Fourteenth application (November 17th): patient had taken a walk, felt very well after it; urine flowed easier and more freely, the involuntary nightly escape was less, feet were warm. The patient was able to walk from his residence to the Royal Library, and, after working for several hours, to return home again on foot. Pain generally only ensued in the course of the winter, during fluctuations of temperature, when especially the great toe of his left foot was affected. The insensibility of the hands occurred only temporarily, and then in never as high a degree as before. The urinary complaints still existed, but were considerably diminished. He continued in this state of health for the next year, using steel-baths, and being enabled to walk great distances without difficulty.

We have already, in the previous chapters, become acquainted with a series of cases cured or improved by galvanizing the sympathetic nerve. They were the following: 1. Paralysis of vasomotor nerves (see Case 1). 2. Primary arterial spasm. 3. Apoplectic paralysis (see Case 87). 4. Cases of progressive muscular atrophy, with or without swelling of the joints (see Cases pages 253 and 299). 5. Neuralgias and spasms of cerebro-spinal nerves, the starting-point of which, as the result of the treatment proved beyond doubt, had to be sought for in an affection of the sympathetic system (see Cases pages 331 and 369). The cases adduced under 1 and 2 can be fully explained by the direct action of the current on the sympathetic system, and the influence of the latter upon the vasomotor nerves, while the favorable results obtained in apoplectic paralysis must be ascribed to the indirect catalytic actions mentioned on page 370 and in other places. It is otherwise with the cures mentioned under 4 and 5; their accomplishment must be explained by the hypothesis of a direct or indirect influence of the sympathetic upon motor and sensor nerves. This hypothesis appears to be plausible, yet no fact can be adduced in proof of it except Remak's experiment quoted on page 80, where he produced the relaxation of the levator palp. sup., and the spasmodic contraction of the orbicularis palp., after having cut the sympathetic nerve in the neck of a cat. We find probable reasons for the relation of the sympathetic system to the motor nerves in the setting in of diplegic contractions, which can be produced in single cases only from the known places of application at the cervical ganglia of the sympathetic (see Case 87), as well as in the repeatedly observed (in progressive muscular atrophy) symptoms, consisting of an increase of circumference, power of function, and excitability of atrophic muscles, in consequence of employing the same method. The relation to the sensitive nerves is confirmed by the repeatedly experienced sensation of the patients during this operation—of their perceiving a passing through or tickling in the arm or leg, sometimes on that side on which the cervical portion of the sympathetic has been brought into the current, sometimes on the opposite side.

With reference to the practice of the method, I think it better to place one conductor on the inner side of the sterno-cleido-mastoid muscle, while the other is applied to that portion of the neck where the respective ganglion is affected by the greatest possible number of currents, than to apply both in the direction of the sterno-cleido-mastoideus. In the first-mentioned method the direction of the current is necessarily rather indifferent.

We shall cite a few more cases belonging to this category.

CASE 86.—Gottfried Kornemann, aged forty-six years, a waiter, after having been exposed to the influence of cold, perceived, for the first time in October, 1860, a feeling of stinging and constriction in his throat, connected with pharyngeal spasm, rendering the act of deglutition impossible for hours. These attacks recurred at uncertain intervals, making the patient feel as if there was something "glued" into the cavity. Soon other disturbances of motion and sensation supervened. They consisted, usually, of a feeling of tension originating in the heels, and thence extending along the vertebral column to the occipital region. He felt as if his head were covered with a cold plate, his chest constricted with a hoop, his abdomen distended, as though air were being continually pumped into it. At times there ensued a state of relaxation and exhaustion, followed by a general trembling, or a feeling of insecurity extended over the whole body, while in the sitting position, of falling off a bench, while walking, of having india-rubber in the joints and under the soles of the feet, which frequently were benumbed. Sometimes visible spasms occurred in the heels, knee-joints, and in the neck, which latter part was so violently affected that the head was turned from the right to the left. Gradually he found it difficult to stand; walking and mounting stairs became impossible. I saw the patient for the first time on May 5, 1865. The starting-point of his affection was undoubtedly the right lateral cervical region, which was greatly swollen, hard, and very painful, especially when pressing upon the place corresponding to the superior cervical ganglion, which pressure also caused simultaneously painful sensations reaching as far as the occiput. The sensibility, when he was touched or pricked with a needle, was intact; the patient could feel correctly without the aid of his sight. As this case depended upon the disappearance of the cervical swelling (producing, according to our diagnosis, the above-mentioned symptoms by pressing upon the cervical ganglia of the sympathetic), a large conductor was placed upon the anterior, and another conductor, corresponding in size to the former, upon the posterior right side of the neck. This treatment having been continued for one and a half years, a resorption of the swelling was brought about, causing a gradual disappearance of all the symptoms of sensor and motor derangement. In this patient, also, the operation produced a feeling of flowing in the arm and leg, especially in the affected right side of the body. After a lapse of six months the patient was enabled to take long walks, and to perform temporarily, in the winter of 1866, his duty of waiting at the table, having been galvanized two hundred and seventy times up to that period. In the course of the year 1867 he presented himself but rarely, the morbid symptoms ceasing one after another.

CASE 87. — Heinrich Struck, tailor, aged twenty-five years and six months, suffered from a severe cold in his nose about eight days ago, which suddenly disappeared, being replaced by a progressive anæsthesia. It began with a feeling of tickling in the sole of the left foot, accompanied by a sensation of cold and numbness. These sensations affected, within two days, the whole left side of the body, extending up to the arm, the anterior portion of the abdominal wall only remaining intact. Irritating ointments had no influence; on the contrary, the disease also attacked, in spite of them and the use of four Russian baths, the whole right side, although in a less degree. In this state he was seen by me, November 10, 1867. There was, especially in the left arm, a feeling of great weakness, the patient being unable to hold a cane with that hand. Neither could he, in consequence of the anæsthesia, take small substances off the table, or button his coat with this arm. Touching the skin with the finger or the needle was felt but slightly. Every attempt to separate the fingers and to bring them near each other again, was followed by incorrect movements. He also had a sensation of tension in all the joints of the upper and lower extremities, those of the left side being more affected, as was the case with the other symptoms.

I employed the full strength of the electric brush in the first two applications—the temporary improvement disappearing before the next sitting. In the next three applications, the use of the constant labile current, from the brachial plexus to the hand, and in the thigh, in a corresponding manner, gave no result whatever. I now resolved to galvanize the sympathetic nerve. Galvanization of the right cervical sympathetic nerve produced diplegic contractions in the arms and legs; usually, however, not till the actions had continued for some time, and to a higher degree in the first applications than at a later period. Galvanization of the left cervical sympathetic had either no result or but a slight one, while at other points they could not be produced at all in the well-nourished and muscular patient. Together with the application of the positive pole to the right cervical sympathetic, there occurred a strong perspiration in the left axilla and *vice versa*. After the first applications, made in the beginning, daily, the feeling of tightness disappeared from the right side; it took, however, a much longer time before the insensibility of the left side, especially of the arm and hand, decreased. For this reason the treatment had to be continued, with frequent interruptions of two and three days, till January 10, 1868, before the patient again became able to work, and no rapid improvement took place until very strong currents (up to thirty-eight elements) were employed, the negative electrode being usually applied to the lumbar or sacral region.

Dr. Drissen observed the following case:

CASE 88.—A. G., eighteen years of age, after having lifted a very heavy weight, noticed a heaviness and stiffness of his arms, which gradually increased, especially on the right side, thence extended to the fingers, making it impossible for him to write. He also was affected by neuralgic pain in the course of the median and ulnar nerve. After a six weeks' peripheral treatment with the constant current had not only done no good, but also, according to the patient, rendered him still worse, he applied, on the 25th of November, 1865, to Dr. Drissen, who, upon an examination, found the deltoid, biceps, and extensor muscles of the right forearm to be hard, and Valleix's pressure points on the median and radial nerves painful. He but imperfectly, and with great exertion, succeeded in raising the arm, bending the elbow-joint, or stretching and bending the fingers, which were usually in a state of semiflexion. The application of a current of eighteen elements, with the positive pole, upon the fossa subclavicularis sinistra, and with the negative pole on the right from the second to the third cervical vertebra, caused a feeling of warmth in the right arm. At the second application there ensued strong spasms of the biceps, rendering the elbow-joint free: in the third application, the deltoid also moved spasmodically. Under this treatment the patient improved gradually, and was discharged perfectly cured, January 20, 1866.

During this treatment, the right arm was twice treated by the peripheral method by way of experiment; he became worse each time the following day. The internal administration of strychnine, continued for six days, caused no increase of diplegic contractions (as mentioned by Remak), but was followed, on the eleventh day, by spontaneous convulsions, accompanied by a return of the neuralgic pain.

Of all kinds of paralysis, the nervous and muscular kinds offer the most favorable field for the employment of both the interrupted and the constant electric current. The method is different according to the situation of the paralysis, either faradization or galvanization of the nerve or muscle being performed. The latter may be made, as above (page 145) explained, extramuscular or intramuscular.

Concerning the choice between the interrupted and constant current in each individual case, peripheral paralysis, if at all capable of amendment, seems usually to be most accessible to that current for which the muscles have retained the irritability. This trial, however, must not be undertaken till the latter part of the second week after the beginning of the paralysis, inasmuch (as is shown in Case on page 244 and Case 33) as in nervous paralysis no derangement ensues before this time in the electric action of the paralyzed muscles. At that period, peripheral paralysis, in which the intermittent current produces more or less muscular contraction, is treated with it; those cases, however, in which the faradical excitability is lost and the galvanic preserved, with the battery current—while in the majority of cases where the reaction for both kinds of current is still existing, although in a less degree, both induction and battery current may be used successfully. If the physician, as is usually the case, has but the induction apparatus, he must, in order to avoid over-irritation, bear in mind what has been said about it, pages 64 and 157, that is, he must employ currents of medium strength, rarely interrupted, the applications being of short duration. As soon as the electro-muscular contractility increases, the strength of the current is to be decreased. If, however, he possesses contrivances fit for the generation of both kinds of currents, he will combine them in many cases with advantage, either by improving the reaction for the intermittent by passing through a constant current (see page 61), or, after having, by means of galvanization, rendered the nerve more capable of conduction, by exciting through faradization the paralyzed or asthenic muscles more strongly.

If we examine more closely those cases of paralysis in which the reaction after the induction current is perfectly extinct, but that of the battery current preserved, we may conveniently divide them into two groups. To the first belong those, in which the contractions following the galvanic irritation have sunk under the normal standard ; and to the second those exceeding the normal standard. For the first group, comprising, according to all observations made about it, single cases of traumatic nervous paralysis, cases of rheumatic facial paralysis, paralysis of the soft palate, etc., we may accept Neumann's opinion (see page 61), that, as soon as the vitality of a nerve or muscle has sunk, there ensues a stage in which the constant current, if applied longer than a moment, produces on the paralyzed muscles and nerves the effect of irritation which cannot be obtained through induced currents of a momentary duration. According to our experience so far, the disturbance of nutrition of the injured nerves in peripheral paralysis, beginning from the slightest and advancing to the highest degree,[1] is recognized by the following differences in the reaction : First degree. Motility limited or suspended, excitability normal for intermittent and constant currents. Second degree. Faradic and galvanic contractility diminished. Third degree. Excitability extinct for the faradic current, preserved for the galvanic current in both nerve and muscle. Fourth degree. Excitability of nerves extinct for both kinds of current, but muscular irritability preserved for the constant current. Fifth degree. Both nerves and muscles are entirely deprived of excitability for both kinds of the electric current. This

[1] See Ziemssen, *l. c.*, p. 109.

division, however, does not comprise all the existing forms of this disease; thus I treated a facial paralysis of a little boy where neither galvanization nor faradization of the nerves or muscles could produce weak convulsions, which only could be accomplished through reflex action from the trigeminal nerve by rapidly passing a small conductor along the muscles. Thus, in the later stages of traumatic paralysis, the faradic returns before the galvanic excitability, or, in rare cases of paralysis, caused by lead-poisoning, the galvanic excitability of single muscles has suffered more than the faradic. Finally, paralysis, in consequence of lead-poisoning, or injury, may have been removed long ago, while the electric irritability is still more or less reduced, or even entirely extinct.[1]

With regard to the second group, however, the characteristic feature of which consists of convulsions after galvanic irritation, considerably exceeding the normal state, to which belong a great number of cases of rheumatic facial paralysis, lead-poisoning, and also single cases of progressive muscular atrophy, I must maintain my opinion,[2] pronounced

[1] This variety of cases, not yet thoroughly investigated, of the muscular action following the use of the constant current, the number of which is still further increased through the absence or predominance of contraction at the opening and closing of the circuit, prevents us making good use of the galvanic current for the diagnosis of paralysis as extensively as with the faradic current, for which reason we have given it but a passing notice in the eighth section.

[2] A. Eulenburg, also convinced by the observation of a case of facial paralysis, lately informed me that he fully agrees with my view in regard to the nature of these spasms. I cannot but pronounce my decided doubt about the manner in which both A. Eulenburg (Zur Therapie der rheumatischen Facial-Paralysis. Deutsches Archiv. für klin. Medecin. 1866. Band II. Heft I.), and especially Ziemssen (Die Electricität in der Medicin. 1866. Page 99), have refuted my opinion by simply denying, as not existing, every thing not observed by themselves in a comparatively small number of cases. Thus, Eulenburg says that in his cases the excitability for the galvanic current did not decrease as the symptoms improved; what I maintained to happen in my cases, also, that the convulsions observed by him were under no circumstances spasmodic. Ziemssen even said that the quality of the contraction of both facial halves, according to his observations, was the reverse of what I had pronounced it.—Before form-

in the Berliner Med. Gesclschaft, at the occasion of a lecture on facial paralysis,[1] namely, that such cases are the result of reflex spasms.

In cases of lead-poisoning[2] and of progressive muscular atrophy marked by an unusually high degree of reflex excitation, the setting in of reflex spasms after the use of weak galvanic currents can easily be explained. It is different with regard to facial paralysis above referred to. Here there occur: 1. Cases in which neither through the intermittent nor through the constant current do spasms result from the excitation of the motor points, these spasms rather ensuing, and usually very intensely, from the excitation of the places of exit of the trigeminal branches in the face.[3] 2. Cases, in which both the employment of a battery current of eight to ten elements, and the application of one conductor to the neck or behind the neck, the other being placed upon any other place of the face, cause unusually active contractions, while every single muscle thus placed in a state of convulsion is perfectly indifferent to the direct influence of a much stronger current, in which also, with the progressing improvement, a constantly increasing number of elements must be added in order to obtain the same result. 3. Cases, in which a current of few elements (six to eight), when directed to the muscles of the paralyzed side, produces contractions at the opening and closing of the circuit, while they do not occur on the sound side until sixteen or twenty elements are added, and even then the symptoms are decidedly milder than on the paralyzed side (cases of Baierlacher, Schultz, Neumann, etc., etc.). It can hardly be doubted that the cases mentioned under 1. and 2. are reflex spasms, the oc-

ing a definite opinion, the greatest care ought to be exercised in the treatment of such subtle questions.

[1] See Deutsche Klinik. 1864. No. 2.
[2] See A. Eulenburg, Beiträge zur Galvano-pathologie und Therapie der Lähmungen. Berl. klin. Wochenschrift. 1868. No. 2.
[3] See Runge, Facialis-Lähmung und Constanter Strom. Deutsche Klinik. 1867. Page 99.

currence of which, in the skin of the face, is especially facilitated by its large supply of sensitive nerves, and the frequent anastomoses between the trigeminal and facial nerves, although we are at a loss to find the centre causing the reflex action. The cases, however, mentioned under 3. may, perhaps, be explained in a different manner.

After these general remarks, we shall treat of some especially remarkable forms of peripheral paralysis.

The treatment of peripheral facial paralysis frequently offers, even to the most skilful specialist, the greatest difficulties, in case the perfect integrity of the function of the muscles, and of the expression of countenance, is desired to be obtained. The causes for this opinion, hardly to be opposed at the present time, are the following: 1. Nowadays the antiphlogistic treatment, even in cases where the paralytic condition is preceded by symptoms of irritation, periostitic pain, etc., is frequently neglected, thus preventing the resolution of the exudation. 2. This exudation into the aqueductus Fallopii is, in nearly every case, the cause of peripheral facial paralysis, producing, more or less, by pressure, a destruction of the nerve-fibres, if it be not of a serous but of a more plastic nature. 3. Most of the facial muscles have but one firm point of attachment to the bone, while the other point lies in the skin, causing contractions, or at least deformities in the expression of countenance, unless perfect contractility is restored. Consequently contractions exist not only in facial paralysis, treated by the intermittent, but also in cases treated by the constant current, and even in those undergoing no treatment whatever, although it cannot be denied that the improper use of the induction current may facilitate their formation, especially if the healthy muscles are irritated with too long applications of rapidly-repeated currents. The formation of such contractions may be recognized by the following premonitory symptoms: 1. By an unusually rapid return of tonicity in a muscle shortly before paralyzed. 2. By spasm affecting the muscles spontaneously or after mechanical irritation, such as rubbing, kneading. These symptoms ensuing, the current is to be reduced or entirely suspended for some time, and the treatment directed merely to the diseased nerve. If the contraction is already plainly in existence, a stable battery current of ten to twenty elements is passed through it, or single powerful induction shocks are employed for the purpose of releasing it. These methods are best combined with the use of mechanical means to stretch the contracted muscles, as recommended by Erdmann, or the introduction of a wooden ball between the cheek and maxillary bone. Spasms sometimes occur in such cases, symptoms, as it were, of a reviving vitality of the muscles. These spasms allow a favorable prognosis, as then a cure is usually more quickly accomplished by treating nerves and muscles with the constant current. 4. The symptoms accompanying paralysis, and still more, the spasmodic phenomena following the use of the different currents and methods of application, require the most careful attention during the treatment. In this regard, the following therapeutic principles are to be kept in view:

1. If the reaction to the intermittent current is more or less well preserved at the end of the second week after the beginning of the paralysis, a primary moderately strong intermittent current is to be directed upon the single muscles, a course which must be especially recommended, if all the muscles have not suffered equally in their electro-muscular contractility. The facial nerve, however, may be irritated either directly by means of a thin electrode placed behind the ear, by the mastoid process and the articulation of the lower maxillary, or indirectly, as recommended especially by M. Rosenthal, through reflex action from the trigeminal nerve, by applying the copper-pole to the mucous membrane of the cheek and drawing the zinc-pole over the paralyzed muscles or the respective nerve-branches. 2. In those cases, also, where the electro-mu......duced to a minimum, a good resul............ough

the induced current, although only after a longer course of treatment, if care is taken to diminish the strength of the current in proportion to the gradually-increasing electro-muscular contractility. However, the constant current is generally preferable in these cases, if both kinds of currents are at the disposition of the practitioner. 3. But, in those cases in which the intermittent current produces no spasms whatever, while they are caused by the battery current, directed either to the nerve or to the muscle, the constant current is indicated. This, however, must usually be applied to the facial nerve itself, as correctly mentioned by Baerenwinkel,[1] especially in those forms of facial paralysis known, on one hand, by the want of any reaction after direct muscular irritation; and, on the other hand, by the setting in of extensive reflex spasms, after applying one conductor to the neck, etc., and the other to any other part of the paralyzed side. After this the spastic muscle may be attacked by stable currents, if direct irritation is followed by undoubted contractions. Here the intermittent current can only be usefully employed at a much later period, after voluntary motion has been recovered, the muscles, however, still being relaxed and deprived of their tone. Cases of this kind generally allow but an unfavorable prognosis, for, although frequently recovering without leaving deformity, a long course of treatment may always be expected. 4. Finally, cases of facial paralysis occur, followed by contractions or clonic spasms, and usually not on the paralyzed, but on the opposite healthy side, contractions, the origin of which can hardly be explained except by supposing that the irritation of a motor fibre is, under certain circumstances, by an increased irritability, conducted to the centrum, and thence transmitted to homologous parts of the other side (Remak). In this type of paralysis, in neuritis (see Case on page 328, and Case 61), the constant

[1] Zur Casuistrik der doppelseitigen Facial-Lähmungen, etc. Archiv für Heilkunde viii., Jahrgang, 1867, page 71, et seq.

current is to be directed to the inflamed nerve. This paralytic condition is ordinarily recognized by an unusual inclinanation to form permanent contractions, so much so, that shortening of single paralyzed muscles takes place soon after the beginning of the paralysis, where the paralytic condition is probably caused by a neuritis facialis.

We have, under Nos. 29 and 30, reported two cases in which the paralytic state, induced probably by a serous exudation, and possessed of a more or less normal electro-muscular contractility, was rapidly cured through the use of the intermittent current. We now furnish a series of more difficult cases.

CASE 89.—Carl A., merchant, thirty-five years of age, always healthy, contracted, on May 24, 1860, a severe cold, by standing in a doorway, in a heated state, with his coat off. On the next afternoon he noticed that he was unable to whistle. He paid, however, no attention to it, and went into the country, but awoke, on the 26th, with a complete facial paralysis of the left side. After having used cantharides, ointment of veratrine, lye, and Russian baths, for three weeks, he came to my office on June 15th. In the local symptoms of the paralysis, as yet no favorable change had taken place, there was no trace of voluntary motion in the affected muscles, the electro-muscular contractility being almost entirely extinct. Patient complained of a continual buzzing in his left ear. During thirty applications, made till August 15th, when I suspended the treatment on account of a journey, his condition had improved so far that he was able to perform the function of eating and drinking, he could also corrugate the left side of the forehead, and draw the angle of the mouth upward and outward. The left wing of the nose, however, was still lower than the right, the sulcus naso-labialis filled out, the eye could not be closed except with the aid of the zygomaticus major muscle, neither could the patient whistle, in consequence of the atrophied condition of the muscular fibres of the left part of the orbicularis oris. When I saw the patient again, after my return on the 6th of October, his condition was generally improved, all the muscles were more developed, he was able to purse the mouth and to whistle, while the buzzing in the ear had also disappeared. But now the left nasal wing was higher than the right one, the sulcus naso-labialis was more distinct on the left than on the right side, a feeling of tension followed the motions of the left side, which extended from the upper-lip to the eye, caused, like the symptoms just mentioned, by a contraction of the left levator angularis which could be felt from the inner surface of the mouth, like a tendinous cord. Through this muscle a constant current was directed, the use of which diminished the contraction considerably, so that after the tenth application, October 29th, there existed but slight traces of it.

Baierlacher, whose merit it is to have first directed attention to the different action of the intermittent and constant currents in facial paralysis, reports[1] the following case:

M. B., a factory-girl, came under his treatment, suffering from a lateral facial paralysis of eight weeks' standing. Induced currents of great strength caused but a very slight reaction. The application of the induced current for three weeks improved neither electro-muscular contractility nor the power of voluntary motion. Then Baierlacher tried the constant current of fifteen elements of Bunsen, by placing one electrode on the trunk of the facial nerve, and the other on the muscles of the cheek. Immediately after the first closing of the circuit, a strong spasm took place in all the muscles supplied by this nerve. After the third time a remarkable improvement was noticed, and after four additional applications the patient left, satisfied with the result. Baierlacher saw her again after half a year, and did not find the slightest deformity.

CASE 90.—Miss Mary S., aged twenty-two years, was

[1] See Beiträge zur therapeutischen Verwerthung des galvanischen Stromes. Baierisches aerztliches Intelligenzblatt, 1859, No. 4.

attacked by a violent pain in the ears on August 27, 1863, after having spent the entire previous evening in the garden, exposed to a cold gust of wind. This was followed the next day by paralysis of the right side of the face, with gastric derangement, which latter kept her in bed for a week. After this the earache was replaced by a dull headache; besides, the patient was so much reduced, that her attending physician, Dr. Boehr, did not permit her to come to my office till October 6th. The paralysis had then become complete. The induced current localized on the muscles and facial branches of the right side of the face produced no trace of spasmodic contraction, although she experienced a strong pain during the irritation; a constant current of ten elements, however, localized in the same manner, produced strong contractions at the closing and weak ones at the opening of the circuit, such as hardly occurred on the sound side after the application of twenty elements. In consequence of these results, the battery current was employed. October 30th (twelfth application): The lower eyelid and the wing of the nose are again a little raised; the patient draws the mouth less on the left while laughing. Now only a current of sixteen elements is necessary to produce a strong spasm; the muscles also begin to react mildly to the intermittent current. November 30th (twenty-ninth application): The naso-labial groove is more distinct, the mouth less distorted; the eye can be nearly closed, and the forehead corrugated. The galvanic excitability has still more decreased, while the faradic irritability has improved considerably, and on that account the induced current is hereafter used. Under this treatment the improvement advanced till the end of December (fortieth application), so that nothing remained but a slight distortion of the mouth during laughing, and a stiffness of the lower-lip, caused by a slight rigidity of the triangularis menti, which disappeared during the months of January and February, 1864, after the current had been applied to this muscle six times more.

CASE 91.—Mrs. T., a phlegmatic, anæmic person, married for two years, but having no children, was affected with paralysis of the right side of the face, on May 30, 1867, after having suffered from neuralgic pain in the right side of the head for several days, while the sense of taste and sensibility of the right half of the tongue were also deranged. Patient came to my office on June 10th. The examination gave the following result: No muscular reaction after the application of powerful intermittent current; no reaction after a constant current was passed directly through the muscles, yet a very distinct action of the facial muscles, surpassing that of the sound side in strength, extent, and precision, followed the use of 8-10 elements, one conductor being placed on the neck, the other on any part of the right side of the face. These symptoms indicated a long course of treatment, which view was fully confirmed. After the twelfth application (July 2d), made, as usual, by placing one conductor on the place of exit of the facial nerve, the other on the pes anserinus, taste returned, and the disturbance of sensation disappeared in the right half of the tongue; yet the first contraction, on directly acting on the paralyzed muscles, did not happen until after the twentieth application (July 22d), when it was observed in the levator labii superioris and triangularis menti, while no reaction followed the examination by means of the intermittent current. When I interrupted, August 23d (forty-third application), the treatment on account of a journey, the forehead could be slightly corrugated, the zygomatic muscle acted somewhat, and the eye could be totally closed to within one line. I saw the patient again on October 10th. Concerning the movability of the muscles, her condition had rather improved, but there existed now rigidity in the levator labii sup. alæque nasi, in the zygomaticus and triangularis, which was but little noticed when the patient kept quiet, as was usually the case with her, but appeared the more striking in laughing, opening the mouth, etc. This necessitated a modification of the method heretofore employed, it being now necessary, besides galvanizing the facial nerve, to galvanize especially the contracted muscle. At the end of December (sixty-seventh application), the movability of all the muscles was perfect, but the rigidity was plainly perceptible to both the eye and the touch. March 3, 1868 (eighty-fifth application): the rigidity is hardly noticeable, yet the expression of the countenance appears somewhat unnatural while the patient laughs, shows her teeth, etc.; while blowing, the right cheek is less puffed out than the left. The reaction to the direct influence of the constant and interrupted currents is still a little reduced on the right side. The contractions appear to be stronger on the left than on the right side, if the positive conductor is placed on the neck and the negative on either cheek.

CASE 92.—Mrs. V. R., aged forty-six years, had first suffered from rheumatic pain in the left shoulder. After about eight days she lost the sense of taste in the right half of the tongue, which felt as if it were scalded. A few days afterward (April 22, 1864), she noticed—perhaps in consequence of a new cold to which she was exposed—on the 20th, about noon, a constant trembling of the upper-lip; on the same evening, a certain difficulty of motion of the mouth; and on the following morning, a paralysis of the right side of the face. Her physician, Dr. Klaatsch, after having employed leeches and other derivants, placed her under my charge on May 14th. The paralysis was still nearly complete, pressure behind the angle of the lower jaw painful, the alienation of taste still existing, also a buzzing noise in the right ear, and spasm of the left side of the upper-lip to the inner angle of the eye; reaction to the intermittent current somewhat reduced. In this case, where the paralysis was probably caused by a neuritis, and where, in addition, the existing spasms of the left side demanded an especial care in the choice of the means of excitation, a weak constant current was used by placing the + conductor behind the angle of the lower-jaw, and applying the — conductor for a short time upon the several muscles. After five applications (May 18th), a decided improvement was visible in closing the eye, in the position and motion of the eye, and in the decrease of the spasmodic convulsions, when a slight indisposition of the patient made necessary a short interruption of the treatment. When the treatment was resumed, on May 23d, the spasms could no more be noticed; the taste was nearly normal; there appeared, however, now distinct traces of rigidity in the right levator labii sup. alæque nasi, and in the triangularis menti. After ten more applications, these, together with the other symptoms of paralysis, were reduced to such an extent that we allowed the patient to return to her country-seat on May 5th, expecting that they would soon disappear without any further treatment. After four weeks, every morbid symptom had vanished except the buzzing in the ear.

With regard to the treatment of the so-called rheumatic paralysis of the muscles of the eye, I refer to page 151 for the method. In Case 76 I have already reported a successful treatment of paresis of the upper oblique muscle through the induced current. I shall now communicate a case of paresis of the abducens, cured through the constant current.

CASE 93.—Our honored colleague, Professor Traube, aged fifty years, after having been exposed to various changes of temperature, and after suffering from rheumatic pain in the right side of the head, noticed diplopia first on October 3, 1867. The examination showed the existence of a paresis of the right abducens, with a defect in the movability of about one line in comparison with the left eye. A rapid increase of the paralysis as well as of the convergent strabismus followed, so that the defect of motion amounted to three lines on the 8th of October. Toward the middle of October the affection had attained its 'height. There was a strong convergent strabismus of the right eye; the line of vision could hardly be turned over the middle of the palpebral fissure to the right; in order to correct the diplopia in the median line, and at an objective distance of 15″, prisms of nearly 40° were necessary. The treatment consisted of depletion by means of Heurtloup's blood-suckers, a diaphoresis, and mild aperients. From November 8th, up to which time his condition had not changed materially, the iod. of pot. and the constant current were employed. The patient being in a state of great nervous irritability, the latter was used in such a manner as to pass a current, generated from but six to eight elements, from the outer angle of the eye toward the temporal region, for about three minutes. It was several times ascertained that immediately after the application of the current a decrease of the convergence ensued; so that if, for instance, the region of the binocular simple vision in the median line extended to 7″ from the root of the nose before the application, immediately afterward a prolongation of this line to 8″ and farther could be proved. In the beginning a gradually, and from the first days of December a rapidly-increasing improvement ensued, so that we were able to terminate the treatment on December 11th (twenty-seventh application), every trace of paralysis having disappeared at the end of December.

Schulz,[1] having a case of paralysis of the branches of the motor oculi, supplying the levat. palp. sup. and rectus inferior, kept for two minutes the positive conductor of a constant current of eight elements of Daniell on the upper eyelid, placing the negative on the hard palate. Although the pain was very violent, the patient was able to move the upper eyelid better after the first application. On the next morning the diplopia of five months' standing had disappeared, the ptosis alone still continuing. Schulz be-

[1] Ueber Anwendung der Electricität bei Paralyse der Augenmuskeln. Wiener Med. Wochenschrift, 1862, No. 16.

lieves that the galvanic current acted in this case cata
lytically upon an exudation situated about the nerves.

I have communicated, on page 262, one of the most
interesting cases of traumatic paralysis, cured by Duchenne
through faradization. I am now so fortunate as to be able
to report a similar, perhaps not less striking case, which I
cured in a comparatively short time by means of galvanization.

CASE 94.—Carl Pretzer, seaman, aged twenty years, fell,
September 15, 1866, off the mast, fifteen feet high, upon the
deck, receiving a dislocation of the right arm interiorly.
No attempt at reduction could be made until the ship
arrived at Helsingör, September 20th, when reduction was
tried for three days in succession, but without result, in
spite of the use of the pulley and of chloroform. The arm
rested on the thorax, the forearm was supined, the hand extended. Finally, on the 27th, twelve days after the accident,
the dislocation was reduced in Copenhagen. But the arm
appeared to be completely paralyzed, violent pain extended
along the supra- and infra-spinatus nerves, thence following
the course of the median nerve into the fingers, especially
the thumb. Soon the muscles became greatly emaciated,
those of the shoulder becoming atrophied at the beginning
of October, followed soon by atrophy of the muscles of the
arms and hands. The patient came for the first time to my
office on October 24th, when the following condition was
found in the completely-paralyzed extremity: perfect atrophy of the supra- and infra-spinatus muscles, relaxation of
the deltoideus, showing an intervening space of 4 to 5′′′, between the humerus and the acromion, an equal atrophy of
the muscles of the arm and hand, contraction of the biceps
and pectoralis minor, inclining the forearm to the upper-
arm at an angle of 75°, while it rested firmly on the thorax,

whence it could be removed only with very great pain, sensibility reduced equally everywhere without being entirely suspended; pain was continual, especially in the daytime, even if the arm was carried in a sling. The intermittent current produced great pain, but only weak contractions; the constant current, however, caused the patient less pain, and produced, by using thirty to forty elements, distinct muscular contractions. After fourteen days, the rigidity of the biceps was greatly diminished, the upper-arm could be removed more than 6" from the thorax, and passive motion and extension of the forearm were less painful; the nutrition of the muscles of the shoulder had improved, noticed especially by the lesser protrusions of the acromion and spina scapulæ; spontaneous pain was less frequent, and then only temporary. On November 27th, the patient was able to raise the arm almost to a right angle, to make slight supination, to stretch the fingers somewhat, the sensibility of the arm also having perfectly returned. December 15th: patient was able to raise the upper-arm to an angle of 120°, and extend the forearm, pronation and supination were free, the fingers could be extended, adducted, and abducted. The muscular tissue of the whole arm had increased, the reaction to the intermittent current was better, yet its influence was so painful that we continued using the battery current. December 29th: the upper-arm was raised to an angle of 150°, and kept for some time in this position, every motion of the fingers was made without difficulty, but the power of closing them was still absent. In the month of January, the strength of the hand increased under the use of labile descending currents, enabling the patient to hold larger substances, to write, and to shake hands; the reaction to the intermittent current improved gradually, although its use was still very painful and unpleasant for the patient; the nutrition of the muscles increased visibly, allowing us to send the patient to his home on January 31st, after having applied the constant current eighty-nine times, believing that he soon would enjoy the full use of his arm again. Privy-Councillor Wilner repeatedly convinced himself of the rapid and surprisingly successful result of the treatment.

After the Danish and Prusso-Austrian wars in 1864 and 1866, a number of officers, suffering from paralysis of the ulnar, tibial, peroneal, crural, and other nerves, in consequence of gunshot wounds, were placed under my care by Surgeon-General von Langenbeck. These cases frequently gave me occasion to prove the extraordinary power of electricity (in the shape of the intermittent and constant currents) for the restitution of the power of motion and sensation, as well as for the frequently rapid increase of the nutrition of paralyzed muscles. I cannot omit at least to mention a case of total paralysis of the left arm with complete atrophy of all the muscles of the shoulder, arm, and hand, caused by a gunshot wound through the upper lobe of the lung, tearing entirely the brachial plexus. A treatment of fourteen months, although not rendering the arm perfectly fit for use, yet improved the patient sufficiently to make him fit for military service, allowing him to serve in the war of 1866. He was able to use the left arm without difficulty while riding on horseback.

Cases of paralysis following acute diseases (scarlatina, measles, typhus, dysentery, etc.) show the most contrary symptoms with regard to the electric influence, the electric irritability remaining frequently intact after they had existed for years, while it was reduced or entirely suspended in other more recent cases. The reason for this difference may be found in the circumstance that, in spite of the coincidence of the paralytic cases with regard to pathogenesis, yet the localization of the paralyzing process may be different: for instance, a cerebral one in one case, and a myopathic in another. In accordance, the treatment must naturally be different—in the first case we might perhaps expect a good result by galvanizing the cervical sympathetic nerve; while in the latter, a treatment applied directly to the affected muscles may prevent their gradual degeneration and restore their functional power. A similar state exists with regard to paralysis caused by syphilis or toxicological influence (lead-poisoning), as here, especially in cases of intact electric action, the central portions of the nervous system form the local starting-point of the paralysis, while in those cases of reduced or suspended electro-muscular contractility, nerves and muscles are affected directly. The peripheral syphilitic paralysis offers a fruitless field for the electric process; at least I have not met with any material success in any cases treated by electricity.

CASE 95.—Hugo Forster, aged sixteen years, suffering from fits of convulsive laughter since his fifth year, was taken sick with typhus in September, 1857, being under medical treatment for ten weeks in Bethanien. During convalescence, which lasted for months, the patient noticed a remarkable weakness of the whole right side of the body, from the face down to the feet. The right side was colder and less sensitive; pain ensued in the right shoulder and upper-arm, especially on a change of temperature; the right arm was considerably emaciated, and could only with difficulty be raised at the shoulder-joint; neither was the patient able to hold small substances, nor to write.

When he visited me for the first time, July 31, 1858, he was of a very anæmic appearance; his pulse was weak, and the right hand trembled when extended. The deltoideus was especially emaciated in its posterior portion; the right arm and hand were also greatly atrophied. The external and internal interosseous muscles, as well as the muscles of the ball of the thumb, were also atrophied, and the hand, especially in the first and second fingers, had assumed a claw-like shape (paralysis of the ulnar nerve). Consequently he was unable to straighten the fingers, or approach them to each other completely, or separate them;

neither could he flex the thumb, nor place it in opposition to the rest of the fingers. Patient is able to get hold of a pen, but not to keep it, in consequence of the bending inclination of the index-finger. The shoulders are painful, the arm is cold and benumbed. The electric examination gives the following results: sensibility is reduced on the whole right side of the body, the right side of the tongue included; the reaction of all the muscles of the same side is less energetic; the deltoideus, the external and internal interossei, the opponens and flexor brevis pollicis, and the extensor indicis proprius, are especially inactive. I restricted the employment of the electric treatment to the arm in the beginning, and faradized the skin and muscles. After the twelfth application (August 10, 1858), the arm was stronger, the hand warmer, the pain less; patient could separate the fingers better, and write for a short time. Twenty-second application (September 29th), improvement progressing, fingers could be nearly straightened and approached to each other, and the cutaneous sensibility was better. Patient was again able to resume his duties as a clerk, although every exertion of the arm, especially continued writing, tired him. These duties also prevented him from pursuing a regular course of treatment, and I did not see him again till October 20th. The muscular power had then increased, and he was now able to write all day. Twenty-ninth application (April 3, 1859): Forster had been electrified only five times in the last six months. The improvement still continued: the hand could be straightened, all the motions of the thumb and little finger were performed, the nutrition of the muscles of the shoulder and arm was increased, and the temperature was also better. The electro-cutaneous sensibility of the right side of the body was, however, still diminished, the right side less warm, the nutrition of the muscles and the electro-muscular contractility less good than on the corresponding portions of the left side. For this reason, daily scrubbing with a brush was recommended.

Case 96.—W. Schultze, thirty-five years of age, a painter by trade for sixteen years, of short, muscular stature, was taken with lead-colic for the first time in 1842. Till 1850, he had been attacked seven times, each attack lasting eight to ten days, and restricted to an obstinate constipation and severe abdominal pain. The last less violent attack occurred in August, 1850, after which he returned to his usual occupation, when he noticed, toward the middle of September, a considerable decrease of strength in the right arm, being obliged to support the right with the left arm after hardly half an hour's work. He continued to work for three weeks, his strength steadily failing, until the most violent pain in the shoulders, arms, and back, becoming almost unbearable during the night, connected with symptoms of paralysis in the right forearm and hand, prevented him from doing any further labor. From the 9th of November he was treated with Russian baths and irritating ointments. This diminished the pain somewhat, but, the paralytic symptoms still persisting, he applied to the Charité Hospital, February 1, 1851. After having been treated in that institution for a month with sulphur-baths, irritating embrocations, and internal remedies, without any success, he again tried the Russian baths—having, in the meanwhile, been discharged from the hospital—without experiencing the slightest relief from their continued use. When he came to my office, May 3, 1851, the following symptoms existed: motion of the right shoulder was perfectly free, on straightening the arm a continued pain ensued, which did not cease until the arm was lowered. If the patient attempted to seize any thing, the hand closed spasmodically, preventing him even from eating without help. The arm being bent at the elbow, he was able to open the hand with great difficulty, with the exception of the thumb and middle finger, which bent inward, and were incapable of any active motion. There existed, consequently, in this case, a paralysis of the extensor muscles, especially of the extensor communis digitorum, the por tion running to the middle finger being more particularly affected, as well as the extensor muscles of the thumb. The predominating affection of these muscles caused every attempt to take a pen to be followed by a symptomatic writer's paralysis. Pain ensued but temporarily, and became only permanent whenever he leaned on the affected arm. The electric treatment was followed in this case with such a surprisingly rapid success, that after the third application, of about twenty minutes, the patient was able to hold a pen, and to write his name and address, although with a trembling hand. After the fifth application, his handwriting was considerably improved; after the eighth, it was perfectly steady. This change in the handwriting was indeed very surprising. After the thirteenth sitting, the patient was able to paint the walls of a large hall, working for nearly eight hours without interruption. In the few following applications, the induced current was employed mainly for the removal of the neuralgic pain in the upper and lower arm, and was followed by an equally good result.

A new attack occurring in December, 1852 (see Case 39), the cure was much slower.

The following is briefly the above-mentioned case of Eulenburg:

N., three years a painter, small and pale-looking, had the first attack of colic a year ago; this was followed by a second, more violent, in August of the current year, which, being soon removed, the well-known symptoms of lead-palsy, preceded by violent spasms, appeared, according to his account, rather suddenly, first in the right and then in the left arm. Patient was faradized, on account of the paralysis, every day since August 17th, without any therapeutic success, however, and finally without any reaction of the paralyzed muscles. Eulenburg found, on examining the patient, November 20, 1867, both forearms considerably atrophied, especially on the dorsal side, and slightly pronated; all the joints of the wrist and fingers were flexed, and an active extension of the hand and fingers only to a very slight extent possible; supination of either arm impaired, the other muscles of the arm acted normally. The examination with the induction apparatus showed the faradic contractility of the extensor muscles of the right and left arm to be reduced in the highest degree, and absolutely suspended in the extensor digit. comm. and extensor carpi rad., even when using the maximum strength of the current. Galvanic exploration of the paralyzed muscles, however, showed the excitability to be perfectly intact and far exceeding the normal standard. The treatment with the galvanic current being continued (four applications a week), a rapid increase of voluntary motility, a return of the faradic contractility, and a still increasing irritability in the paretic muscles ensued. This irritability was manifested in three directions: in the steady increase of galvanic irritability, in the existence of slight spasms after a slight mechanical insulation (for instance, after stroking with a sharp-bordered substance, or, still better, after a moderate pressure with the finger on the muscles themselves, or their motor points), and, finally, the setting in of diplegic contractions. I had occasion to see the patient in the middle of February, when he had already recovered the full energy in the use of the extensor muscles.

Remak[1] mentions yet a third method, by which he improved the functional power of paralyzed arms, especially in patients suffering also from lead-colic, namely, by the action of the constant current on the cœliac plexus.

The electric irritation of the diaphragm and the other muscles of inspiration is indicated, in cases of poisoning by coal-gas, and in the apparent death of new-born children (see Chapter II. of this section, "The use of electricity in Midwifery"), in asphyxia caused by chloroform, in poison-

[1] Med. Central-Zeitung. 1862. Page 546.

ing through gas, carbonic acid, and other poisons endangering life, and especially by impairing and stopping respiration. The cases of this kind, which were partially followed by good results, have been well compiled by Ziemssen, who deserves great credit for having perfected Duchenne's method.[1] In this work, we find, besides Ziemssen's own cases, some especially interesting ones of Friedberg and Mosler. Ziemssen's method of operation, of which I approve unconditionally, is as follows: The electrodes, which here are best made of metallic buttons furnished with a thick cushion of fine sponge, are thoroughly moistened. They are then, after ascertaining that the strength of the current is sufficient to produce a powerful contraction of the muscles of the ball of the thumb, placed firmly on either side of the neck, over the lower end of the scalenus anticus muscle, on the outer border of the sterno-cleido-mastoideus, which is to be pressed a little inward, thus enabling the operator to affect with the current not only the phrenic nerves, but also, in consequence of the large surface of contact, the other inspiratory muscles (scalenus anticus, sterno-cleido-mastoideus), or their nerves originating from the brachial and cervical plexus. An assistant fixes the head, shoulders, and forearms. The duration of a single irritation is that of a deep, quiet inspiration, that is, about twenty seconds; the expiration is aided by an assistant who presses strongly and broadly on the abdominal wall from below upward. After a number of irritations, a pause is made, in order to observe whether spontaneous respiration begins. If no inspiratory motions follow the faradization after the first irritation, an increase of the strength of the current becomes the more necessary, as the irritability of the nerves of respiration sinks very soon in dangerous cases of asphyxia. If the irritability of the phrenic nerves for the induction current is already lost or near it, Ziemssen advises, if possible, the employment of the constant current by way of experiment.

[1] See Die Electricität in der Medicin. Dritte auflage, 1866, p. 174-197.

I have myself used the faradization of the muscles of inspiration without result once, but very successfully twice. In a case of poisoning by charcoal, I succeeded, after short exertion, in reviving the person; in a second, where death threatened every moment in consequence of severe diphtheria, I also avoided a fatal termination with the above-specified method.

The following is the last-mentioned case:

CASE 97.—I was called, on the advice of Dr. Riese, to Mr. L., aged twenty-one years, who suffered from a severe attack of diphtheria after scarlatina. He had passed through it as far as the local symptoms were concerned, but was in danger of dying in consequence of great prostration. I found the patient half asleep, in bed, and apathetic to the highest degree, his lips pale, and the temperature low. Respiration was superficial, pulse small and intermittent (the fourth beat was absent), in short, death could be expected any moment. I immediately began artificial respiration through faradization of the phrenic nerves and the inspiratory muscles by means of a strong current. The result was surprising: the thorax expanded visibly, the lips had color, respiration became deeper, the pulse rose, its intermissions ceased, and the temperature of the skin increased. After having faradized twice for five minutes, with an intermission of five minutes, I left the patient after half an hour, as both respiration and pulse remained in the same favorable condition, he having, in the mean time, become somewhat more lively, and also swallowed a few teaspoonfuls of wine. When I saw him again at 8 P. M., his condition, in regard to respiration, pulse, and temperature, was perfectly satisfactory. Still I faradized the patient once more on his express desire. On the next morning he was out of danger, and finally recovered entirely.

Friedberg's[1] case of asphyxia from chloroform is the following:

[1] See Virchow's Archiv. 1859. Vol. xvi., page 527, et seq.

Otto Krause, aged four years, was put under the influence of chloroform for the operation of removing an encysted tumor of the left lower eyelid, when, suddenly, a short, rattling inspiration ensued, after which, breathing ceased. For from two to three minutes, attempts were made to restore him by means of rubbing, the introduction of a sponge over the epiglottis into the larynx, etc., when the features appeared like those of a dead person, the lower jaw falling down. Artificial respiration through a methodic compression of the abdomen not having the slightest success, Friedberg faradized the diaphragm by placing one of the electrodes of the induction apparatus of Du Bois-Raymond upon the phrenic nerve, and applying the other to the lateral wall of the thorax in the seventh intercostal space, pressing it deeply against the diaphragm. This faradization was made alternately on the right and left side, the circuit remaining closed each time for the duration of a deep inspiration. After the current had thus been interrupted ten times, the first weak but plainly-perceptible spontaneous inspiration happened, which was soon followed by a second and a third, the face also reddening, and the radial pulse becoming perceptible. Soon, however, the breathing and the contractions of the heart again became weaker, convincing Dr. F. that he could not yet desist in his exertions. As every thing depended on removing rapidly the chloroform-gas accumulated in the lungs, he now tried again the methodic compression of the abdomen, and this time so successfully that, with the simultaneous use of external stimulants, the child had sufficiently recovered, in twenty minutes from the beginning of the asphyxia, to undergo the operation.

In the use of the secondary induction current for the cure of incontinentia urinæ, three methods are successfully employed: 1. The application of the — conductor over the symphysis pubis, and the + conductor to the sacral bone or perinœum (see Case 98). 2. Introduction of a sound, covered with caoutchouc, into the bladder, and the other probe-pointed excitor into the rectum, through which method Erdmann succeeded in permanently curing a patient, after nine applications, who had suffered from incontinence for three years. 3. Introduction of a similar sound, furnished with a brass ring a quarter of an inch wide, into the urethra, only as far as the ring reaches, and closing the current by placing the + conductor immediately over the symphysis. The last-mentioned method depends probably upon a reflex action produced by the sensitive nerves of the urethra on the motor nerves supplying the muscular fibres of the pars membranacea urethræ (through which part the bladder is closed most promptly).

CASE 98.—Student H., aged nineteen years, a corpulent, plethoric young man, suffered, since his sixteenth year, from frequent pollutions, for the alleviation of which he went much among women. He first noticed, in the winter of 1855, that even when pressing strongly on the bladder, he was obliged to wait a long time for the passage of the urine, or that, it did not pass at all in spite of a strong pressure. In such cases he drank a great deal of white beer, which was always followed by an evacuation of urine. This desire to pass water became less noticeable in course of time, allowing him to drink six or more glasses without being troubled in the least. The bladder was naturally more and more distended, the muscular coat relaxed, and, finally, symptoms of paralysis of the bladder supervened, after an attack of gonorrhœa at the end of March, treated by the usual means.

Professor von Baerensprüng ordered irritating ointments to be rubbed over the region of the bladder, and the internal use of cantharides, and, after failing in his efforts, sent the patient, on May 18th, to my office for electrical treatment. A treatment of eight weeks (forty-three applications) caused the desire to urinate to become spontaneous, especially in the morning and in the course of the day, when the urine was passed promptly, and with a sufficient jet; only in the evening the desire was less frequent, and even then the bladder was emptied, although only after pressing down for some time. At the end of December, the patient, having left Berlin in August, informed me by letter that he had fully recovered without the further use of medicines.

I was also successful in curing permanently, in a short time, three cases of nocturnal incontinence of urine (enuresis nocturna), that obnoxious evil, so frequently defying every medical treatment. It had existed in these cases till the thirteenth and fourteenth year.

Three boys, Otto F., Paul D., and Hermann R., all pupils of Kornmesser's Orphan Asylum, suffering since their seventh year from this affection, were sent to me by Dr. Hildebrandt. In Paul D., the enuresis ceased after the first application, in Otto F. it occurred more rarely in the first fourteen days; only on Hermann R. the treatment did not seem to have any perceptible influence in the first weeks, yet twenty-two applications cured him entirely. A fourth case failed after a long-continued treatment.

Seeligmueller[1] reports the following case:

Miss Caroline B., aged twenty-two years, daughter of a physician, suffered, from her early childhood, from incontinence of urine by day and night, every possible remedy having been employed in vain. Although, at first, intermissions in the disease occurred of a monthly and even quarterly duration, the evil finally became worse. For the last half year, before the patient came under the care of Dr. S., the disease increased so much that her mother had to wake her every night two to three times regularly to urinate, in spite of which the enuresis frequently occurred. It was natural that the unhappy girl, being deprived of every enjoyment of life, became very low spirited.

[1] See Correspondenzblatt des Vereins der Aerzte im Regierungsbezirk Merseburg. 1867. No. 7.

On April 14, 1867, the electrodes were held for the first time by a midwife, for five minutes, in the manner mentioned (3), Dr. S. directing the strength of the current, and employing a degree sufficient to be plainly felt by the patient, without causing her any pain. On that day the patient, having the day previous been forced to go to the closet every quarter of an hour, was obliged to urinate but twice, passing the night without any desire whatever. When she came to Dr. S.'s office for the third time, April 16th, she declared herself to have perfectly recovered. After the fourth application (April 17th), the catamenia appeared, regular as usual, and, although she was not electrified, the improvement continued till April 22d, in the afternoon, when she again perceived some weakness in the bladder. From the 23d to the 26th the patient had four additional applications, after which she returned to her home. As enuresis nocturna had occurred but twice up to May 30th, she came again to Halle for four additional applications from June 10th to 13th. Since that time no relapse has taken place—at least not by September, 1867, when Dr. S. reported the case. The patient had improved greatly in bodily health, and freely participated in all the pleasures of life.

Only such cases of paralysis of the laryngeal muscles are naturally amenable to the use of the electric current which are caused by an alteration of the nerves. They consist of the following classes: 1. A complete inflexibility of the vocal cords. 2. Where aphonia is caused by a more or less deficient closing, or only a suspended or altered vibration of the vocal cords. 3. Where slight exertion is soon followed by a fatigue of the organ of voice, the feebleness or absence of sound depending upon an asthenia of the muscles of the glottis.

If the laryngoscopical examination shows a case to belong to the third kind, the current may be passed percutaneously by placing a large positive conductor on the neck, and a small negative one on the region of the upper and lower bones of the thyroidean cartilage, and connecting them with quite a strong intermittent or, still better, constant current. The same method is to be tried in cases of complete paralysis of the voice belonging to the first category, which failing, recourse must be had to Ziemssen's method, described on page 152, of direct irritation of the respective laryngeal muscles. For the treatment of the second class, however, happening frequently in young girls as an hysterical symptom, or in men in consequence of mental emotion or the influence of cold, existing for months, and even years, in spite of the use of every possible remedy, I cannot too strongly urge the employment of the induction current directed to the larynx, in the shape of the electric moxa, on account of the certain and surprisingly rapid success following it.

In proof of this assertion, the following cases are quoted:

CASE 99.—Miss Mary O., twenty-nine years of age, healthy during childhood, suffered, in her thirteenth year, in the spring of 1844, from vomiting each time after taking any kind of food, and did not recover until in the fall, after the use of the sea-bath. In her sixteenth year she had chlorosis, suffering besides from frequent headache on the left side for nearly a year. In July, 1860, again frequent vomiting ensued, without any known cause—at first only after dinner, later also after breakfast, and finally whenever she took food, especially in the liquid form. At New Year her voice became suddenly very weak, and, from the 4th of January, absolute aphonia ensued. After the useless administration of dissolvents and derivants (croton-oil, blisters, etc.), the patient was advised to place herself under my care, March 26th, of the same year. I applied the electric pencil, with the greatest possible intensity of the current, directly to the larynx, until the patient cried out loud in consequence of the extremely violent pain. The voice immediately returned, the aphonia having been entirely removed.

Case 100.—Miss R., aged eighteen years, was engaged, for two years, to a military officer, who did not obtain the consent of his parents until lying on a sick-bed. Half a year ago she visited her future parents-in-law. While there she was probably subjected several times to mental emotions of various kinds—at least, having heretofore enjoyed good health. She returned, at the end of December, 1865, to her home, having become nervously affected to the highest degree. She began to cough, lost flesh, her voice became weak, and disappeared completely at the end of January, 1866, and she was believed to be affected with a pulmonary disease. On March 28th the despairing patient applied to Professor Traube, who found the lungs to be perfectly normal, and in the larynx only a gaping of the vocal cords without any vibration. He then turned the patient over to my care. After the electric moxa was applied once, Miss R. had recovered the full use of the voice, Professor Traube convincing himself, the following day, of the perfectly normal function of the vocal cords.

Case 101.—Franz H., thirteen years old, a patient of Dr. Hammer, having been exposed to a cold on the 9th of January, while dancing, was taken with pain in the left side of the larynx, losing also his voice. After the use of the tartar-emetic ointment and warm cataplasms, pain and aphonia disappeared, enabling the patient, on February 1st, to go to school again, but only for eight days. Since that time he was absolutely speechless, and remained so in spite of every remedy employed, until a permanent cure was effected, on March 22, 1864, by a single application of the electric moxa to the larynx.

Case 102.—Rev. W., from Hanover, thirty-three years of age, was attacked, March, 1861, by pneumonia and subsequent bronchitis, after having exerted his voice too much while speaking in a cemetery in cold, stormy weather. The application of leeches, with a long-continued after-bleeding, was followed by the loss of speech, which, after the use of whey and sea-bathing, still continued, allowing him only to speak with great difficulty a few words aloud, when the voice ceased immediately. This condition of his voice caused the patient, in May, 1862, to consult Professor Traube, who, after ascertaining, by means of the laryngoscope, that kind of paralysis of the vocal cords where the pars ligamentosa forms an elliptical fissure, sent the patient to my office for the purpose of electric treatment. After the first application of the moxa, the patient was able to speak louder and for a longer period. A repeated use of the moxa, and the simultaneous subcutaneous faradization of the laryngeal nerve, enabled Mr. W. to read aloud for some time, and he left with the full use of his voice.

CASE 103.—Miss H., of Halle, aged twenty-three years, suffered from a severe laryngeal catarrh, in consequence of a cold contracted in May, 1859. Aphonia followed, changing first in intensity, and finally continuing without interruption. Neither the mountain air nor a long sojourn on the Geneva Lake, in the spring of 1861, restored her voice, until, after having been hoarse for two and a half years, she was cured through the inhalation of sulphur-vapors in Langenbruecken, in August, 1861. But this recovery lasted only a short time. The patient, having returned to her home, lost her voice, after three weeks, she being able only to speak a few words aloud at long intervals, until even this ceased, and she became entirely aphonic in February, 1862. Professor Traube found both vocal cords paretic, forming a wide gaping fissure upon every attempt of modulation. Patient came to my office May 20, 1862. The voice did not return immediately on the use of the electric moxa, yet she was able to speak to Professor Traube in a loud voice after a few hours. The sound of the voice was weaker in the morning during the first days; after each faradization, however, it was of a full timbre, and continued thus after thirteen applications. In accordance with this improvement, a gradual approximation of the vocal cords took place too. At the end of May, 1865,

I was informed that the patient had recovered the full use of her voice.

II. ELECTRICITY IN DISEASES DEPENDING UPON ANOMALIES OF SECRETION AND EXCRETION.

A. *Rheumatic Exudations.*

If we start, with regard to the origin of rheumatic affections, from the opinion now pretty generally adopted, that the secreting function of the skin is deranged through a sudden change of temperature, in consequence of which the retained cutaneous secretions cause a change of the constituent parts of the blood and lymph, the effects of which change are either restricted to the starting-place, or which also may affect other tissues predisposed to it on account of their anatomical and chemical formation, the already known effects of the electric current, both the interrupted and the continued, will explain to us its use in rheumatic affections. This is caused partially by the increased secretion of the perspiration ensuing after the employment of the interrupted current in consequence of the irritation of the contractile fibres of the connective tissue, partially through the influence of the currents on the blood and lymph vessels, which, being first dilated under the use of the current, bring again into circulation the stagnating blood and lymph cells, and absorb exudations in consequence of the free circulation caused by it.[1] The employment of the interrupted current also produces the same effect by increasing the energy of the vascular walls, thus causing stronger contractions; or, finally, through the chemical process ensuing, probably, in consequence of the transmission of liquids within the tissues influenced by the current, which action is more intense by the use of constant batteries than with the magneto-electric appa-

[1] Remak, *l. c.*, page 290.

ratus, and again more intense with the latter than with the Volta-induction apparatus.

Concerning the method itself, rheumatism of the skin is usually soon removed through cutaneous faradization. In rheumatic callosities (see Note, page 271), one of the moistened conductors is placed upon the induration itself and the other applied in its vicinity, it making no difference which apparatus is used. The rheumatic articular inflammations and exudations are most suitably treated by passing as strong a current as possible for from five to ten minutes transversely through the joint; and it will be of advantage to frequently change the direction of the currents, as recommended especially by Fromhold, which not only diminishes greatly the painfulness of this method, but also renders a long-continued application possible. Remak, believing that a transmission of liquids takes place from the positive to the negative pole, advises the connection of the positive electrode with the inflamed surface, the negative pole being placed in its vicinity, but without the irritated joint; the direction of the current, however, respecting the position of the electrodes, is to be reversed, if the inflammation is accompanied by symptoms of a serous secretion. This method is especially indicated in acute rheumatic or traumatic affections of the joints with an extraordinarily increased sensibility, where we soon are able to find out whether electricity is applicable to such a case, without incurring the risk of augmenting the danger of the inflammatory process. For if the use of a moderately-strong current, showing a deviation of the needle from 20° to 25°, causes, after one or two minutes, not only no decrease but rather an increase of pain, the electric treatment is not yet applicable, a previous local antiphlogistic treatment being necessary. On the other hand, in those cases in which the application of electricity is followed by a perceptible alleviation of pain and a feeling of decided relief, the inflammatory process soon ceases, followed by a rapid absorption of the inflammatory products, prognosticating, in fact, an early cure, happening sometimes after one or a few additional applications.

Besides this catalytic action, the current passed transversely through the joint performs another no less important part, of causing anæsthesia of the joint. This result is the more to be valued, as, in spite of the visible diminution of the exudation, free motion is frequently impaired by the continued hyperæsthesia. In addition, this method removes, sometimes permanently, the most violent and long-continued pain at once, as if by a charm, even if the chronic exudation still continues. Thus, I treated a phthisical patient of Dr. Riese, suffering from inflammation of all the joints of the fingers, of the wrist and elbow-joint of the left arm, existing for several months without any known cause. In this case, a single transverse passing through of the induction current removed, immediately and permanently, the most violent pain following the slightest touch or motion, or, occurring spontaneously, especially in the night. In addition to the articular inflammation of the joint, or without it, there are found inflammatory exudations at the places of insertion of single muscles (especially at the insertion of the biceps and coraco-brachialis muscle to the coracoid process), rendering the joint completely immovable through their extraordinary tenderness, and frequently also causing radiating pains and motor reflex symptoms, all of which are frequently cured by directly acting on the painful portion of the joint. Exudations in the joints of the hands and fingers developed after fractures of the bones in consequence of plaster-of-Paris dressings, and of the immovability of the respective joint, lasting frequently for months, thus rendering the arm useless for years and even forever, also yield often to the same method of treatment, especially if there are directed at the same time single powerful shocks to the contracted flexors, and strong induction currents upon the semiflexed extensors.

CASE 104.—Friedrich Herm, a weakly man, of fifty-five years of age, was taken, about six weeks ago, with pain in the right shoulder-joint, which ceased somewhat on using the arm, but became so intense whenever he kept quiet or lay down, that he was unable to raise the right hand without supporting it with the other. The pain ensuing, especially, on pressure of the coracoid process, increased for the next three weeks to such an extent, that it was absolutely impossible for the patient to raise the hand or forearm, preventing him from doing any kind of work and even from eating. Sulphur-baths rendered him still worse, but the repeated application of leeches at least alleviated the tenderness. When the patient came to my office, July 14, 1857, he was unable to move the elbow farther than three inches. Every effort to do so, anteriorly or laterally, was prevented by a violent pain, originating in the pointed end of the coracoid process immediately at the place of insertion of the biceps muscle. At this spot I felt a soft exudation, touching which, caused the patient to cry aloud. The deltoid as well as the other muscles of the upper arm, was emaciated. I employed the induction current, placing a smaller conductor on the painful place and a larger one on the deltoid muscle. After an action of about ten minutes, I had the pleasure of observing in the patient a considerable diminution of pain and an easier motion of the arm. After the second application, he was able to raise the arm anteriorly to an angle of 60°; after the third (July 10th), to a right angle. The exudation was materially reduced, a strong pressure with the finger caused but little pain. After the eighth application, July 26th, the patient resumed his work. A few additional applications sufficed to cause the complete resorption of the exudation.

CASE 105.—Mr. L., pianist, slipped while walking, in the middle of February, 1860, saving himself from falling down entirely only by projecting stiffly the left arm, so that the surface of the hand bore the whole weight of the body. In consequence of this fall he had pain in the wrist-joint, which he tried in vain to alleviate by cold compresses and liniments. The pain increased whenever he played on the piano, extended soon into the little and ring fingers, and finally prevented him from playing altogether. On examining him, on March 13th, I found an exudation, about as large as a pea, between the os magnum and the metacarpal bones of the little and ring fingers, causing, on pressure, besides the local pain, another, radiating to the little and ring fingers. On placing one of the moistened conductors on the exudation, and the other upon the corresponding metacarpal space, decrease of pain ensued after a few minutes. After four applications, the patient was able to play on the piano for an hour at a time, and to appear the next week in a concert. The induced current was also employed in this case.

CASE 106.—Mr. F., merchant, aged forty-one years, always healthy, was attacked, in the spring of 1855, with rheumatic pain in the left arm, for the removal of which he went to Töplitz. The result was so far favorable, as the pain was absent during the winter, returning, however, again, and causing him to revisit the baths of Töplitz in 1856. Here the patient allowed a jet of warm water to fall upon the temporarily-painful elbow-joint, thus causing, or at least increasing, an inflammation of that joint. Soon after his return the joint became swollen, stiff, and painful, preventing every attempt of stretching the bent arm. In the spring of 1857 the swelling and stiffness increased, every involuntary motion, the slightest touch of the left arm, produced the most violent pain, which occurred also during the night, whenever the patient lay on the left side. I found, on June 8, 1857, the elbow-joint considerably swollen, especially in the condyles, and more so in the internal condyle. Pressure on these parts, and on the groove between the inner condyle and the olecranon, caused a violent pain. The forearm was bent toward the humerus at an angle of about 70°, extension being impossible. Partly cutaneous faradization, partly a passing of currents through the joint, partly increased extension by faradizing the triceps muscle, acted so favorably that the pain was greatly diminished June 11th (fourth application), and an extension to 100° became possible, fifteenth application (July 1st); tenderness entirely gone, the swelling is reduced, especially in the external condyle. The internal condyle is still greatly swollen; the arm can be extended to an angle of 130°. The treatment terminated with the twenty-ninth application, when the arm could be extended to 170°. Pain had not returned; the arm was perfectly useful; the swelling was considerably reduced.

CASE 107.—Lieutenant R., of Stettin, aged twenty-six years, was affected, eleven weeks ago, probably in consequence of a cold, with pain in the right maxillary joint, rendered worse through every attempt at chewing, but also continuing without exercising the affected parts. After the pain had yielded, within three weeks, to local depletion, poultices, and the use of the unguentum Neapolitanum, the left articulation was affected in the same manner, but in a less degree; here, also, pain gradually ceased, leaving, however, an incomplete anchylosis of both maxillary articulations, for the removal of which Dr. Nagel advised the employment of electricity. On May 1, 1857, the patient could hardly separate the jaws to the extent of a finger's breadth; lateral motion, as well as motion of the lower jaw anteriorly, was impossible; every attempt to do this, or to open the mouth farther, caused a dull pain in the joint, extending into the ear. In this case one of the moistened conductors was placed on the maxillary joint, at the external border of the cheek, the other being applied, through the mouth, to the condyloid process of the lower maxillary bone, and thus kept for several minutes. Immediately afterward, the jaws could be separated to the extent of one-fourth inch, but this improvement was only of short duration, for, on the next morning, the contraction of the masseter muscles made it impossible to put the thumb into the mouth. After six applications, however (May 7th), slight lateral motion was observed, becoming pretty easy after twelve applications (May 16th); the patient now being able to chew solid food without pain, and to move the lower jaw about two lines forward. The eighteenth application terminated the treatment, the patient having recovered the full use of both joints.

CASE 108.—Nina S., aged nine and a half years, was affected with a swelling of the left knee, after having passed through an attack of scarlatina, in April, 1859, or, perhaps, in consequence of a cold. Iodine ointment was employed for two years, without any result. Having afterward used, with comparatively little effect, the baths of Baden-Baden, and Pyrmont, she was placed under my care, October 15, 1863. On receiving her I ascertained the following: The left knee was one inch larger in circumference than the right; it was bent to the thigh at an angle of 175°; every attempt to stretch it above this angle caused great pain; the muscles of the left thigh were atrophied; the child limped; no deviation of the spinal column existed. The conductors of a strong induction current were placed crosswise above and below the knee-pan, and kept for several minutes in this position, after which the thigh was extended by faradizing the quadriceps femoris. After six applications (October 26th), a visible improvement was noticed. After the twentieth application (December 1st), the leg could be perfectly straightened, the nutrition of the femoral muscles was perceptibly improved, the swelling of the knee was diminished, and there remained but a slight dragging of the leg. Yet electricity was still employed till February, 1864, making in all fifty-two applications, at which time no other morbid symptom remained, except a slight difference of bulk between the two knee-joints.

CASE 108.—Mrs. Nietner, laundress, forty-two years of age, received a fracture of the radius and ulna immediately above the wrist-joint, April 28, 1867. She was treated by Dr. Wilms with dressings of plaster of Paris, and sent to me, on May 25th, for the purpose of having the stiffness of the joint removed through electricity. I found supination entirely suspended, the wrist and all the finger-joints immovable, the fingers in a state of semiflexion, an attempted passive extension very painful. A battery current, averaging thirty to forty elements, passed first, for two to three minutes, transversely through the wrist, and then through the finger-joints. After eight applications, lasting five to ten minutes each, the wrist was movable upward and downward, supination still impaired, but possible, too. In six additional applications (two per week), the same method was employed, partially-descending labile currents passed now through the extensors, now through the flexors, and finally powerful flexions and extensions, produced by directing the current transversely through the wrist-joint by means of a metallic current changer, thus materially improving the motion of the joint. This treatment enabled the patient, on July 15th, to resume her work as laundress, and to continue it without interruption.

Remak reports, in his Galvano-therapie (page 295), the following case of traumatic affection of the joint:

Michael Hartleib, tailor, thirty-six years of age, fell, March 2d, the sidewalk being slippery, on the right hand, spraining the wrist-joint, rendering it immediately impossible to bend or shut the hand, and passing a sleepless night, in spite of the application of cold water. Remak found, the next morning, the wrist-joint so much swollen, especially on the dorsal surface, hot, and painful, that he was unable to ascertain whether a fracture of bones had taken place. The fingers were also stiff and tumid. He immediately directed labile currents, of thirty elements of Daniell, both through the swelling and through the neighboring muscles, until mild contractions ensued in the muscles covering the dorsal surface. This being continued for five minutes, during which period the patient noticed, from minute to minute, his hand become freer from the swelling and stiffness, every motion of the hand and fingers was restored, enabling him to write his name. The following day (March 4th), he reported having sewn some coarse work, only the handling of the scissors being difficult. A slight swelling was still visible on the dorsal side of the wrist. The former treatment being repeated, the patient reported himself free of every complaint.

In traumatic and rheumatic articular exudations, even in those of long standing, I have repeatedly observed that, after the resorption has been instituted through the electric current, this process progresses spontaneously, even to the perfect removal of the exudation, without the further use of electricity, or any other resolving agent, so that here an after-effect of electricity may be justly said to exist.

B. *Arthritic Articular Exudations.*

We have already, on page 253, treated of a form of gouty articular affection (arthritis nodosa), in which the swelling of the joint is connected with atrophy of the interosseous muscles, which affection can be completely removed by galvanizing the sympathetic nerve. In a second form, too, in which not only the synovial capsule and the ligaments present the appearance of a chronic inflammation spreading to other joints, but where, also, the articular cartilages and surfaces show, at the same time, peculiar changes and malformations (arthritis deformans), the galvanization of the sympathetic system seems also to produce a material improvement. I have, in a stout girl, twenty-four years old, a patient of Dr. Boeger, produced, by the above-mentioned treatment, an increase of temperature, alleviation of pain, diminution of the swelling, and easier motion.

Concerning the true gout (arthritis vera), only internal remedies are to be employed while the disease is in the acute stage; after the fever is gone, and the true gouty nodules remain, it is sometimes possible to insure a cure through the employment of strong constant (derived from forty to sixty elements of Daniell), or through strong induced currents.

I am indebted to the kindness of Dr. Cahen for the following case:

Mrs. S., aged sixty years, a lady of great refinement, became so reduced in circumstances, through the unexpected death of her husband, that she was compelled to perform labors to which she was previously unaccustomed. For ten years she suffered from a gouty affection to such an extent, that finally both wrists, and all the finger-joints, were almost completely anchylosed, through gouty deposits. Every attempt to move the joints caused violent pain, preventing her from doing any kind of work. The finger-joints were enlarged, painful on pressure, and somewhat fluctuating. No hereditary disposition could be ascertained. After the patient had for years in vain employed various internal and external remedies, she applied to Dr. Cahen for an electric treatment. A few years ago she had used the rotation apparatus, experiencing some relief, but suspended the treatment soon after. Dr. Cahen employed induction electricity with the greatest assiduity for half a year, daily without interruption, in such a manner as to enclose for several minutes each single enlargement in the circuit. Soon the painfulness of the joints disappeared, the swellings became gradually less, the movability of the joints increased in proportion, until the patient had, at the end of the treatment, recovered the full use of her hands. No abnormal formations existed in the wrist-joints; the joints of the fingers, however, were thicker than in the normal state; fluctuation was entirely gone; but strong crepitation was heard whenever the joints were rubbed against each other.

C. *Suppressed Secretions and Excretions.*

With regard to the influence of electricity in diseases caused through a derangement of an existing, or through the absence of a normal secretion, we must consider its direct effect upon the non-secreting organ, the exciting influence exercised by the current on the nerves collecting in the respective glands, and to a greater extent the contractions it produces in the muscular-fibres situated in the glands, thus occasioning secretion of the proper material. That the last-mentioned action is the more important, is proved by the following circumstances: 1. The electric current has the power of restoring the suppressed perspiration of the feet, and to promote the secretion of cerumen, while, at least up to the present time, it has been impossible to find nerves in the perspiratory and ceruminous glands. 2. The secretion of milk is independent of the connection of the gland with the intercostal nerves, as proved by the experiments of Eckhard, made by their section. Finally, 3. The intermittent is generally far more efficient than the constant current for the purpose of restoring suppressed secretions. In some cases, where a direct irritation must be avoided as much as possible, it is better to obtain the desired result through reflex action by acting on the skin and its nerves through faradization.

Suppressed perspiration of the feet is soonest restored by faradization.

CASE 109.—August Braklo, merchant, aged twenty-four years, after having worked eight days in a cellar, in which he also slept, felt a stitching pain in both heels, extending thence into the feet, so that every step became painful, especially after having been quiet for some time. Soon both feet began to swell, followed by a suppression of the habitual perspiration and a feeling of numbness in both legs. The patient came to my office, November 24, 1859, after having in vain employed irritating foot-baths, embrocations, and Russian baths, for a month. After the first cutaneous faradization of the feet and legs, the feet became warmer, and the walking easier. After the third application, the feet began to perspire, the swelling diminished, and the pain on making a step disappeared; after the eighth application he was enabled to pursue his usual occupation.

With regard to menstruation, we have already, on page 93, mentioned that it has often been produced or augmented against our intention in consequence of the electric irritation of any portion of the body, especially those near the uterine region. This experience might often be employed with advantage; if this kind of action does not suffice, we may try Schultz's [1] method of cutaneous faradization of the soles of the feet, the legs, or the chest; and, this being insufficient, we may follow the example of Golding Bird, by passing a series of shocks (twelve to fifteen in number) through the pelvis, applying one conductor to the lumbo-sacral region, and the other to the pubic bone or the vagina. Of twenty-two patients suffering from amenorrhœa, fourteen were cured in Guy's Hospital, through this method; of the eight unsuccessful cases, seven were at the same time affected with anæmia, leucorrhœa, or phthisis pulmonum. We read the following case in Guy's Hospital reports, 1822 (page 143):

Miss B., eighteen years of age, of tall stature, suffered, for some time, from amenorrhœa, for the removal of which she employed, in vain, the different preparations of iron. Her general health became worse, appetite diminished, and she became irritable and low-spirited. Iron, soda, and rhubarb, improved her general condition, but the menses were still absent. Then statical electricity was applied, a series of shocks being passed, every other day, through the pelvis. The menses appeared after three weeks, lasting for three days. The treatment was now suspended for three weeks, and applied again three times in the fourth week. Menstruation took place at the normal period, continued five days, and returned regularly. The general health of the patient also continued good.

[1] Die Reflexwirkungen der Induction-Electricität. Wiener med. Wochenschrift, 1855, No. 40.

Similar successful results in amenorrhœa and dysmenorrhœa were obtained by v. Holsbeck and Bitterlin,[1] also by Charles Taylor,[2] Hervieux, Graves, etc.

The impaired secretion of milk may also be improved in two ways, either by allowing the induction current to act, by means of moist electrodes, for several minutes on the gland, or through reflex excitation by faradizing the skin of the pectoral region. Aubert[3] thus treated a woman for an anæsthesia of the skin of the pectoral region, for from ten to twenty minutes, with dry conductors, and who, having been confined seven months before, did not nurse her child, and in consequence had no trace of milk three weeks after delivery. After the third application, a kind of milk-fever ensued, the breast began to swell, and the nipples became moist. After the fifth application, the milk could be readily collected.

Aubert reports, besides,[4] the following case:

A woman, twenty-six years of age, mother of three children, nursed the third one herself for eleven and a half months, when it was taken with pneumonia, and refused the breast. When the child was put to the breast again, the secretion had entirely ceased. Aubert placed wet electrodes alternately upon both breasts, taking care to avoid pain and muscular contraction, by gradually increasing the strength of the current. After the fourth application, the breasts were tense and full, and the child could be nursed again.

In the *Gazette Hebdomadaire*, of January 16, 1857, we find the following case of Becquerel:

A healthy but nervous woman, of twenty-seven years of age, had been nursing six months, having always a full supply of milk. In consequence of violent and repeated mental

---

[1] See Annales de l'Électricité, 1860, page 149.
[2] Lancet, ii., September 9, 1859.
[3] L'Union Médicale, 1857, No. 9.
[4] See L'Union Médicale, September, 1855, No. 116.

emotions, the secretion of milk was reduced to a minimum in the left, and completely suspended in the right breast. It was resolved to bring up the child with the bottle. The child, however, did not thrive, and its health suffered. Becquerel now tried to stimulate the left breast (in which, for eight days, hardly a trace of milk was left) to increased secretion, by allowing a mild, rapidly-interrupted current to act by means of wet conductors, placed alternately on different portions of the breast. After the first application, which caused some inconvenience, but no pain, the lacteal secretion began anew. After the third, it flowed so freely as to be sufficient for the further nourishment of the child. The right gland secreted less, but, the whole amount being sufficient, electricity was no more employed.

Similar cases have been published by Moutard-Martin and Lardeau,[1] by Descivières,[2] and others.

CHAPTER II.

THE EMPLOYMENT OF ELECTRICITY IN MIDWIFERY AND GYNECOLOGY.

THE employment of electricity in midwifery dates from Bertholon and W. G. Herder, the latter of whom recommended contact electricity as a remedy for absent labor-pains.[3] They were followed by Basedon, Stein, and afterward Kilian, who constructed for this purpose his "galvanic obstetrical forceps," consisting of two metals. Dr. Hoeniger, of Zyly, and Jacoby, of Neustadt,[4] first used the induction electricity for the excitement of labor-pains. In our own day, Benj. Frank is the only German physician who, to our knowledge, has thus employed electricity; of English physicians,

---
[1] Gaz. des Hôpitaux, 1859, No. 60.
[2] Gaz. des Hôpitaux, 1861, No. 53.
[3] See his Practical Contributions for the Extension of Obstetrics, 1803.
[4] See Zeitschrift für Geburtshülfe, vol. xvi., page 428. Berlin, 1844.

however, there are Radford,[1] Dorrington, Johnson, Wilson, Mackenzie, Tyler Smith, Dempsey, Barnes, Houghton, etc., who all used electricity as an excito-motor stimulant in cases in which, the pelvis being normal, there existed dynamic disturbances, depending on an absence, weakness, or perverse action of the expelling power, or where long-continuing fits of fainting, or eclampsic accidents, necessitated a rapid termination of the delivery, or where hœmorrhages, caused either by placenta prævia or asthenia of the uterus, required as early a termination of the birth as possible, or an immediate contraction of the womb afterward, or, finally (Barnes), where paralysis of the uterus took place in consequence of the employment of chloroform.

Thus Dempsey[2] mentions a case where, the pelvis being normal, labor had lasted for thirty hours, the very weak contractions having entirely ceased for three hours, and the patient, with short intervals, been in a fainting condition for two hours. Here the first application of the induction current, continued for about five minutes, was followed by drawing-pain in the small of the back; the second, repeated after five minutes, caused energetic contractions of the uterus; and, after forty minutes, during which time the current was employed in this manner four times, for five minutes, a live, healthy child was born. Ergot had been previously in vain administered in large doses.

Benj. Frank[3] mentions a woman, thirty-eight years of age, who had been confined successfully seven times and aborted twice, in whom again, in consequence of a fall on the nates, in the fifth month of pregnancy, abortion had taken place, followed by a considerable loss of blood. The uterine contractions were entirely suspended; the patient, aroused

[1] See Froriep's Notices, 1845, No. 729, and 1846, No. 789.
[2] See Lawrence on the Application and Effect of Electricity and Galvanism. London, 1853, page 53.
[3] Magnet-Electricität zur Beförderung der Geburtsthätigkeit. Neue Zeitung für Geburtskunde, 1846, Band ii., Heft ii., page 370.

from a fainting-fit by sulphuric ether, was bathed in blood, looking more dead than alive. The pulse was small, and could not be counted; the uterus soft below the navel, and still of considerable circumference, and but loosely connected with the cord. After the application of the induction current for several minutes, a strong pain ensued, the uterus contracted, and the bleeding ceased. At intervals of from five to ten minutes, the labor-pains returned; without requiring the further use of the apparatus, the patient revived, and, after half an hour, Frank was able to remove the placenta, causing but a slight loss of blood.

F. W. Mackenzie[1] has stopped bleeding, in three cases of metrorrhagia, through the application of the electric current. In the first case, where a dangerous bleeding was maintained by the incomplete removal of the ovum, defying every known remedy, the use of electricity caused a rapid expulsion of the remaining portions of the ovum, and an immediate stoppage of the blood. In the second case, where, in consequence of placenta prævia, several dangerous hæmorrhages had taken place before the beginning of delivery, a continued current, applied for six hours, prevented not only every loss of blood, but facilitated also the opening of the os, allowing a rapid and, for the mother, safe termination of the confinement. In the third case, where placenta prævia necessitated a speedy delivery, on account of hæmorrhage, the same method was employed for three hours. The bleeding ceased, and the confinement went on so rapidly that a live child was born after a few hours.

Radford[2] believes he has met with good results from the use of electricity in cases of hour-glass contractions of the womb.

According to the above-mentioned observers, electricity fulfils in general the same indications as ergot, and, accordingly, is only to be employed, like it, after the membranes

---

[1] Gaz. Hebdomadaire, du 2 Avril, 1857, No. 14, page 250.
[2] See The Lancet, 1853, vol. ii., No. xxii., page 500.

are broken; it has, however, the following advantages over that remedy: 1. Electricity acts certainly; ergot is frequently uncertain. 2. Its action ensues immediately after its use; that of ergot does not take place for a longer or shorter period afterward. 3. The strength of the electric current can be adapted to the degree of existing irritability, while the necessary dose of ergot can only be approximately determined. 4. The contractions produced by the electric current are more energetic and equal in their direction to the normal contractions, while the use of ergot is frequently followed by irregular, spasmodic contractions, placing the life of the child in danger. 5. The administration of ergot has, according to the experience of Ramsbotham, Wright, and Barnes, frequently an injurious influence on the new-born child; thus Barnes saw, in four cases, in which the birth was accomplished through ergot, the children die from convulsions after a few hours. 6. Electricity can be employed, even in the most extreme cases, in which swallowing is impaired, every medicine ejected from the stomach, and every mechanical interference in the uterus, introduction of the hand, etc., contraindicated on account of the great irritability. 7. Electricity does not exclude the simultaneous employment of other remedies. In opposition to the above-mentioned authors are Simpson and Scanzoni (perhaps in consequence of an unsuitable method), who consider the employment of electricity in feeble contractions and uterine hæmorrhage useless, thus leaving this question still open for a final decision.

Benj. Frank and Golding Bird, the latter especially, in consideration of some cases, in which he brought on an undesigned abortion, through the influence of the electric current, in a supposed suppressio mensium, believe the use of the electric current, for inducing premature artificial labor, to be especially indicated in those cases in which the os has been dilated by means of sponge-tents, or through other methods.

Dempsey used the electric current for this purpose in a case where he desired to induce premature labor at the end of the seventh month, on account of narrow pelvis. After having perforated the ovum, and waited for forty-eight hours for the appearance of labor-pains, he used the current three times, for five minutes, at an interval of ten minutes, until a mild and transient pain took place. No labor-pains ensuing, in spite of this, he returned, after half an hour, to the same method, and electrified three times, with the same intervals. Now regularly-returning pains ensued, delivery progressed normally, and was terminated eight hours after the beginning of the operation.

Berryman[1] used the same method at the end of the eighth month, in a woman with narrow pelvis. After having tried in vain to sever the membranes of the ovum from the uterine walls with the sound, and having also, with the same result, after two days, introduced a flexible male catheter, and kept it inside for an hour, he resorted, after five days, to the induction current. Contractions of the womb immediately followed, producing the easy delivery of a live child.

Concerning the method itself, one conductor is usually applied to the sacral region or the fundus uteri, while the other, furnished with a vaginal conductor,[2] is introduced, through the vagina, to the os. Barnes advises, instead, to apply a conductor to either side of the lower abdominal region. According to the experiments of Mackenzie,[3] the action of the current on the uterine fibres would ensue soonest by passing the current from an upper segment of the spinal

[1] Galvanism in Effecting Premature Labor. Edinburgh Med. Jour. 1862. December.
[2] See the engraving in the Neue Zeitung für Geburtskunde, Bd. xxI., Heft lii., Table 1, Figure 8.
[3] See page 82.

column transversely through the uterus. As the writings of the different authors vary from each other, it will be necessary to decide through an experiment in every individual case, and it will be best, after having moistened the abdominal walls thoroughly, to pass a strong current of the induction apparatus from the fundus uteri to the region over the symphysis.

Lately electricity has been very favorably employed for the resuscitation of new-born children, apparently dead. Upon the recommendation of Hufeland, Struve, Marshall Hall, and Underwood, Gottbold Scholz[1] first made more extensive experiments with electricity, and ascertained, as the result, that no other agency was able to revive the extinguishing spark of life as rapidly and safely as the cautiously-used electric current. Scholz's method consisted in placing one conductor on the neck and the other on the place of insertion of the diaphragm, or the apex of the heart. The same result may be obtained, in a more simple and suitable manner, through the faradization of the phrenic nerves (see page 429). Pernice[2] used this method in five cases of apparent death, of which two failed, but three resulted perfectly satisfactorily, inasmuch as respiration was established and life continued.

The following is the first of Pernice's cases:

After regular labor-pains had taken place till six P. M., dilating the os till eight P. M., to the size of a silver dollar, the water escaped. After a short pause, powerful contractions propelled the head to the floor of the pelvis, but were unable, for five hours, to overcome the resistance offered to the soft parts, by reason of the large size of the head. On account of the decrease of the frequency of the fœtal pulse, the forceps was applied, at half-past one A. M., and the head

[1] Bemerkungen über die Eintheilung des Scheintods der Neugebornen, Guensburg's Zeitschrift, Bd. ii., pages 16–35.
[2] Greifswalder Medicinische Beitraege, Bd. ii., page 1, et seq.

delivered. The child, weighing nearly nine pounds, was apparently perfectly dead, relaxed, the body pale, with the exception of the brow and the vertex, which latter was covered by a considerable swelling. No palpitation of the cord was felt; the sounds of the heart feeble and rare; cutaneous irritation gave no result whatever. The induction apparatus was then applied. After several attempts, he succeeded in striking the phrenic nerve on both sides, and in causing a contraction of the diaphragm; a second contraction was effected after about two minutes. The child was then placed in a warm bath, and faradization repeated after a few minutes. After the current was applied ten times—consequently in about from one-half to three-fourths of an hour—the first independent inspiratory motion ensued, which was repeated after a short time. Irritation of the skin now proved beneficial, and was employed till the complete revival.

The employment of electricity has also met with some success in gynecology. Thus, for instance, a case is reported by B. Dempsey, from the practice of Tyler Smith, in which a uterine polypus, the pedicle of which could by no means be reached by the operator, was, in consequence of the contractions induced by the electric current, expelled sufficiently to make it easily accessible to the ligature, which done, the polypus was removed without difficulty.

Another case was that of a woman of forty-two years of age, who had aborted three times, and borne eight children. The menses had again ceased for six months. At first occasionally, and in the later periods continually, a bloody flow took place from the vagina. For two months the patient experienced a severe burning pain in the abdomen; in the last week anasarca of the legs rendered her condition very deplorable. An increased bleeding surpervening, it was resolved to immediately induce delivery. The examination proved the presence of a tumor, resembling the pregnant uterus, situated more in the right side, and extending to the navel, being firm and elastic, and tender on pressure. Neither placental murmur nor fœtal pulse could be heard. The os was open to the extent of a shilling, the breasts were relaxed. Consequently, the diagnosis was—a dead fœtus, or a diseased ovum. After the application of the electric current, a number of hydatids were evacuated, followed soon afterward, and also the next day, by a still larger quantity.

Finally, the electric current has been used especially by the French physicians Beuvain, Fano, Tripier, Beau, and others, for the removal of chronic swellings of the uterus, and its subsequent descent and dislocation—observations worthy to be investigated, in consideration of the evils so frequently following the use of the sound, and other means usually employed against flexions. Thus, Fano[1] reports the following case:

Mrs. K., aged twenty-nine years, mother of several children, experienced, for eight months, a feeling of heaviness in the abdomen, pains in the right inguinal region, and numbness in the right leg. She also suffered from pain in the renal region, and leucorrhœa, but had neither constipation nor dysuria. The examination showed anteflexion of the uterus. An electric current was employed for five minutes, by placing one pole on the hypogastrium, the other being applied to the collum uteri. The patient felt a tickling sensation, and noticed something rising in the abdomen; immediately after the application, the anteflexion seemed to be diminished and the pain lessened. During the next application, made the following day, the patient felt as if something was moved from the right inguinal region, to the hypogastrium; pain and leucorrhœa were stronger the following day, but the examination made on the day after showed the anteflexion to be reduced. With this, the pain

[1] L'Union méd., 1859, page 134.

and the numbness of the right lower extremity disappeared, and the patient was permanently relieved.

Beuvain[1] obtained a no less happy result in the following case:

Mrs. R., aged twenty-six years, mother of three children, suffered, for four years, from a descensus uteri, and chronic swelling, with ulcerations, against which neither local depletions, nor emollient injections, nor the application of the caustic for weeks, were of any avail. Then, Beuvain directed a galvanic current, generated of four elements of Bunsen, against the granulations and ulcerations.[2] After this painless operation was repeated five times, free menstruation took place without giving her any inconvenience, and when this had ceased, the granulations and ulcerations were removed, and a clean, healthy surface left in their place. In order to raise the descended womb, Beuvain then used the induction electricity for four months, with so favorable a result that the patient was able to walk great distances without any uterine support. All the other symptoms of disease had also disappeared, and did not again return, as Dr. Beuvain was afterward informed.[3]

CHAPTER III.

THE USE OF ELECTRICITY IN SURGERY.

A TREBLE use has been made in surgery of electricity, by employing it: 1. For the purpose of producing heat. 2. Causing chemical effects. 3. As a means of stimulation.

I. ELECTRICITY FOR THE GENERATION OF THERMIC EFFECTS.

Although the thermic action of the continued current has been known for a long time—it being also known that

---

[1] Annales de l'Électricité Méd., 1860, page 43.
[2] See chapter III., section II.
[3] On the operation for uterine polypus, see page 391, et seq.

the degree of heat did not depend on the number but on the extent of surface of the metal plates, and that, accordingly, only one single pair, of very large surface, was necessary for the heating of metal wires; that, in this manner, a degree of temperature could be generated, such as was produced by no other medium, the blow-pipe excepted—yet the employment of electricity for surgical purposes made but slow progress. It was Middeldorpf who recently succeeded, through the improvement of existing and the invention of new methods, in placing galvano-causty on a scientific basis, and securing for it a permanent footing in surgery. Concerning his predecessors, Heider,[1] prompted mainly by Steinheil, conceived, in 1843, the idea of killing the nerves of the dental pulp, by means of the electric heated wire. He employed this method in July, 1845, in such a manner as to insert between the two conducting wires of a very large Grove's element, which could, through a simple mechanism, be united and separated, a fine platina wire, bent in the form of a loop. He then introduced this platina wire cold, the circuit being opened into the proper dental cavity, heated it through the closing of the circuit, and withdrew it, after a few seconds, again cold. Gustav Crussel, the inventor of electrolysis, must also be mentioned, as among the first who appreciated the advantage of the electric cautery, by using, in 1846, the electric heated wire for the removal of a large fungus hæmatodes, situated in the frontal and ocular region; and, finally, John Marshall, who, in November, 1850, destroyed fistulæ in a similar manner.

By this method it was, however, only possible to heat a platina wire, or a platina point, and consequently to act but on a small surface at the same time. Dr. Ellis[2] succeeded, through the following ingenious method, in rendering possible the action on a larger surface, and thus in contriving a *modus operandi* which he employed successfully for the

---

[1] Zeitschr. de Wiener Aertze, Maerz, 1846.
[2] See the Lancet, 1853, vol. ii., No. xiii., page 502.

cauterization of the neck of the uterus, in ulcerations, chronic inflammations, etc. Taking a thick, straight silver catheter, he cut off the upper portion, and slit open the remaining end, thus adapting it for the reception of a porcelain button. Two isolated wires run in this catheter, connected on one end with the poles of a Grove's battery of four to five pairs, and on the other end with a platina wire wound several times around the porcelain button, and heating it to a white heat. After introducing a glass speculum, the porcelain button is applied for a longer or shorter period to the affected part, which first is cleansed by means of a pledget of lint.

If we now turn to the operations of Middeldorpf[1] in this department, we find, above all, that they are due to the greatly improved apparatus for galvano-caustic purposes, as well on the source of heat as on the instrument used for heating. Concerning the source of heat, Middeldorpf employs the battery described and represented on page 101. For cauterization itself, he uses burners, cutting-loop, and heated wire. The burners are usually constructed in the following manner: Two gilt copper wires run through a piece of ebony, connected on their lower ends with the conducting wires of a battery, but receiving on their upper ends a thin piece of platina of different shape, according to the different use. One wire is cut obliquely within the wooden handle, springlike, and at the distance of about ¼''' upward, and can be connected with the other segment by means of a slide, thus closing the circuit. In the dome-shaped burner the two wires protrude 3¾''' from the handle, run along each other without being in actual contact, and receive in front the thin piece of platina, five millimetres broad. In the porcelain burner, a thin-walled, hollow porcelain cap is used instead of the thin platina plate, which is heated by a platina wire wound around it. The burners used for the destruction of the lachrymal duct, or for the cutting of strictures, are

---

[1] See Middeldorpf, die Galvanocaustic, ein Beitrag zur operativen Medicin. Breslau, 1854.

straight or bent, and covered at their point by a small piece of elastic catheter during their introduction or withdrawal. In the galvano-caustic cutting-loop, the most important instrument, the wire is passed through well-conducting, but isolated tubes, allowing the protruding end to become heated; it is moved by a wheel in the tubes, making it possible to shape the loop to every desired size. The heating wires are made of platina, and are introduced into tumors, or drawn through fistulæ, by means of a perforated sound or by needles.

The following are the morbid conditions in which the galvano-caustic has been used by Middeldorpf with extraordinary results: 1. Hæmorrhages requiring the deep and energetic cauterization of large surfaces; bleeding from medullary carcinoma. 2. Neuralgia, when small and restricted portions of tissue can be acted upon easily and safely by means of this instrument. 3. Ulcers on the neck of the uterus difficult to be approached. 4. Carcinomatous tumors when it is desired to avoid the danger of bleeding. 5. Fistulæ which may be either: *a.* Cauterized thoroughly (lachrymal, parotidean, dental-vesicular, recto-vaginal, vesico-vaginal, urinary, etc.), or, *b.* By cauterizing the surrounding parts alone, or with the opening at the same time, thus causing a cicatricial contraction, and their subsequent closing (minute fistulæ of the parotis, of the salivary duct, etc.), or, *c.* By cutting through the fistulæ (intestinal, recto-vaginal fistulæ). 6. Strictures of the urethra where, in the anterior portion of the penis, only the finest bougies can be introduced, and requiring, at the same time, the destruction of the stricture callus. 7. Polypi in general, but especially if they are attached, difficult of access, or entirely inaccessible through the surgeon's knife (uterine, laryngeal, naso-pharyngeal polypi, etc.). 8. Pediculated tumors of the larynx, protruding from the larynx into the pharynx, having a sufficiently large body, and not connected with the glottis. 9. Prolapse of the uterus, or the anterior vaginal wall, etc., where the employment of the dome-shaped burner narrows permanently the vagina through inflammation, suppuration, and cicatricial contraction.

We here give the history of the case which spread most extensively the fame of galvano-causty, and established it permanently by rendering a successful operation possible in a case in which no other operative method could be employed.

A minister, aged forty-two years, heretofore healthy, had been suffering, for two years, from an increasing difficulty in swallowing, and from hoarseness. He occasionally, while coughing, threw up small pieces of flesh, and finally he noticed behind the epiglottis a roundish substance, which his physician supposed to be a polypus. Middeldorpf examined the patient, and found the following: Inspiration audible, expiration pretty free, voice absent, swallowing impaired. If the patient opened the mouth and put out the tongue, there was observed in the bottom of the normally-reddened pharynx the slightly-injected white-yellowish epiglottis, and close behind a pale-red swelling of a dirty, sulphur-yellow appearance, covered by the shining and partially-excoriated mucous membrane, about as large as a walnut, projecting about 3''' over the deepest portion of the middle fissure of the epiglottis, and approaching the pharynx posteriorly. After examining the expectorated piece under the microscope, the diagnosis was "a carcinoma originating in the upper laryngeal region, above the superior thyro-arytenoid cartilage, which grew up to the superior aperture, and then expanded laterally." The prognosis was doubtful, the treatment difficult. On May 20, 1853, Middeldorpf performed the operation in the following manner: The patient sat on a chair, leaning with his head against the breast of an assistant; the battery was placed on a table behind, held in readiness by the assistant, to be closed any moment. The platina-loop, being about one and a half inch in diameter, had a circumference of about a silver dollar. The handle of the instrument being seized with the left hand,

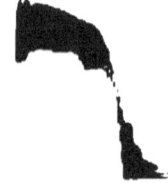

and the index and middle fingers of the right passed through the loop, and separated from each other as far as possible, an attempt was made to pass the loop, with a rapid movement, over the polypus. With a violent retching and involuntary closing of the jaws, the polypus and larynx receded three times, necessitating the prompt withdrawal of the hand. Finally, the tongue, and with it the larynx, were fixed with Museux's hooked forceps, the canula passed down between the swelling and the larynx—the retching still continuing—the loop adjusted, tightened, and the battery closed, and, after a few turns of the wheel, the tumor (weighing 140 gr., 44 millim. broad, 20 millim. thick, and 21 millim. high) was severed, and lying loose in the throat, permitting its removal with the finger. The wire was broken. The operation caused scarcely any pain; ice-water was administered and easily swallowed, respiration was free and inaudible, the voice loud and perceptible, although a little hoarse. The examination with the finger showed the pedicle to have been cut off smoothly, on a level with the walls of the larynx, without injuring the epiglottis.

Concerning the employment of the galvano-caustic method in preference to the knife, the following are the advantages of the former: 1. The condition of the patient is never rendered dangerous by its use. 2. It is but slightly painful during and after the operation. 3. In no case is the operation followed by hæmorrhage, as all the vessels supplying the tumor are swiftly and effectively destroyed. 4. The method can often be employed usefully on parts which are not accessible to the knife of the surgeon on account of their position and extension; a wire can be introduced into the nose, pharynx, œsophagus, larynx, etc. 5. It frequently preserves parts which would have to be removed in operating with the knife. 6. It is especially valuable in those cases where the cauterization of the wound is indicated after the operation.

The electric cautery offers the following advantages for

the hot iron, the rival of which electricity also becomes in the above-mentioned manner: 1. It does not frighten the patient with any preliminary preparations. 2. The success is surer, because the wire is not heated till applied to the place to be operated upon, thus preventing a loss of temperature through previous cooling. 3. The patient is protected against any injury by either its introduction or withdrawal. 4. As the heat is generated only at the point of union of both electrodes, it is possible to introduce the electric cautery into deep cavities, without affecting any surrounding tissue, which can hardly be avoided with the common hot iron. 5. The platina point being very small, the loss of substance, and accordingly the subsequent cicatrix, is likewise comparatively small.

As disadvantages of the galvano-cautery, Middeldorpf mentions: 1. The cost of the apparatus. 2. The easy melting of the wire, unless it lies on soft parts along its whole extent. 3. The breaking of the wire during the cutting, as well as its crossing, thus preventing the heating above the crossing-place; the last-mentioned facts, however, can easily be avoided with proper attention and skill.

Since the publication of Middeldorpf's works, many experiments have been made with the galvano-cautery, especially in Vienna and Paris. Zsigmondi[1] is prominent in having made a large series of galvano-caustic operations, which led him to the following conclusions: This method of operation is of practical value: 1. On account of its hæmostatic action on one side in parenchymatous hæmorrhage, and bleeding in places difficult of approach; on the other side, in patients of a hæmorrhagic or anæmic condition, where every loss of blood must be avoided. 2. Through the use of its caustic effect for the destruction of organic formations, especially where an energetic action is required in small and deep-

[1] Die galvanocaustische Operationsmethode nach eigenen Erfahrungen und mit besonderer Rücksicht auf "Middeldorpfsche Galvanocaustia." Wiener Med. Wochenschrift, 1858 und 1859.

lying points. 3. Through the employment of its ligature-like action in many operations for the removal of polypi, especially in such cases allowing heretofore only ligation on account of want of space, a high place of insertion, or for other reasons. The last-mentioned effect has especially given a permanent place to the use of the galvano-cautery in surgery, whenever a polypus is situated in the pharynx, posterior nares, larynx, and œsophagus, in which the electrically heated wire insures the patient against bleeding, removes the danger of suffocation, in consequence of the tumefaction of the polypus, and renders unnecessary, in some cases, the opening of the respiratory tract. Thus, among others, Neumann and Semeleder[1] operated with the galvanic cautery on a tumor the size of a hen's egg, arising from the base of the skull; for the removal of uterine polypi and other gynecological operations, this method has been recommended by Braun[2] and Von Gruenewald.[3]

If the galvanic cautery has not been, on the whole, employed as extensively as could be expected after its introduction into the profession, the fault lies in part in the costliness of the necessary apparatus, in the technic difficulties of management requiring a careful course of preparation, and, finally, in its deficiency preventing us from keeping the wire every moment at a temperature necessary to avoid its melting or breaking. The first-mentioned evil is remedied by the very cheap apparatus of Stœhrer (see page 102); the latter seems to be avoided by the use of Fromhold's galvano-caustic apparatus.[4]

II. ELECTRICITY FOR CAUSING CHEMICAL EFFECTS.

The chemical action of electricity, used in surgery, depends on the property which the currents possess of decom-

[1] Wiener Med. Wochenschrift, No. 27, 1860.
[2] Wiener Medicinal-Halle, ii., No. 49. 1861.
[3] Petersburger Med. Zeitung, i., pages 1-13 und 55-63, 1861.
[4] See Electrotherapie von C. Fromhold, 1859, page 117, et seq.

posing organic liquids (see page 26), and which, as well as the thermic effect, is produced especially by the constant current. The thermic and chemical effects differ, however, from each other, in obtaining the former through large plate elements, and the latter through a large number of small elements. If two needles, connected with the poles of a battery of the last-named kind, are introduced into a blood-vessel, or into a tumor filled with a liquid, a decomposition of the contents takes place, albumen, fibrin, acids, etc., collecting at the + pole, and watery extracts, alkaline bases, iron, coloring-matter, going to the — pole (see page 89). Then both poles, as ascertained by Crussel, in 1839, through experiments, presented a perfectly different appearance, for if he introduced the conducting wires in opposite directions into the white of a fresh egg, there were, in a short time, formed at the positive pole flakes, which enlarged and thickened more and more, and were attached, with a certain degree of toughness, to the point of the wire, causing a regular process of consolidation, while at the negative pole the albumen became thin, losing its peculiar viscid quality in the vicinity of the point of the conductor, thus inducing a process of liquefaction. The same chemical process may be effected, in a more precise manner, by introducing but one pole into the liquid, and closing the circuit by placing the other pole on the surface of the body, when different indications may be fulfilled, according to the introduction of the positive or negative pole. On these effects are based the methods employed for the cure of varices and aneurisms by galvano-puncture, as well as the electrolytic treatment of some tumors, etc.

A. *Galvano-puncture in Varices and Aneurisms.*

The treatment of varices and aneurisms through the electric current, by needles introduced into the interior of the vessels, is not new. Scudamore first directed the attention of the profession to the faculty of the continued current of causing a rapid coagulation of the blood. Guérard, 1831, Pravaz, and Leroi d'Etiolles, deduced from it the possibility of a coagulation of the blood in aneurismatic sacs. Petréquin, of Lyons, obtained, in 1846, the first favorable result in aneurisms; Bertani and Milani, in 1847, in varices.

Concerning the method itself, a bandage or tourniquet was generally placed around the limb to be operated on, for the purpose of diminishing the supply of blood, and then two straight needles, one to two inches long, one from above downward, the other from below upward, were slowly introduced into the enlargement of the vessel in such a manner as to separate their points a few lines from each other. Which done, the conducting wires of a Voltaic pile (consisting of thirty to sixty pairs of plates, if an aneurism, and of from twenty to thirty pairs, if a varix was to be operated upon) were attached to the heads of the needles, which were furnished with flat rings, and turned from each other; the needles being kept in this position for from ten to twenty minutes. Ciniselli and Petréquin believed the application of the tourniquet to be useless and harmful. Petréquin frequently changed the direction of the needles, in order to obtain a nucleus of fibriform coagula, around which the coagulation could then take place faster and be completely finished in from ten to twenty minutes.

By using this method, the operation was successful in some cases, remaining in others without a result. In rare cases coagulation of the blood followed immediately after the operation, but usually not till after several days. Thus it happened that some, seeing that coagulation did not ensue till after some hours or days, thought this process to be a consequence of an inflammation of the vascular walls, from the introduction of foreign bodies. In four individuals, for instance, on whom Schuh[1] operated thirteen times for varicose veins, a cure did not take place till several days had passed—while others considered it a chemical effect

[1] Zeitschr. der k. k. Gesellschaft der Aerzte zu Wien, June, 1856.

caused by the action of the electric current on the blood, especially because they found that, if the needle connected with the negative pole is withdrawn after the operation, bleeding follows, explained by the separation of the serum or the salts at the negative pole, while the withdrawal of the other needle, around which fibrin, albumen, etc., are deposited, causes no bleeding, or but a very slight loss of blood.[1] It is only recently that the exertions of Baumgarten and Wertheimer[2] have made it possible to solve these doubts, and place the method of operating on a sure basis. For the numerous experiments made by them on animals invariably gave the following results: 1. If the needle connected with the negative pole was introduced alone into the blood-vessel, while the other needle was applied to the surrounding parts, no coagulation took place. 2. The introduction of both poles produced a slow, rather weak, and rarely perfect coagulation. 3. The introduction of the positive pole alone, with the application of the negative pole to the neighboring parts, always brought about a rapid and complete coagulation.

Malgaigne gave to the experimenters an opportunity to try the method on the human subject. The case furnished was that of a young girl, who for some time had been suffering from a varicose degeneration of the large and small veins of one upper extremity up to the acromion, whence the evil seemed to spread over the trunk. The volume of the limb had increased to twice its normal size. As a predisposing cause, only an extraordinary thinness of the venous membranes could be considered. In this case, where the patient had either to be left to her fate or her life placed in jeopardy through the cauterization or ligation of so many veins, electro-puncture, made as described sub. 3, gave some very remarkable results. Baumgarten and Wertheimer introduced

[1] See Rapporto della Commissione che a fatto gli sperimento sull' électropunctura, etc., Annal. univers., Jan., 1847, page 219.

[2] Ueber Galvanopunctur bei Aneurysmen und Varicen. Gaz. des Hôpitaux, 1852, No. 72.

in three sittings, at an interval of two to three days each time, about ten needles into the most extended veins, placed a conductor, connected with the negative pole, into the hand of the patient, at the same time connecting all the needles with the positive pole. The operation caused but little pain. After a few minutes the needles were removed, when, in place of the dilated veins, full, resistant cords were felt, a sure sign of complete coagulation. After a month, the greater portion of the veins was obliterated and the volume of the limb considerably reduced; only then those veins, heretofore of normal size, began to dilate a little, which circumstance can exercise no influence on our opinion of this *modus operandi*. Thus galvano-puncture appears to offer a sure method for the successful treatment of aneurisms and varices, and also appears to avoid the danger of phlebitis following the methods formerly employed.

The following is, according to Steinlin,[1] the chemical process ensuing in this method: The salts in the serum of the blood maintaining the albumen, fibrin, and casein in solution favor the coagulation of these substances on account of their decomposition through the electric current. The acids formed in consequence of this decomposition go to the positive pole, and these form, with the metal of the pole—needles—metallic salts, which precipitate the albumen, etc., thus causing a firm coagulation at the positive pole. Consequently the metal of which the needles consist has a considerable influence on the rapidity with which coagulation of the blood takes place. If the needle attached to the positive pole is made of platina, coagulation occurs slowly; if the platina needle is furnished with an iron point, this process ensues more rapidly, and more rapidly still if a zinc needle, or, on account of its brittleness, a steel needle, covered with zinc, is introduced. For this reason Steinlin recommends for his operation the use of the last-mentioned kind of needle, which is to be connected

[1] Galvanopunctur bei Varicositäten und Aneurysmen. Zeitschr. der k. k. Gesellschaft der Aerzte zu Wien, 1858, Heft iv.

with the positive pole of the pile, while the negative pole is, by means of a platina plate, or a sponge moistened with a solution of salt, placed near by on the skin, the conducting power of which is improved by a dilute acid or a solution of salt.

I was fortunate enough to cure permanently, through galvano-puncture, the case of aneurism described below, but must also remark that the final favorable result is perhaps not to be ascribed to galvano-puncture exclusively, inasmuch as digital compression was also employed.

CASE 110.—Mr. R., a druggist of Herrnhut, aged fifty-two years, noticed for the first time, about twelve years ago, that the left knee was always warmer than the right, and that, at the same time, there existed also a small swelling in the middle of the knee-pan. About ten years later he struck the left knee very violently against a hard, angular substance, causing great pain and swelling of the joint. Through rest and the use of lead-water applications, the symptoms of irritation disappeared within eight days, the swelling being also diminished, but since that time pulsation was plainly perceived on either side of the patella, to which symptom the patient did not, however, pay much attention, causing him, nevertheless, to cover the knee with a compressing india-rubber bandage. In spite of this, the swelling gradually increased until, in the last years, pulsation could also be plainly felt in several dilated arteries in the vicinity of the patella—a group of symptoms causing the patient to go to Berlin for the purpose of consulting Dr. Wilms. He recommended the employment of galvano-puncture for the obliteration of the aneurism, which here undoubtedly existed, and sent the patient to my office, June 20, 1855. I found the following symptoms: The tumor was covered by skin of normal color, and easily moved; it covered the knee-pan to three-quarters of its extent, and thence extended partially to both sides, especially to the inner side, and partially upward, into the muscular tissue of the quadriceps femoris. Pulsation could not only be felt on different points of the patella, but was also visible to the eye; the temperature was also considerably increased.

The operation was made for the first time on the 30th of June, 1865, by introducing as deeply as possible three needles, connected with the positive pole of Remak's zinc-carbon battery, into the most prominently-pulsating places of the tumor, while the negative conductor, covered with flannel and linen, measuring one and a half inches in diameter, rested on the thigh above. After the needles were kept in this position for half an hour, the current having the strength of twenty elements, they could only with a certain degree of force be extracted from the firm coagulum. No bleeding followed, nor was there any pain felt during the operation, a slight burning at the zinc pole excepted.[1] Upon Dr. Pirogoff's request, who was present at the operation, this, as well as the next three operations, was followed by a digital compression of the femoral artery at the beginning of the lower third of the thigh, made for twenty-four hours alternately by three attendants. The galvano-puncture was repeated on the 6th, 15th, 21st, and 29th of July, with the difference that the number of needles introduced on July 6th was three; on the 15th and 21st, ten; on the 29th, five; they always remaining in the vessel for half an hour. It was found that coagulation was less firm if ten needles acted simultaneously; at least,

[1] According to Fromhold (*l. c.*, page 110), the galvanic current must be of sufficient strength to form, in one minute, a coagulum of the size of a bean, at the positive pole, if tested with albumen taken from a fresh egg and placed in a saucer, and, besides, to cause a deviation of 25° of the magnetic needle. He also advises to connect each time but one needle with the positive conductor, allowing the galvanic current always to act for two minutes, and continuing the same method with each successive needle. I prefer the method employed by me of allowing the current to act continually at the same time on a larger number of needles (which, however, ought not to exceed five or six in number), for the reason that I have never, under these circumstances, observed the slightest bleeding follow the removal of the needles (the same happened also in another case of aneurism on the volar surface of the hand, the final result of which I regret to be unable to report), while Fromhold mentions the bleeding as not a rare result of his method.

after the operations made on the 15th and 21st, the withdrawal of one or the other needle was followed by a slight bleeding, which did not occur in the first, second, and fifth operations, after the introduction of a less number of needles. The long intervals between the single applications were necessary, on account of the patient feeling very much affected after each compression, and the thigh being very tender, in a considerable extent, to every touch. The pulsation in the tumor, however, became less each time, the coagulation in the blood-vessels rendering, at the same time, the tumor so firm and hard that the introduction of five needles was made only with some difficulty, on July 29th. When the patient left Berlin, August 8th, a very weak pulsation could be felt only at the upper part of the tumor, the volume of which was also considerably reduced. Concerning the further course, I was informed that, in the next days after the patient's departure, an abscess formed in the fibro-cellular tissue, on the lower inner border of the patella, in consequence of the suppuration of some needle-wounds, from which a few teaspoons of bloody pus were discharged, and which then healed within a week. Otherwise the patient, in a letter dated March 27, 1868, expressed his great satisfaction about the permanently happy result of the treatment, adding, finally, the following: "There exists but a moderate swelling, of about two inches in diameter, with a very weak pulsation. I always wear an elastic bandage around the knee, and I have but a few times perceived a sensation of heat, after exerting the knee considerably, while travelling in the mountains, but felt no pain or other inconvenience."

B. *Electrolytical Treatment of Strictures, Exudations, Tumors, Ulcers, etc.*

Crussel[1] was the first to use electrolysis for the removal of strictures, exudations, ulcers, etc. He was followed

---

[1] Die Electrolytische Heilmethode. Neue Med.-chir. Zeitung, 1847, No. 7. Med. Zeitung Russlands, 1847 und 1848.

by Willebrand, Spencer Wells, Ciniselli, etc. Lately this method has been revived by Scouteten and Tripier[1]—by the latter especially in the treatment of the obliterated lachrymal sac, the constricted Eustachian tube, and of stricture of the urethra, but most of all by Althaus, of London,[2] who, at the same time, tried to generalize this method, and to extend it to the treatment of serous exudations, strictures, wounds, and ulcers, and to tumors, especially those having soft contents. According to Althaus, two factors enter into the effect of the negative pole on animal tissues : 1. The mechanical effect of the liberated hydrogen, which can be seen, under the microscope, to rise in numberless vesicles, to penetrate the minutest parts of the tissues, and to separate their fibres. 2. The chemical effect of the free alkalies (potash, soda, and lime), generating with the hydrogen at the negative pole, and corroding the parts chemically. For the operations themselves Althaus used a battery, consisting of fifteen elements of Daniell, for the introduction into the tissues, a needle of gold or gilt steel attached to the negative pole, or various modifications of the needle in the shape of a fork, with two, four, six, eight teeth, or a dull blade, etc., while the circuit was made by applying to the skin a sponge, connected with the positive pole.

In the following we shall report the noticeable results of the electrolytical method for the treatment of the above-mentioned diseases, discussing briefly, at the same time, the other methods of electricity employed for their removal :

1. In strictures of the urethra, Willebrand, following Crussel's example, introduced, as far as the stricture, a metallic sound, furnished with an india-rubber covering, from which only a conical silver point protruded, connecting it with the negative pole of a battery, while the conductor at-

[1] Arch. gén., 1866, page 18.
[2] See Vorlöufige Mittheilung über meine electrolytische Behandlung der Geschwülste und anderen chirurgischer Krankheiten. Deutsche Klinik, 1867, Nos. 34–36.

tached to the positive pole was placed in the patient's hand. The sound was kept in this position daily for ten, or, at most, twenty minutes, a cure being effected in eight to ten days. Wertheimer has resumed these attempts, and Jaksch[1] reports having seen the catheter fixed on the stricture, and connected with the negative pole, glide easily over the constricted spot after ten minutes. To this, authorities in Paris, for instance Leroi d'Etiolles, have objected, as the same result could be obtained, without the use of electricity, by quietly pressing on the stricture, yet the rapid results obtained by Tripier, through the employment of galvanism, speak against the correctness of this assertion. For Tripier proceeded in the following manner: He pressed a thin metallic olive (made of platina—gold, copper, or any other metal resisting the action of electrolysis), connected with the negative pole, against the stricture, moving it farther against the constricted place, in proportion to the destroyed tissue, while the positive pole was kept fixed to the pelvis. The result was striking, for, usually, a cure followed after one or a few applications; whether it remained permanently, Tripier was unable to say at the time of publishing his report.

2. If we now consider the exudations, we shall speak in contradistinction to the firm rheumatic and gouty articular exudations, the treatment of which has been mentioned on page 439, *et seq.*, of the serous exudations, which have become an object of electrolytical treatment, especially in the form of hydrocele, or of dropsy of the joints, or of an accumulation of liquids in cysts. After Lewis, Travers, Hack, etc., had tried simple acupuncture in the treatment of hydrocele, Schuster[2] seems to have been the first who, in 1839, cured hydrocele and similar affections by means of electro-puncture, and delivered a report on his method to the Academy in 1843. The method is distinguished

---

[1] See Prager Vierteljahrsschrift für die pract. Heilkunde, 1851, Bd. iii, page 188.

[2] Bull. de Thérap., 1839, Février, Mars, pages 174, 225.

before others, serving the same purpose, through the simplicity, safety, and slight painfulness. It consists of two acupuncture needles entering the swelling at opposite sides sufficiently deep so that the opposing points are near to each other. These needles are then connected with a Voltaic pile of thirty to forty elements, the current being allowed to act in three or four applications, about ten minutes each time. The hydrocele disappears immediately; the remaining œdema of the scrotum after a few days.

Burdel,[1] Delstanche,[2] Lehmann,[3] Thevissen,[4] etc., have likewise employed the induced current, with favorable results.

Burdel reports the following case:

A man, fifty-three years of age, had suffered for three years from a voluminous hydrocele of the left side, for the removal of which two insect needles were introduced, and connected with Bréton's rotation apparatus. Vermicular motions ensued in the scrotum, accompanied by pains extending into the kidneys. After the gradually-increased current had acted for twenty minutes, the swelling was reduced to about one-third of its volume, and had disappeared entirely the next morning.

At the end of a month, however, it had reappeared, and he was then electrified for three-fourths of an hour; the swelling again vanished and did not return—at least, it had not reformed when Burdel published this case (nine months after the operation).

Lehmann's case was as follows:

A man, fifty years of age, whose right testis had become atrophied, in his early youth, from a blow, had a hydrocele on the left side, measuring eleven and a half inches in circumference. Lehmann employed Du Bois's apparatus, by

[1] Union Méd., 1859, No. 13.
[2] Journal de Bruxelles, 1859. Juillet.
[3] Deutsche Klinik, 1859, No. 37.
[4] Annal. de l'Électricité Méd., 1860, No. 4.

introducing both needles into the tunica vaginalis, changing the poles after ten minutes, and operating half an hour in all. Immediately after the operation the skin was œdematous, the tunica vaginalis less tense, and no disagreeable sensation present. The scrotum was wrapped up in wool, and a suspensory bandage applied, enabling the patient to walk about. In the evening the œdema increased; the serum in the tunica vaginalis, however, decreased. On the following morning the œdema was less, and the liquid in the serous cavity reduced to about one-half; the patient took a ride of ten miles. No œdema existed the next morning, the liquid within being reduced to one-fourth. After four applications, a perfect cure took place.

Benedikt[1] reports several cases of articular dropsy, cured by means of galvanization, either with or without the use of acupuncture needles.

Josa, a student of medicine, had contracted a hydrops genu et burs. muc. patellæ on both sides, which, in the following winter, was removed through the galvanization of the joints, and did not again return.

Johann Jokesch, a servant, aged thirty-four years, with constitutional syphilis, suffered, fifteen months ago, from articular rheumatism, and has now hydrops genu on both sides. Galvanization through the joint made no material change; galvano-puncture, however, caused a complete cure in four applications.

These cases encourage, at any rate, a more frequent employment of galvano-puncture in articular dropsy; it will be, however, more practical then to connect all the introduced needles with the negative pole of the battery, and to place a larger conductor, attached to the positive pole, upon some near portion of the skin.

In addition to the treatment of serous transudations, electricity has also been used, sometimes with advantage, for the removal of the more plastic exudations within the cornea,

[1] Electrotherapie, 1868, page 177.

Willebrand being the first to employ electricity for this purpose.[1] He placed a fine round silver button, furnished with a silk-covered handle, and connected through a wire with the negative pole of a single galvanic element, upon the middle of the cornea, while the patient put a small plate, attached to the positive pole, into his mouth. Soon a feeling of stitching-pain and of burning took place in the eye, the conjunctiva reddened, an effusion of tears ensued, but these symptoms soon yielded to the application of cold water. The disintegrating process once begun, it proceeded uninterruptedly, without the further use of the apparatus. Willebrand has used this method in four cases, of which two are reported to have been cured, and the others to have been improved materially. Von Graefe (see the report cited in the note) considers these assertions to be well founded. For having, in cases in which exudations existed in both eyes, employed electricity on one side and tincture of opium and lapis infernalis on the other, seems to have accomplished his purpose sooner with electricity.

I myself presented,[2] at a meeting of the "Gesellschaft für wissenschaftliche Medicin," April 21, 1856, a patient, sent to me by Prof. von Graefe, in whom, after four months' employment of the induced current, a considerable exudation on the cornea was resorbed sufficiently to allow the patient to recover the normal length of vision, while before he could, with the left eye, read large print only at the distance of one and a half inches, the right being entirely useless. Although exudations in the cornea are frequently resorbed, in the course of time, without resorting to irritating agencies, yet in this case the improvement became so marked, from the first week of the use of electricity, that it must be

[1] Although Willebrand speaks of scars of the cornea, he means exudations, a mistake excusable on his part, he not being a professional man (see Sitzungsbericht der Gesellschaft für wissenschaftliche Medicin vom 16. August, 1852, in der Deutschen Klinik, 1852, No. 39, page 445, or in der Med. Central-Zeitung, 1852, No. 68.

[2] See Med. Central-Zeitung, 1856, No. 34.

ascribed mostly to the electric treatment, a fact confirmed repeatedly on presenting the patient at Graefe's clinic. The method used in this case, which avoided every irritation of the highly-inflamed eyes, consisted in placing a wet sponge, connected with the negative conductor, on the closed eye, and placing the moistened positive conductor in the patient's hand, allowing the current to act thus daily for from ten to fifteen minutes.

3. Concerning the dispersion of tumors, attempts were some time ago repeatedly made to remove, with the electric current, infiltrations in lymphatic glands, goître, ganglia, and similar swellings. Thus de Haën applied in vain the shocks of an electric battery to lymphatic tumors situated in the necks of two young girls; Mauduyt, Sigaud de Lafond, and Massé, however, obtained better results. Duchenne has twice removed lymphatic swellings of the neck through cutaneous faradization. Boulu[1] used metallic disks, which he attached to two opposite sides of the tumor, then passing through them the magneto-induction current, by means of moistened conductors. In this manner he obtained a cure in two and improvement in four cases. Of the first two mentioned, one was that of a young man, thirty-two years of age, affected with a swelling of the left parotis, of the size of an orange, which first appeared two years ago, after an attack of rheumatic pains. Electricity effected a complete cure in two months. The other case was that of a young man, aged seventeen years, who was freed, within three months, of a parotideal tumor of the left side, of about the size of an egg, which had existed for ten years. Demarquay also[2] removed, through galvanism, a swelling of the submaxillary gland, of the size of an egg, which had continued, in spite of every medical agency, by

---

[1] Du Traitement des adenites cervicales par l'Électrisation localisée. Union Médicale, 1856, No. 63.
[2] De quelques cas heureux d'application de l'électricité. Gaz. des Hôp., 1855, No. 85.

introducing two needles transversely and two needles vertically into the margin of the tumor, and then connecting alternately the transversal and vertical needles with the pile. The operation was hardly at all painful, and the swelling disappeared in the course of a month, after twelve applications. A. Becquerel,[1] however, and others, maintain that electricity has no influence whatever on glandular swellings.

I am able to oppose this opinion decidedly. I will now report two cases, in the first of which I dispersed an infiltration of lymphatic glands, of the size of a hen's egg, while in the second case I reduced to a minimum the greatest tumor probably ever treated with electricity.

CASE 111.—Miss N., aged twenty-nine years, applied to me, November 13, 1867, upon the advice of her physician, Dr. Simonsohn, for the purpose of getting rid, through electricity, of a glandular swelling, the size of a hen's egg, situated on the left side of the neck. Its posterior part was covered by the sterno-cleido-mastoid muscle, which was raised above the level, and it extended upward to the angle of the lower jaw, having been noticed at least two years previously. It grew but slowly during the first year and a half, and increased rapidly to its present size in the last six months, disfiguring the patient considerably. During the first eight applications a constant current, causing a deviation of the needle of 25°, was passed transversely through the swelling. No noticeable reduction of the tumor seemed to take place. I then, by way of experiment, tried a powerful secondary induction current, passing it likewise transversely through the tumor. Continuing this for ten minutes, the result was so remarkable that I resorted thereafter to the same method. Up to the 22d of December (twentieth application), the swelling was reduced to one-third of its former size. Since that time the decrease of volume was much slower, requiring, till March 31, 1868,

[1] Traité des applications de l'Électricité à la Thérapeutique méd. et chir., Paris, 1857, page 314.

forty additional applications, of the same duration, to make the tumor sufficiently small not to be perceived by the eye, while an induration, of the size of a peach-stone, could still be felt by the finger.

CASE 112.—Miss F. P., aged twenty-two years, strong and healthy, began menstruating in her fifteenth year. The catamenia appeared quite regularly in the first few years, but failed afterward, frequently for two months and more. Having been attacked, in the fall of 1857, by rheumatic pains in her right shoulder, a swelling appeared, without any known cause, on the right side of her neck, which was first supposed to be a parotitis, and treated accordingly, by simply covering it. It, however, neither disappeared nor suppurated, and at last it assumed the size of a child's head, and became of a stony firmness within four weeks, being situated between the head and the scapula. Cataplasms, the internal and external administration of iodine, mineral baths, etc., were in vain employed. After the patient had, in the summer of 1858, used forty-five baths in Kreuznach, etc., she was advised by Drs. von Langenbeck and Ries to apply to me, for the purpose of trying electricity, as a last resort, every known remedy having failed, and an operation also appearing to be inadmissible. The two medical gentlemen frequently convinced themselves of the favorable success of this treatment. The tumor, terminating angularly, filled the space between the lower jaw, the mastoid process, and the inferior semicircular line of the occipital bone; thence extending posteriorly to the spinal column, which it displaced to the left side, ending anteriorly in the middle of the neck, and reaching inferiorly to the shoulder-blade, where its limits could not be exactly defined. As a consequence, the scapula protruded farther than normally from the chest, the patient being unable to approach its upper angle nearer than three and its lower angle nearer than two and a half inches to the vertebral column. The swelling not being, however, attached to any bone, was, especially in its lower portion, of a stony firmness. The circumference of the right cervical half was about fourteen, that of the left six inches. The right sterno-cleido-mastoid muscle could not be defined, the tumor overlooked the supraclavicular region, the clavicle was completely covered, the head inclined to the right continually, making any motion to the right completely impossible. The expression of the whole face appeared to be somewhat idiotic.

I passed the induced current transversely through the tumor for from one to one and a half hours at a time, by means of brass plates, covered with sponge. After having made fifty-six applications, I presented the patient, at the end of August, 1859, to Dr. von Langenbeck, who found the tumor reduced one-half; it was also less hard, especially at its upper part, those parts to which the conductors were applied appearing to be softer after each application. The tumor gradually decreased until it had hardly one-third of its former volume, after one hundred and forty-two applications (November 30, 1860). The circumference of the right cervical half was now only ten and a half inches; the sterno-cleido-mastoideus could now be perceived, even in the usual position of the head; the clavicle, the supraclavicular, and aural regions were free; the head was straight, and could be moved somewhat to the right side. The spinal column no more bulged to the left, the shoulder region was freer. The tumor had decreased most in its antero-posterior diameter, less in the lateral direction. The treatment was continued, with frequent interruptions, till July, 1862, two hundred and seventy-three applications having been made in all. The improvement progressed without interruption, but it was ascertained, through carefully measuring the tumor each time, that it remained stationary during the suspension of the treatment, which occurred every year for several months. When the treatment was finished, the transverse diameter of both sides of the neck differed hardly two inches. The head could be turned to the right without difficulty, the supraclavicular fossa was perfectly free, the difference of both sides of the neck appearing only in the broad and not in the deep diameter. The face had assumed a pleasanter expression. As a proof of these facts, I caused the patient to be photographed before and after the treatment. The patient subsequently married, and became a happy mother. The swelling has remained the same, but perhaps it may have been diminished a little.

Althaus[1] has removed, through electrolytical treatment, the following kinds of tumors: 1. A nævus of the eyelid. 2. A papillary swelling in the axilla. 3. A molluscum of the right eyelid. We shall report briefly the first two cases:

1. A lady, aged twenty-eight years, had a congenital nævus, of the size of a pea, on the right lower eyelid, for the removal of which she applied to Mr. White Cooper, who introduced, July 23d, a needle, attached to the negative pole of a battery composed of ten cells, into the right half of the swelling, while Dr. Althaus closed the circuit by placing a moistened electrode on the skin of the neck. The needle having been withdrawn after two minutes, without the loss of a drop of blood, the right half of the nævus appeared to have shrunk, while the left half was unchanged. On July 26th the operation was repeated, with the same satisfactory result, on the left side, thus removing the nævus entirely.

2. A lady, twenty-seven years of age, consulted Dr. Althaus, November 21, 1866, on account of a highly-vascular papillary swelling in the axilla, which was first observed in the beginning of 1865. It had rapidly increased during the last months, measuring now, in its broadest portion, one-third of an inch in length and one-fourth of an inch in width. Dr. Althaus introduced a needle, connected with fifteen cells of the battery, into the basis of the swelling, allowing the current to act for three minutes. After having operated for a few seconds, a remarkable change took place in the swell-

[1] L. c., page 323.

ing, it losing its flesh-color and becoming white, as if frozen. After the withdrawal of the needle, the circulation in the tumor had apparently completely ceased. During the operation slight pain was felt, afterward none, neither was there any loss of blood. On November 23d the swelling had entirely withered, appearing like a thin brown leaf, having hardly any connection with the skin. For this reason the operation was not repeated. One week after the operation, the scab fell off, and after four weeks neither a cicatrix nor a reddening of the skin, nor any sign whatever, could be noticed of the former tumor.

4. If we finally direct our attention to the galvanic treatment of ulcers, we find Crussel[1] basing his electrolytical treatment of ulcers upon the following observation. He found that, by connecting two metal plates with the poles of a battery, and placing them on two different parts of the body, the plate connected with the positive pole acted like an acid, that is, consolidating; while the other plate, attached to the negative pole, acted like an alkali, that is, liquefying. If he had to treat a simple ulcer, he covered it with a metal plate, attached to the positive pole, connecting the negative with the hand or foot of the patient. Soon a skin was formed, which covered the ulcer for several days, when it fell, leaving the ulcer smaller, which finally healed, after the repeated use of the same method. If Crussel covered a suppurating cancer with a metal plate connected with the positive conductor, a coagulated layer was deposited upon its surface, which remained there like a firm scab. After it fell off, the ulcer appeared to be cleaner, more reddened, and less painful, showing a tendency to heal. In syphilitic ulcers, electrolysis acts similarly to other caustics, nitr. of silv., etc., with this difference, however, that the application of caustics causes the formation of a scab, which does not come off till after twenty-four hours, leaving behind a wound which requires several days for its healing, while the early

[1] See Neue Med.-Chirurg. Zeitung, 1847, page 235.

application of the electrolytical method heals the ulcer usually within twenty-four hours.

Dr. Kyber, physician to the Marine Hospital in Cronstadt, has thus treated ten soldiers affected with syphilis; Dr. Rosenberger, physician-in-chief to the hospital for syphilitic women in St. Petersburg, also treated fifty syphilitic patients in the same manner. In forty-one the ulcers healed entirely, while in the remaining nine other means had to be employed. Kyber asserts that the use of galvanism is more suitable in cases where the number of primary ulcers is not too large, and where their size, situation, and form allow the metallic conductors to touch their surface completely.

Spencer Wells,[1] judging from a similar observation, covered torpid, waxy, relaxed ulcers with the zinc-plate of his galvanic arch (page 95), and found them, after three days, to have a healthy surface. Deep ulcers, with indolent granulations, were covered by him with the copper or silver plate, after the removal of which they began to heal, with a healthy granulating process. He remarks that, after trying the most different methods of treatment, he found galvanism to be the best agent for causing a healthy, even granulation. He frequently saw deeply-excavated ulcers covered with granulations in twenty-four hours, which, after forty-eight hours, had grown to a level with the surrounding skin, beginning to cicatrize, which process was soon finished through coldwater dressings. He especially mentions cases, occurring not unfrequently in sailors, where ropes, thrown forcibly around a limb, tear out circular pieces of skin, connective tissue, fascia, and muscles, exposing the bones of the extremity as does a burn. Even in those cases, in which the use of the most different means caused hardly a trace of granulations, covering the wound, for twenty-four hours,

[1] Bemerkungen über Heilwirkungen des Galvanismus aus der Praxis des Dr. Cogevina in Corfu.; Oppenheim's Zeitschrift, 1849; Schmidt's Jahrbücher, Band 64, page 161.

the silver plate, caused conical granulations to spring up, so that, in a comparatively short time, the ulcer healed.

Becquerel, taking into consideration the secretion of the ulcer, covers it with the plate connected with the positive pole, if the secreted liquid is of an alkaline reaction, and applying the plate attached to the negative pole if there is an acid reaction.

C. The Galvanic Current for the Solution of Vesical Calculi.

After Gruithuisen had proposed to dissolve vesical calculi through the action of the Voltaic pile, Prévost and Dumas[1] experimented first outside of the animal body. For this purpose they placed a dry, fusible stone, weighing ninety-two grains, in a vessel filled with water, connected it through platina wires with the poles of a pile consisting of one hundred and twenty-five pairs, and found that the mechanical action of the gases, formed through decomposition of the water, amounted, by renewing the charge every hour, to twelve grains in the first twelve hours; that the stone was softened, and fell asunder on the slightest pressure, after an additional action of sixteen hours. They also experimented on animals. The apparatus consisted of an elastic sound, enclosing two platina conductors, isolated from each other, which were covered with silk, except on their ends. The termination of each conductor was fastened to a small ivory hemisphere, on the flat surface of which the platina lay bare, and was to be applied to the stone. Both hemispheres, when placed in apposition, formed a button, which closed the opening of the sound. By means of such an instrument, they introduced a fusible stone into the bladder of a bitch, which they then dilated through injections of tepid water, preventing reflux by closing the opening of the sound; which done, the conductors were connected with the poles

[1] Annales de Chimie et de Physique, 1823, vol. xxviii., page 202, et seq.

of a battery, consisting of one hundred and thirty-five pairs of plates. After a few movements, the animal remained quiet, and bore the action of the current for an hour. On withdrawing the sound, plain traces of disintegration of the stone could be perceived. The same experiment was repeated for six consecutive days, in the morning and evening, for an hour, until the stone became so fragile that they had to desist from further introducing it. When they killed the animal, after a few days, the bladder was found to be perfectly normal, and without any injury. These authors add that the same method could be employed for the solution of numerous vesicular calculi, consisting of saline combinations, but not in such concretions formed exclusively, or nearly so, of uric acid. They also add that an addition of diluted nitric acid would probably facilitate the action of the galvanic pile more than pure water.

H. Bence Jones,[1] proceeding from the supposition that, as the continued current is able to decompose a solution of the nitrate of potash in potash and nitric acid, probably urinary calculi placed between the electrodes of a galvanic battery would be attacked by the potash at the negative pole, and by the nitric acid at the positive pole, brought first a compact piece of stone formed of uric acid in a saturated solution of nitrate of potash between the electrodes of a Grove's battery of ten pairs. The liquid was soon boiling, and, after three hours, the stone was reduced to one-half its size. He now tried a more diluted solution, kept at the temperature of the human body, and found that, under these circumstances, there were dissolved in one hour:

  2–9 grains of uric acid.
  2–25 grains of phosphate of lime.
  ½–2 grains of oxalate of lime.
  1–2 grains of a mixture of uric acid and oxalate of lime.
  4½–5½ grains of a mixture of oxalate and phosphate of calcareous earth.

[1] On the Dissolution of Urinary Calculi in Dilute Saline Fluids at the Temperature of the Body by the Aid of Electricity. Philosophical Transactions, 1858, pages 201–216.

These results, at least, were obtained in stones which had been removed long ago from the bladder, and consequently were very dry. The less dry the stones, the faster, the less dilute the solution of nitric acid, the slower the operation proceeded. It may be assumed that stones in the bladder are easier dissolved than those which are for a long time without the bladder and very dry, because in the first case the electric current is more capable of penetrating the substance itself and of acting on it, while in the latter case, it can act only on the surrounding liquid. Up to the present time, a proper instrument is wanted for this operation in the human body. The instrument must, according to Bence Jones, fulfil the following indications: 1. The stone must through it be isolated in the bladder. 2. The mucous membrane of the bladder and urethra must not be attacked by the chemical process. 3. A contrivance must be adopted which on one side keeps down the temperature of the liquid in the bladder, and, on the other side, provides for the escape of the gases developed in the bladder.

D. *Electricity for the Removal of Poisonous Metals from the Organism.*

Verqués and Poey, in Havana,[1] have used continued currents for the removal of poisonous metals from the organism. Verqués made the first experiment on himself, 1852. He had, while gilding and silvering by galvanism, contracted a malignant ulceration on the dorsal surface of his hands, which defied all means of treatment. He then dipped his hands into an electro-chemical bath connected with the positive pole of a Voltaic pile. After fifteen minutes a metallic plate, connected with the negative pole, was covered with a thin layer of gold and silver; after the use of a few such baths, the ulcers healed radically. The electro-chemical bath

[1] Mémoire sur une Nouvelle Application de l'Electrochimie à l'Extraction des Métaux Introduit et Séjournant dans l'Organisme. Compt. Rend., de l'Acad. des Sciences, 1855, No. 5; Gaz. Méd. de Paris, 1855, No. 16.

is prepared in the following manner: In a metallic tub isolated from the floor, a long bench is placed which again is isolated from the tub. The patient is now put into the bath, his arm being held by supports attached to the bench. The tub is filled with acidulated water, nitric acid being used, if mercury, gold, or silver, is to be extracted, and sulphuric acid, if lead is to be extracted. As soon as the patient is sitting in the bath, the tub is connected with the negative pole of a pile of from ten to thirty carbon and platina elements having a diameter of forty millimetres, and a height of two hundred and seventeen millimetres, while he himself takes the positive pole, furnished with a conductor, the handle of which is covered by lint (in order to avoid the violent burning), alternately into the right and left hand. In this position the current enters through the arm, circulates from head to foot, and is neutralized on the walls of the tub or on the plate of the negative pole. Poey has thus extracted a large quantity of mercury from a man's femur and tibia, which were supposed to have contained the metal for fifteen weeks. The acidulated water is said to become negative electric and to be decomposed, so that gas-bubbles are seen to rise. The metallic spots varied from microscopical smallness to the size of a pea. The extracted metal is found again in three forms: 1. On the walls of the tub; 2. In the atmosphere of the room, in consequence of the evaporation caused by the heat generated through the operation; 3. In the water contained in the tub.

Caplin, of London, repeated these experiments. Dr. Meding, of Paris,[1] placed a patient, suffering for years from mercurial poisoning, in a bath containing eight hundred litres of water and one kilogramme of nitric acid. The negative pole of a Bunsen's battery of twenty pairs was attached to a copper plate immersed in the isolated tub, and the positive pole put in the hand of the patient, who was also isolated

[1] Tageblatt der 32 Versammlung deutscher Naturforscher und Aerzte in Wien. 1856, No. 7, page 150.

from the tub. After the fifth bath, which lasted for one hour, subnitrate of mercury was found on the bottom of the tub, which could be proved by testing with iodide of potash and hydrosulph. of ammon. A gray-greenish precipitate on the negative plate was changed, by rubbing it with the finger, into a distinct amalgam, which disappeared again by heating over the fire. Finally, the microscope proved the peculiarly sprinkled mercurial globules of that form assumed by the rapidly-deposited galvanoplastic precipitate.

III. ELECTRICITY AS A STIMULANT IN PSEUDOARTHROSIS.

The results of the treatment of pseudoarthrosis are, on the whole, not very satisfactory. The rubbing of the fractured surfaces against each other, the forcible stretching and bending, to break the adhesions, and to produce an irritation; finally, the acupuncture, made in such a manner as to leave the needles introduced between the fractured ends for five or six days, give rarely the desired result, and soon the seton and ligature, or the drilling of the fractured ends, and the introduction of pieces of ivory or bone, or, finally, the introduction of wires, have been tried. As, however, seton and ligature frequently cause suppuration and necrosis of the fractured ends, as the introduction of metal pegs, ivory nails, etc., produces often no formation of callus, but rather absorption of bone, one method deserves mention which is perfectly free from danger, and yet effective in single cases, namely, electropuncture.

Thus, Heidenreich,[1] reports the following case which occurred to Burmann: A transverse fracture of the tibia and fibula had not united after four weeks. Burmann then applied a suitable bandage, and then passed the electric current daily, for half an hour, through the fracture, by means of two needles, introduced on opposite sides. Suppuration, formation of callus, and recovery followed.

[1] Elemente der Therapeutischen Physik, 1854, page 279

Hall[1] united through the same method, in the York County Hospital, a fracture of the lower portion of the thigh, which had occurred a year ago, and remained ununited. He introduced a needle on either side of the thigh into the space between the fractured fragments, and allowed the continued current to pass through for some time. The operation was repeated daily for fourteen days, and resulted in recovery.

Hahn, of Stuttgart,[2] reports the following case: a young man suffered from a separation of the femoral epiphysis (perhaps fracture of the neck) in consequence of a fall on the right hip, which resulted in the formation of a false joint, for the treatment of which, bandaging and irritating means were employed in vain. H. resorted to electropuncture; he placed two needles between the fragments, passing the induction current of the rotation apparatus through them daily for from fifteen to twenty minutes. No improvement being noticed after eight days, he employed the constant current, when, after the sixth application, inflammation kindled up around the needles, followed within ten weeks by a union of the fractured parts.

[1] Medical Times and Gazette, November 12, 1853, page 30.
[2] Zeitschrift für Wundärzte und Geburtshelfer, Band xiii., Heft 2.

APPENDIX.

Since the publication of the first American edition of this work, the Galvano-Faradic Manufacturing Company of this city has introduced a number of remarkably efficient and elegant instruments for use in electro-therapeutics. A detailed description of some of the more important of these will probably not be considered out of place.

PORTABLE ELECTRO-MAGNETIC BATTERY. (Fig. 26.)

A. *Battery Rod*—to its lower extremity the zinc plate, a, is fastened. By means of the hinge b, the rod can be laid over horizontally when the battery is not in use, thus securing the zinc from dropping down into the exciting fluid. The *punctuations* on the rod indicate the depth to which the zinc is immersed in the fluid, when the rod is down, and consequently the battery power obtained; it can be secured at any point by the binding screw. Should the rod become tarnished by the acid, its conducting power will be diminished; this is restored by its head, c, coming in contact with the spring, Fig. 1.

The *disk*, D, against which the platina point, b, plays, where the electric spark is evolved, in time becomes oxidized, which interferes with the perfect working of the machine. This disk can be rotated, so that a fresh surface of the metal will be presented to the platina point, and its action instantly restored.

The *adjusting screw*, e, must always be arranged to maintain the platina point in its proper position. When required to effect this purpose, loosen the set screw, d, turn the screw e until the desired point is reached, which is evidenced by the action of the machine, then tighten the set screw as before.

The *hammer*, D, is enclosed between the prongs of the fork, C, which control its vibrations. If the fork be pushed downward, the hammer vibrates slowly; if it be elevated, its prongs limit the lateral space for the vibrations, and their rapidity will be increased. By this contrivance the interval between each shock can be increased or diminished as desired. If the fork should lean too much to either side it can be readjusted by the set screw, Fig. 2. The primary current can be instantly changed to the secondary, or *vice versa*, by means of the rheotrope, E, without removing the conducting wires.

494   APPENDIX.

A fragmentary opening in the *hydrostat* exhibits the interior of the cell with the zinc, a, and carbon, $b\ b$, elements. Between the covering, 7, and rim of the

Fig. 24.

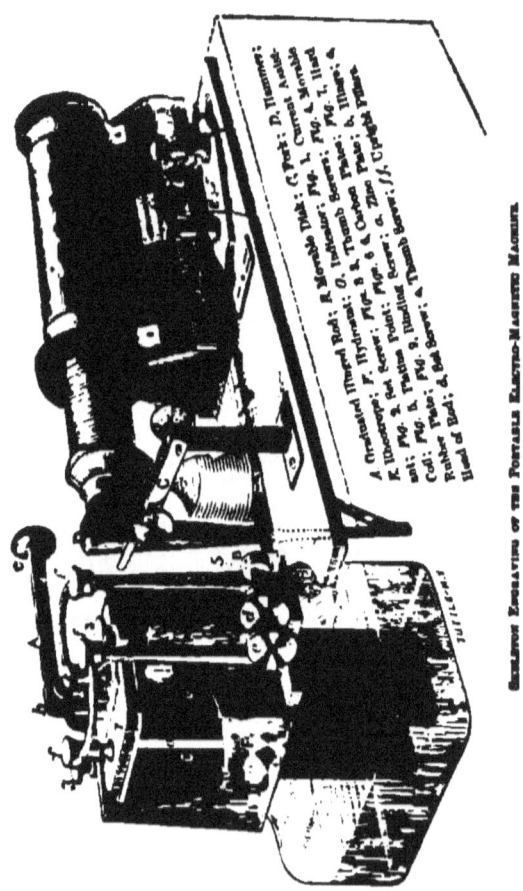

cell, soft rubber packing is placed. The hydrostat is fastened down by the screws, s; this prevents the liquid being spilled, keeps the cells in their places, and impedes the evaporation.

Fig. 27.

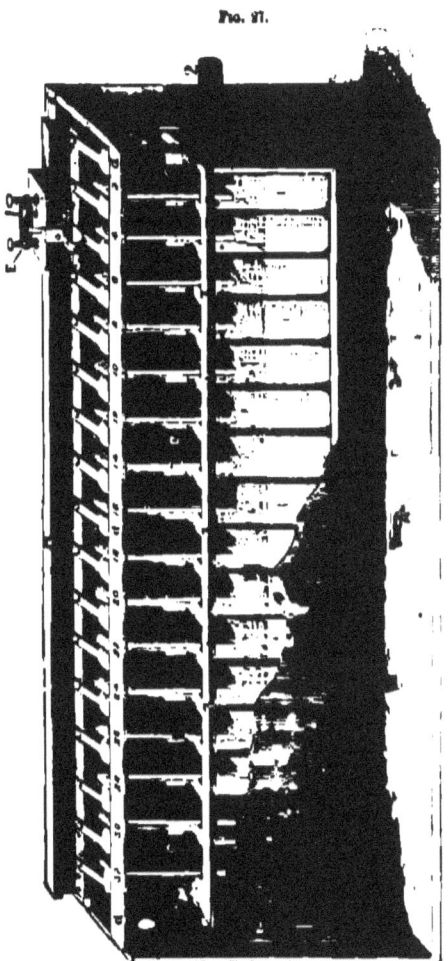

28-Cell Portable Galvanic Battery (Skeleton Representation).

The *scale* beneath the coil is intended to assist in keeping a record of the electricity applied at each setting.

This brief description of the Portable Electro-Magnetic Machine illustrates several very important improvements, each of which contributes to its marked superiority, efficiency, and convenience. There are four sizes of these machines, each contained in a black-walnut or mahogany case.

PORTABLE GALVANIC BATTERY. (Fig. 27.)

A designates the outer box. B, an inner case wherein are lodged the cells which contain the battery fluid. There are handles attached to the case by which it can be removed when required. The projecting keys, 2 2, at each end pass, through openings in the outer box, into the case, by which means it can be elevated or let down, and retained in position by turning them at right angles. They can be set so that a part or the whole of the elements can be immersed in the exciting fluid, thereby governing the strength of the galvanic current obtained.

From the central beam, C, the elements, $b\ c$, are suspended by metallic supports. On the beam is the commutator, E, by which the polarity of the current can be instantly changed, or its flow suddenly stopped. Through this commutator the current passes to the electrodes; it can be moved along the beam. When it is opposite figure 2, on the slat, the current from two cells is obtained, when opposite 4, thus from four cells, and so on to thirty-two cells. The zinc plates are well amalgamated and the carbons remarkable for durability and power.

The *galvanic hydrostat*, 3, 3, 3, consists of a plate of gutta-percha firmly attached to the inner case. A flange of it extends down into each cell. Separate openings are also provided, through which each of the elements passes. This confines the battery fluid, secures the coils and plates in position, and cleanses the latter from all deposits when they are moved up or down, prevents evaporation and maintains the strength of the battery fluid.

The portable galvanic battery is an adaptation of Stöhrer's, with the additional arrangement for controlling the strength of the current by immersing the elements to a greater or lesser degree in the battery fluid. The attachment of the hydrostat is also a valuable appendix, as it prevents the splashing over of the fluid, secures the cells and elements in their places, cleanses the plates from all deposits, prevents evaporation, and thus renders the battery fluid more enduring and of greater constancy.

There are three sizes: eight, sixteen, and thirty-two cells, put up in mahogany or black-walnut boxes.

LARGE PERMANENT GALVANIC BATTERY.

Some time since my attention was drawn, in another connection altogether, to the simplicity and efficiency of Hill's cell as a generator of a constant and most equable galvanic current. After an examination of its construction and action, I was satisfied that, for medical purposes, it was vastly superior to every other form of element which had come under my observation. At my suggestion, the Galvano-Faradic Manufacturing Company of this city has constructed, under the superintendence of Mr. Bartlett, a permanent battery, which, for office or hospital use, is of inestimable value. When erected, it becomes, as its name implies, a permanent fixture. Two of these have been made, one for myself, and the other for the New York State Hospital for Diseases of the Nervous System.

The cells used for this battery have been hitherto applied to telegraphy. They possess, however, in an eminent degree, the peculiar qualities that are essential for a galvanic battery for therapeutic purposes. The battery itself is simple in construction, easily managed, exceedingly economical, utilizing almost all the materials consumed.

Each cell contains about half a gallon of fluid. A disk of sheet-copper is laid flat on the bottom of the cell. To the under side of this is affixed a copper wire, covered with gutta-percha. The copper sheet forms the *negative plate*; the insulated wire which rises to the top of the cell, the *positive pole*. Two or three inches below the upper margin of the cell is suspended, by a brass hanger, a thick, disk-shaped plate of zinc, concave on the lower side, with a round aperture in the centre. This is the *positive plate*. To the hanger is attached a binding screw, and this forms the *negative pole*. Three cells *in situ* are represented in Fig. 28.

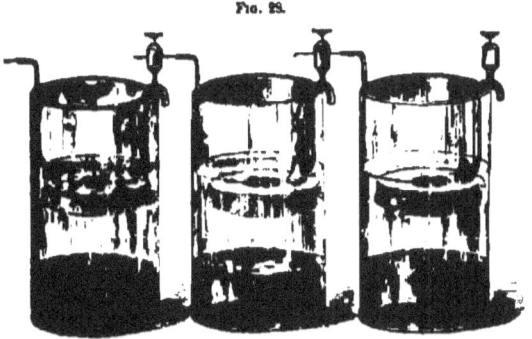

Fig. 28.

The body of the battery fluid is formed of a solution of sulphate of zinc. Occasionally, as required, crystals of sulphate of copper are dropped through the central aperture in the zinc to the bottom of the fluid. These dissolve, and produce a layer of blue liquid, which covers the copper. Thus, we have copper in the bottom of the cell, immersed in a solution of copper, zinc suspended above, immersed in a white liquid, the solution of zinc. (*See* engraving of these cells.) The mode adopted in other batteries to separate the fluids consists in using a

498   APPENDIX.

porous diaphragm, or cup, within, and surrounding which are placed dissimilar metals and fluids. The porous septum, it was thought, would allow the current to pass, and yet prevent the admixture of the diverse elements. It has, however, been demonstrated that, when two such liquids, and even two gases, are thus separated, they will invariably become mixed. In this battery, without the intervention of any diaphragm, the denser liquid, the blue, remains in the bottom of the cell, the lighter one overflows and rests upon it; thus arranged, there is less liability to diffusion or mixing than if the two liquids were placed side by side, in vertical columns, with a porous partition between them.

The central aperture in the zinc plate also admits the introduction of a hydrometer to measure the density and strength of the liquid. Provision is likewise made for preventing too rapid evaporation of the fluid. The occasional addition of a little water, and every three or four days dropping in a few crystals of sulphate of copper, is nearly all that is required in the management of this battery. Further directions for its preparation, *modus operandi*, and care, may be obtained from the manufacturers.

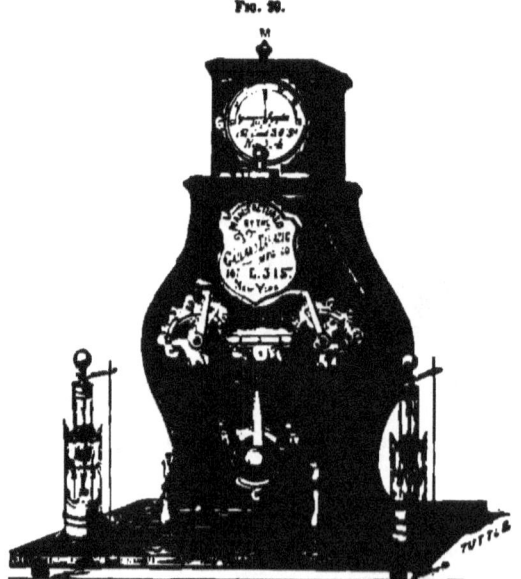

FIG. 29.

FIG. 29 represents Mr. Bartlett's "Improved Galvanic Regulator for Hospital Batteries," uniting current-selector, commutator, galvanic-current interrupter, current modifiers, and galvanoscope, in one construction, which is a very decided advance upon the similar instrument of Siemens and Halske.

The current selectors (A1, A2) enable the operator to bring into action any number of cells, from one to sixty. If we desire to use the current from twenty-four cells, we turn the winch A2 to 20, A1 to 4; while, if we wish to use only eight cells, the winch A2 is moved to the letter O, the winch A1 to 8. When both winches are at O, there is no current passing. The commutator (C) changes the *polarity* of the current. When it points vertically, the current ceases to pass. When the winch of the commutator is on N (normal), the positive current passes through the binding-post (C), and the negative through the binding-post (Z). If the winch rests on R (reversal), the positive passes through Z and the negative through C. The galvanic-current interrupter controls the interruptions of the current—by turning the knob J to the left, the current is interrupted; when the knob is turned to the right, the current flows on uninterruptedly.

The current-modifiers (V V) weaken or intensify the strength of the current. By elevating the rod, or piston, of that on the right, the current flowing from the binding-post (Z) is weakened. Hence, if the winch of the commutator (C) is resting on N, the positive current only will be modified; if the rod on the left side be at the same time raised, the negative current will also be controlled, and *vice versa*. Thus either current separately, or both conjointly, can be modified at pleasure.

The *Galvanoscope* (G).—If the conducting-pole cords, or electrodes, are placed in contact with any part of the body, and the stopper (S) be removed, the strength of the current will be denoted by the extent of the deviation of the needle from the point 0. On the knob (M), above the galvanoscope, there is a small magnet-rod. If the circuit be open, and the needle deviates from the point 0, it can be replaced by turning the knob to the right or left.

The whole arrangement forms a most complete and indispensable galvanic battery for hospitals, combining constancy, and every requisite accompaniment for regulating the current. It reflects great credit on the enterprising manufacturers.[1]

GALVANO-CAUSTIC BATTERY. (Fig. 80.)

The engraving represents the *American galvano-caustic battery*. It consists of four capacious cells, in each of which are four large zinc and three carbon plates, suspended by hangers, and connected with each other, in parallel rows, by means of stout copper wires. These can be lowered or elevated by the lifting screw so as to increase or diminish the heat as required. Bellows are provided to aërate the exciting fluid when it becomes inconstant or inert. From this apparatus no noxious or unpleasant gases are evolved. It is the most powerful, reliable, and effective, galvano-caustic battery ever manufactured in the United

[1] The foregoing account is taken from the second edition of my "Treatise on Diseases of the Nervous System" in which this battery was originally described. It was also the subject of a short article, by me, in the New York Medical Journal for November, 1870.

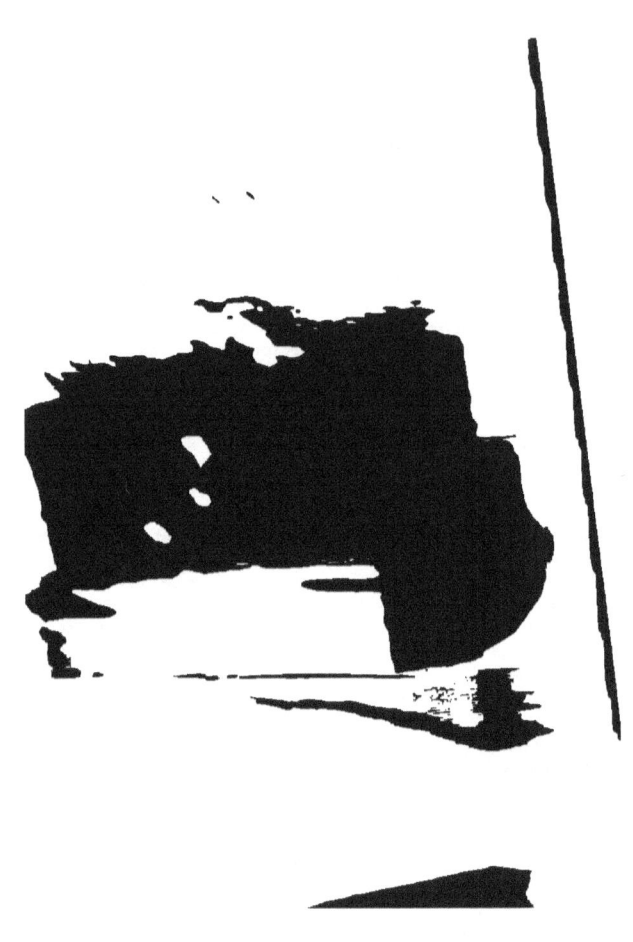

APPENDIX. 501

Fig. 81 represents a case manufactured by the Galvano-Faradic Company, containing all the *galvano-caustic electrodes, in situ.* The galvano-cauter, with its insulated handle, the galvano-moxa, galvano-caustic loop, galvanic knife, galvanic curette, etc., etc. These electrodes are a credit to our home-manufactured articles. They cannot be excelled.

Among the many novel and useful electrodes produced by the Galvano-Faradic Manufacturing Company are the following:

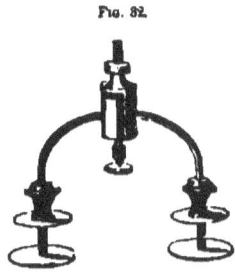

Fig. 82.

Dr. A. Murray's *double-stem disk*, which conveys both the positive and secondary currents, can be advantageously applied in many cases where Duchenne's double-cup electrode is inapplicable.

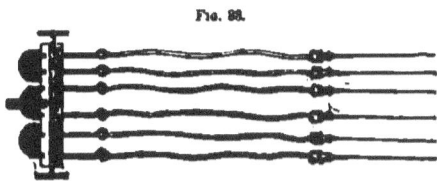

Fig. 83.

Murray's *serres fines.* This is an admirable arrangement for needles. From the bar are suspended six insulated wires, which are secured by thumb-screws. Attached to the lower extremity of each is a platina or steel needle. One or more can be inserted directly, or, owing to the flexibility of the conducting wire, laterally, or at a distance from each other. The entire arrangement screws on the universal or interrupted handle through which the current is conveyed.

The same inventor also offers a double-stem, adjustable *ovarian electrode* (Fig. 84) for application to both ovaries at the same time.

APPENDIX.

Fig. 84.

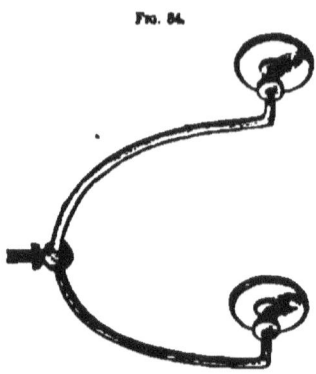

Powell's *spinal electrode* (Fig. 85), for self-application, enables the patient to apply electricity, without assistance, along the whole course of the spinal column.

Fig. 85.

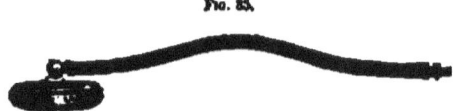

Powell's *rheotome*, or self-acting interrupter of the galvanic current, forms a portion of the *regulator*, as heretofore described. It is also arranged separately, and can be used with any galvanic battery. Slow or rapid interruptions, as desired, can be obtained without the intervention of a third party. These interruptions are, therapeutically, of the utmost importance. No galvanic battery is complete unless provided with this additional instrument.

INDEX.

A.

Accessory Effects of the Current, 92.
Action of the Current on Motor Nerves and Muscles, 44.
Actions of various Muscles, 162.
Advantages of different Forms of Apparatus, 120.
American Apparatuses, 123.
Anæsthesia, 224.
Anatomy, Physiology, and Pathology, Electricity in its Application to, 187.
Aneurisms and Varices, Galvanism in, 463.
Animal Electricity, 35.
Apparatus, American, 123.
—— Advantages of different Forms of, 120.
—— Baierlacher's, 123.
—— Du Bois-Reymond's, 125.
—— Duchenne's, 120.
—— Galvanic, 97.
—— Keil's, 116.
—— Modification of Du Bois's, 131.
—— Neef-Wagner, 119.
—— Saxton-Ettinghausen, 114.
—— Stöhrer's, 117.
—— Voltaic Induction, 113.
Applications, various, 166.
Arm, Irritation of Nerves of, 148.
Arthritic Articular Exudations, 447.
Ataxia, Locomotor, 223.
Auditory Nerve, Irritability of, 72.

B.

Baierlacher's Apparatus, 123.
Battery, Fromhold's, 109.
—— Grenet's, 108.
—— Middeldorpf's, 100.
—— Remak's, 106.
—— Stöhrer's, 102.
—— Stöhrer's large, 104.
—— Thomson's Polarization, 111.

Bladder and Testicle, Excitation of the, 156.
Blood, Effect of the Electrical Current on the, 62.
Blood-vessels and Lymphatics, 89.
Bones, Effect of the Electric Current on the, 92.
Brain and Spinal Cord, Electrical Excitation of the, 74.
—— Excitation of the, 160.
Brain, Electrical Excitation of the, 72.

C.

Calculi, Galvanic Current for the Solution of Vesical, 457.
Cases, 162.
—— of Cerebral Paralysis, 192.
Case of Cerebral Paralysis, 195.
—— of Hysterical Paralysis, 204.
—— of Lead Paralysis, 181.
—— of Locomotor Ataxia, 217.
—— of Rheumatic Paralysis, 183.
—— of Traumatic Paralysis, 184.
—— " " 210.
Cautery, Galvanic, 461.
Cerebral Paralysis, 192.
—— " 174.
Changes produced by Paralysis, 193.
Chemical Effects of Galvanism, 467.
Constant Currents, Induction and, 422.
Constant Current, Laws of, 49.
—— Paralyzing Action of, 62.
—— Phenomena of the, 60.
Constant Currents, Relations of Induced and, 61.
Constant Current, Therapeutics of the, 154.
Constant and Interrupted Currents, Methods of Using, 139.
Contact Electricity, 11.
Contractility, Electro-Muscular, 46.
Contractions, Reflex, 153.
Cornea, Opacities of the, 479.

INDEX

Curative Agent, Electricity as a, 305.
Current, Accessory Effects of the, 92.
Current Variation, Phenomena of, 45.

D.

Deafness, 343.
Diagnosis, differential, 201.
—— Electricity in, 188.
Differential Diagnosis, 201.
Digestive Organs, Excitation of the, 82.
Diplopia, 421.
Du Bois-Reymond's Apparatus, 125.
Duchenne's Apparatus, 120.
Duchenne's Method of using Constant Currents, 140.

E.

Eckhard's and Pflüger's Observations, 63.
Effect of the Electric Current on the Bones, 92.
—— on the Skin, 90.
Electrical Excitation of the Brain, 78.
—— of the Brain and Spinal Cord, 74.
—— of the Spinal Cord, 76.
Electricity and the Nerves of Sense, 68.
—— Animal, 35.
—— as a Curative Agent, 305.
—— as a Stimulant in Pseudoarthrosis, 421.
—— Contact, 11.
—— for the Generation of Thermic Effects, 460.
—— for the Removal of Poisonous Metals from the Organism, 452.
—— Friction, 2.
—— in Diagnosis, 188.
—— Induction, 30.
—— Importance of, in the Diagnosis and Prognosis of Paralytic Affections, 180.
—— in Gynecology, 458.
—— in its Application to Anatomy, Physiology, and Pathology, 167.
Electricity in Midwifery, 453.
—— in Midwifery and Gynecology, 452.
—— in Surgery, 460.
—— Nerve and Muscle, 37.
—— of Organic Muscles, 83.
Electrodes, 137.
Electro-muscular Contractility, 44.
—— Sensibility, 47.
Electrotonus, 41.
—— Phenomena of, 55.
Excitation of the Bladder and Testicle, 154.
—— of the Brain and Spinal Cord, 160.
—— of the Digestive Organs, 82.
—— of the Iris, 85.
—— of the Heart, 86.
—— of Laryngeal Muscles, 153.
—— of the Nerves of Special Sense, 165.
—— of Organic Muscles, 81.
—— of Respiration, 149.

Excitation of the Special Senses, 155.
—— of the Sympathetic, 97.
—— of the Urinary and Sexual Organs, 84.
—— Excretions and Secretions suppressed, 448.
Exudations, Arthritic Articular, 447.
—— Galvanism in Plastic, 473.
—— Galvanism in Serous, 476.
—— Galvanism in Strictures, Tumors, Ulcers, etc., 474.
Exudations, Rheumatic, 439.
—— Traumatic, 445.
Eye, Irritation of Muscles of, 151.

F.

Facial Nerve, Irritation of, 146.
—— Paralysis, 402.
Friction Electricity, 2.
Fromhold's Battery, 102.

G.

Galvanic Action and Temperature, 48.
—— Apparatus, 97.
—— Cautery, 461.
—— Current for the Solution of Vesical Calculi, 457.
Galvanic Treatment of Ulcers, 485.
Galvanism, Chemical Effects of, 467.
—— in Plastic Exudations, 473.
—— in Serous Exudations, 476.
—— in Strictures, 478.
—— in Strictures Exudations, Tumors, Ulcers, etc., 474.
Galvanization of the Sympathetic, 402.
—— in Varices and Aneurisms, 463.
General Remarks, 187.
Glosso-Laryngeal Paralysis, 301.
Gronet's Battery, 103.
Gynecology, Electricity in, 458.
—— and Midwifery, Electricity in, 452.

H.

Heart, Excitation of the, 86.
History of Medical Electricity, 1.
Hysterical Paralysis, 203.

I.

Importance of Electricity in the Diagnosis and Prognosis of Paralytic Affections, 180.
Impotence, 345.
Indirect and Direct Irritation, 150.
Incontinence of Urine, 432.
Induction Apparatus of Pixii, 113.
—— and Constant Currents, 409.
—— Electricity, 30.
Infantile Paralysis, 214.
Interrupted and Constant Currents, Methods of using, 139.
Iris, Excitation of the, 85.

INDEX 505

Irritability of the Auditory Nerve, 72.
—— Observations on, 64.
—— of the Olfactory and Gustatory Nerves, 73.
—— of the Optic Nerve, 71.
—— Relations of, 67.
—— of the Skin, 69.
Irritation of Facial Nerve, 144.
—— Indirect and Direct, 150.
—— of the Motor Nerves, etc., 142.
—— of Muscles, 143.
—— of Muscles of Eye, 151.
—— of Muscles of Larynx, 152.
—— of Nerves of Arm, 143.
—— of Nerves of Lower Extremity, 149.
—— Reflex and Sympathetic, 154.
—— of the Skin, 141.
—— of Skin and Muscles, 144.
—— of Vagus Diaphragm, etc., 147.

K.

Keil's Apparatus, 116.

L.

Laryngeal Paralysis, 435.
Larynx, Irritation of Muscles of, 152.
Laws of the Constant Current, 49.
Lead Paralysis, 281.
—— Paralysis, 427.
Locomotor Ataxia, 216.
—— Ataxia, 898.
—— Ataxia, Cases of, 217.

M.

Marshall Hall's Observations, 191.
Medical Electricity, History of, 1.
Metals, from the Organism, Electricity for the Removal of Poisonous, 482.
Methods of Using Interrupted and Constant Currents, 139.
Middeldorpf's Battery, 100.
Midwifery, Electricity in, 453.
——, and Gynecology, Electricity in, 452.
Modification of Du Bois's Apparatus, 183.
Motor Nerves, Irritation of the, 142.
—— and Muscles, Action of the Current on, 44.
Müller's Experiment, 39.
Muscles, Actions of various, 168.
——, Excitation of Laryngeal, 153.
——, Irritation of, 143.
——, Spasm of the Facial, 859.
Muscular Atrophy, Progressive, 237.
—— Paralysis, 267.

N.

Neef-Wagner Apparatus, 119.
Nerves of Lower Extremity, Irritation of, 149.
Nerve and Muscle Electricity, 87.

Nerves, Paralysis of certain, 177.
—— of Sense, Electricity and the, 68.
—— of Special Sense, Excitation of the, 165.
Nervous and Muscular Paralysis, 403.
—— Paralysis, 254.
Neuralgia, 807.

O.

Obscure Muscular Paralysis, 285.
Observations, Eckhard's and Pflüger's, 63.
—— on Irritability, 64.
——, Marshall Hall's, 191.
——, Remak's, 145.
——, Todd's, 193.
Organic Muscles, Electricity of, 85.
—— Muscles, Excitation of, 81.
Organism, Electricity for the Removal of Poisonous Metals from the, 482.
Olfactory and Gustatory Nerves, Irritability of the, 73.
Opacities of the Cornea, 479.
Optic Nerve, Irritability of, 71.

P.

Paralysis, 872.
——, of Adults, Spinal, 229.
——, Cerebral, 192.
——, Cerebral, 197.
——, Cerebral, 376.
——, Case of Cerebral, 195.
——, Cases of Cerebral, 199.
——, Changes produced by, 198.
——, Hysterical, 203.
——, Case of Hysterical, 204.
—— of Certain Nerves, 177.
——, Facial, 412.
——, Glosso-Laryngeal, 300.
——, Infantile, 218.
——, Laryngeal, 435.
——, Lead, 427.
——, Lead, 281.
——, Case of Lead, 181.
——, Muscular, 267.
——, Nervous, 254.
——, Nervous and Muscular, 403.
——, Obscure Muscular, 285.
——, Case of Rheumatic, 183.
——, Secondary, 424.
——, Spinal, 229.
——, Spinal, 243.
——, Spinal, 383.
——, of the Sympathetic, 547.
——, Traumatic, 422.
——, Case of Traumatic, 184.
——, Case of Traumatic, 210.
——, Writers', 364.
Paralysing Action of the Constant Current, 62.
Phenomena of the Constant Current, 40.
—— of Current Variation, 45.

Phenomena of Electrotonus, 55.
Pixii, Induction Apparatus of, 112.
Poles, Positions of the, 152.
Progressive Muscular Atrophy, 287.
Pseudoarthrosis, Electricity as a Stimulant in, 421.

R.

Rapid and Slow Interruptions, 157.
Reflex Contractions, 153.
—— and Sympathetic Irritation, 154.
Relations of Induced and Constant Currents, 81.
—— of Irritability, 67.
Remak's Battery, 106.
—— Observations, 145.
Respiration, Excitation of, 429.
Rheumatic Exudations, 432.
Rheumatism, 440.
Rosenthal's Law, 52.

S.

Saxton-Ettinghausen Apparatus, 114.
Secondary Paralysis, 414.
Secretions and Excretions suppressed, 443.
Senses, Excitation of the Special, 155.
Sensibility, Electro-muscular, 47.
Skin, Effect of the Electric Current on the, 90.
——, Irritation of the, 141.
——, Irritability of, 69.
—— and Muscles, Irritation of, 144.
Spasms, 343.
Spasm of the Facial Muscles, 368.
Spasm, Vaso-motor, 347.
Spinal Cord, Electrical Excitation of the, 74.
Spinal Paralysis, 335.
—— 209.
—— 243.
—— of Adults, 229.
Stöhrer's Apparatus, 117.
—— Battery, 102.
—— large Battery, 104.
Strictures, Galvanism in, 475.

Strictures, Galvanism in Exudations, Tumors, Ulcers, etc., 474.
Suppressed Secretions and Excretions, 443.
Surgery, Electricity in, 460.
Sympathetic, Blood-vessels and, 88.
Sympathetic, Excitation of the, 72.
—— Galvanization of the, 402.
—— Paralysis of the, 347.

T.

Temperature, Galvanic Action and, 42.
Tetanisation, 49.
Therapeutics of the Constant Current, 158.
Thermic Effects, Electricity for the Generation of, 460.
Thomson's Polarization Battery, 111.
Todd's Observations, 193.
Torticollis, 370.
Traumatic Exudations, 445.
—— Paralysis, 422.
Tumors, 480.
—— Galvanism in Strictures, Exudations, Ulcers, etc., 474.

U.

Ulcers, Galvanism in Strictures, Exudations, Tumors, etc., 474.
—— Galvanic Treatment of, 485.
Urinary and Sexual Organs, Excitation of the, 84.
Urine, Incontinence of, 432.

V.

Vagus, Diaphragm, etc., Irritation of, 147.
Varices and Aneurisms, Galvanism in, 463.
Various Applications, 156.
Vaso-motor Spasm, 347.
Voltaic Induction Apparatus, 112.

W.

Writers' Paralysis, 364.

THE END.

MEDICAL WORKS

PUBLISHED BY

D. APPLETON & COMPANY.

Barker on Sea-Sickness. 1 vol., 16mo. 75 cents.
Bellevue and Charity Hospital Reports. 1 vol., 8vo. Cloth, $4.00.
Bennet's Winter and Spring on the Mediterranean. 1 vol., 12mo. Cloth, $3.50.
Davis's (Henry G.) Conservative Surgery. Cloth, $3.00.
Elliot's Obstetric Clinic. 1 vol., 8vo. Cloth, $4.50.
Flint's Physiology. (Vol. 4 in press.) 8vo. Cloth, per vol., $4.50.
Huxley & Youmans's Physiology and Hygiene. 1 vol., 12mo. $2.00.
Johnston's Chemistry of Common Life. 2 vols., 12mo. Cloth. $4.00.
Letterman's Recollections of the Army of the Potomac. 1 vol., 8vo. Cloth, $2.00.
Lewes's Physiology of Common Life. 2 vols., 12mo. Cloth, $4.00.
Maudsley on the Mind. 1 vol., 8vo. Cloth, $3.50.
Meyer's Electricity. 1 vol., 8vo. Cloth, $4.50.
Niemeyer's Practical Medicine. 2 vols., 8vo. Cloth, $9.00.
Sayre's Club-foot. 1 vol., 12mo. Cloth, $1.25.
Tanquerel's Treatise on Lead Diseases. Cloth, $2.00.
Tilt's Uterine Therapeutics. 1 vol., 8vo. Cloth, $3.50.
Vogel's Diseases of Children. 1 vol., 8vo. Cloth, $4.50.
Flint's Manual on Urine. 1 vol., 12mo. Cloth, $1.00.
Van Buren on Diseases of the Rectum. 1 vol., 12mo. $1.50.
Barnes's Obstetric Operations. 1 vol., 8vo. $4.50.
Hammond's Physics and Physiology of Spiritualism. 1 vol., 12mo. $1.00.
Neftel on Galvano-Therapeutics. 1 vol., 12mo. $1.50.
Hammond's Diseases of the Nervous System. 1 vol., 8vo. $5.00.
Billroth's General Surgical Pathology and Therapeutics. 1 vol., 8vo. Cloth, $5.00.
Maudsley's Body and Mind. 12mo. Cloth, $1.00.
Stroud's Physical Cause of the Death of Christ. 1 vol., 12mo. $2.00.
Peaslee on Ovarian Tumors.
Neumann on Skin Diseases.
Combe on the Management of Infancy. 1 vol., 12mo. $1.50.
Sir J. Y. Simpson's Complete Works. Vol. I. $5.00. (Vols. II. & III. in press.)
Barker on Puerperal Diseases.
Howe on Emergencies.
Markoe on Diseases of the Bones.

⁎ Any of these works will be mailed, post free, to any part of the United States, on receipt of the price. Catalogues forwarded on application.

D. APPLETON & CO.,
549 & 551 Broadway, New York.

THE
NEW YORK MEDICAL JOURNAL,

EDITORS,

JAS. B. HUNTER, M. D.,
WILLIAM T. LUSK, M. D.,

Is published monthly; each number contains 112 pages, making two large octavo volumes yearly, of nearly 700 pages each.

THE VOLUMES BEGIN IN JANUARY AND JULY.

Terms, $4 per annum. Specimen numbers sent by mail on receipt of 25c.

Since its Enlargement, the New York Medical Journal contains more Reading Matter than any Monthly Medical Journal published in this Country.

THE JOURNAL OF
PSYCHOLOGICAL MEDICINE:

A QUARTERLY REVIEW OF

Diseases of the Nervous System, Medical Jurisprudence, and Anthropology,

EDITED BY

WILLIAM A. HAMMOND, M. D.,

Professor of Diseases of the Mind and Nervous System in the Bellevue Hospital Medical College,

Is published quarterly, each number containing not less than 208 pages, making one large volume annually.

THE VOLUME BEGINS WITH THE JANUARY NUMBER.

Terms, $5.00 per annum. Specimen numbers, by mail, $1.00.

CLUB RATES.

N. Y. MEDICAL JOURNAL and Appletons' New Weekly Journal....$7.00
PSYCHOLOGICAL   "   "   "   " 8.00
N. Y. MEDICAL JOURNAL and PSYCHOLOGICAL JOURNAL............ 8.00

PREMIUM PORTRAIT.

As a premium to new subscribers to either of our Medical Journals at the regular subscription rate, we will send a magnificent line and stipple engraving, size 19x24 inches, of the distinguished physician, the late Dr. JOHN W. FRANCIS. This engraving is eminently adapted to adorn the parlor of the physician. The price of the portrait alone is $3.

Payment in all cases must be in advance.

Remittances should be made by postal money order or check to the Publishers,

D. APPLETON & CO.,
549 & 551 Broadway, New York.

Letterman—Medical Recollections of the Army of the Potomac.

By JONATHAN LETTERMAN, M. D., late Surgeon U. S. Army, and Medical Director of the Army of the Potomac. 1 vol., 8vo, pp. 194. . . . . . . Cloth, $2.00

"Surgeon Letterman has succeeded in giving a very interesting, not to say fascinating book. He writes in a perspicuous, elegant style, and we venture to assert that but few who open his volume of medical annals, pregnant as they are with instruction, will care to do otherwise than finish them at a sitting."—*Medical Record.*

"The whole book (which may be considered a graceful and affectionate tribute to the zeal and ability of the many who 'evinced their devotion to their country and to the cause of humanity without hope of promotion or expectation of reward') is written in a pleasing style, and will awaken many kindly associations in the memories of those who shared with our author the varying fortunes of the 'dear old Army of the Potomac.'"—*N. Y. Medical Journal, Sept., 1866.*

Davis—Conservative Surgery.

Conservative Surgery as exhibited in remedying some of the Mechanical Causes that operate injuriously both in Health and Disease. By HENRY G. DAVIS, M. D. Elegantly printed on tinted paper and handsomely illustrated. 1 vol., 8vo, pp. 314. . . . . . . Cloth, $3.00

Dr. Davis has enjoyed rare facilities for the study and treatment of certain classes of disease, and in this line has achieved a well-deserved reputation. The now approved methods of treating of hip-joint disease are all based upon Dr. Davis's method and appliances. In this volume he brings together the result of his experience, and has made a book both interesting and valuable to the Surgeon.

"Dr. Davis, bringing as he does to his specialty a great aptitude for the solution of mechanical problems, takes a high rank as an Orthopedic Surgeon, and his very practical contribution to the literature of the subject is both valuable and opportune. We deem it worthy of a place in every physician's library. The style is unpretending but trenchant, graphic, and, best of all, quite intelligible."—*Medical Record.*

Gosse on the Microscope.

Evenings at the Microscope; or, Researches among the Minuter Organs and Forms of Animal Life. By PHILIP HENRY GOSSE, F. R. S. Beautifully illustrated with upward of one hundred Engravings on wood. 1 vol., 12mo, pp. 480. . . . . . Cloth, $2.50

In order to relieve as much as possible the dryness of technical description, a colloquial and familiar style has been given to the work, without, however, sacrificing the precision essential to science. The objects selected for illustration are common things, such as any one placed in tolerably favorable circumstances may reasonably expect to meet with in ordinary research. Instructions on microscopic manipulations, and the selection, securing, and mounting of objects for examination, are given with a view of facilitating the work o beginners.

Nightingale—On Nursing.

Notes on Nursing. What it Is and What it is Not. By FLORENCE NIGHTINGALE. 1 volume, 12mo, pp. 140.
Cloth, $0.75

D. APPLETON & CO.'S MEDICAL PUBLICATIONS.

Flint's Physiology.

The Physiology of Man, designed to represent the existing State of Physiological Science as applied to the Functions of the Human Body. By AUSTIN FLINT, Jr., M. D., Prof. of Physiology and Microscopy in the Bellevue Hospital Medical College, Fellow of the New York Academy of Medicine, etc., etc.

Vol. I. Introduction. The Blood; Circulation; Respiration. 8vo. Cloth (tinted paper). . . . . $4.50.

Vol. II. Alimentation; Digestion; Absorption; Lymph, and Chyle. Cloth (tinted paper). . . . . $4.50.

"Before the issue of the first part we entertained the opinion in common with others that there was no room for a text-book on physiology, and that a physician of his (Dr. F.'s) learning and acquirements could more advantageously employ his time in experimental research than in writing a systematic treatise. Dr. Flint has convinced us that we were mistaken. In this view. We accept the two volumes already issued as evidence of what we may expect in the remaining part of the series. We regard them as the very best treatises on human physiology which the English or any other language affords, and we recommend them with thorough confidence to students, practitioners, and laymen, as models of literary and scientific ability."—*N. Y. Medical Journal, Oct., 1867.*

"The treatise of Dr. Flint is as yet incomplete, the first two volumes only having been published; but if the remaining portions are compiled—for every physiological work embracing the whole subject must be in a great measure a compilation—with the same care and accuracy, the whole may vie with any of those that have of late years been produced in our own or in foreign languages."—*British and Foreign Medico-Chirurgical Review.*

"The second of the series has just been published, and is now before us. It treats of the great function of Nutrition under the several heads of Alimentation, Digestion, Absorption, the Lymph, and Chyle. Upon these topics the author bestows the same judicious care and labor which so eminently characterize the first volume. Facts are selected with discrimination, theories critically examined, and conclusions enunciated with commendable clearness and precision."—*American Journal of the Medical Sciences.*

"Judging from the able manner in which this volume is written, the series, when perfected, will be one of those publications without which no library is complete. As a book of general information, it will be found useful to the practitioner, and as a book of reference, invaluable in the hands of the anatomist and physiologist."—*Dublin Quarterly Journal of Medical Science.*

"The work is calculated to attract other than professional readers, and is written with sufficient clearness and freedom from technical pedantry to be perfectly intelligible to any well-informed man."—*London Saturday Review.*

"From the extent of the author's investigations into the best theory and practice of the present day the world over, and the candor and good judgment which he brings to bear upon the discussion of each subject, we are justified in regarding his treatises as standard and authoritative, so far as in this disputed subject authority is admissible."—*N. Y. Times.*

"The complete work, judging from the present instalment, will prove a valuable addition to our systematic treatises on human physiology. The volume before us is executed with conscientious care, and the style is readable and clear. It is a volume which will be welcome to the advanced student, and as a work of reference."—*London Lancet.*

"These excellent monographs offer the most complete summary of the physiological knowledge of our day yet written in America. They are brought down to the most recent advances of the science, and include the results of a number of original experiments."—*Philadelphia Medical Reporter.*

"The leading subjects treated of are presented in distinct parts, each of which is designed to be an exhaustive essay on that to which it refers."—*Western Journal of Medicine.*

"The interesting feature of the work is a recital of typical experiments, which are timely and judiciously introduced to impress the facts upon the mind of the reader. It is printed in elegant style, and may be considered a model in the typographical line."—*Med. Record.*

"We have found the style easy, lucid, and, at the same time, terse. The practical and positive results of physiological investigation are succinctly stated, without, it would seem, extended discussion of disputed points."—*Boston Medical and Surgical Journal.*

"To those who desire to get a concise, clear, but at the same time sufficiently full résumé of the existing state of physiological science, we heartily recommend Dr. Flint's work. Moreover, as a work of typographical art, it deserves a prominent place upon our library shelves."—*Medical Gazette, N. Y.*

D. APPLETON & CO.'S MEDICAL PUBLICATIONS.

Elliot's Obstetric Clinic.

A Practical Contribution to the Study of Obstetrics and the Diseases of Women and Children. By GEORGE T. ELLIOT, Jr., A. M., M. D., Prof. of Obstetrics and the Diseases of Women and Children in the Bellevue Hospital Medical College, Physician to Bellevue Hospital and to the New York Lying-in Hospital, etc., etc. 8vo, pp. 458. . . Cloth, $4.50

This volume, by Dr. Elliot, is based upon a large experience, including fourteen years of service in the lying-in department of Bellevue Hospital of this city. The book has attracted marked attention, and has elicited from the medical press, both of this country and Europe, the most flattering commendations. It is justly believed that the work is one of the most valuable contributions to obstetric literature that has appeared for many years, and, being eminently practical in its character, cannot fail to be of great service to obstetricians.

"The volume by Dr. Elliot has scarcely less value, although in a different direction, than that of the Edinburgh physician (Dr. Duncan, *Researches in Obstetrics*). The materials comprising it have been principally gathered through a service of fourteen years in the Bellevue Hospital, New York, during the whole of which time the author has been engaged in clinical teaching. The cases now collected into a handsome volume illustrate faithfully the anxieties and disappointments, as well as the failures and successes, which are inseparable from the responsible practice of obstetrics—a line of practice which, under difficulties, demands the greatest moral courage, the highest skill, and the power of acting promptly on a sudden emergency. Dr. Elliot's favorite subject appears to be operative midwifery; but the chapters on the relations of albuminuria to pregnancy, ante-partum hæmorrhage, the induction of labor, and the dangers which arise from compression of the funis, are all deserving of careful perusal. The pleasure we feel at being able to speak so favorably of Dr. Elliot's volume is enhanced by the circumstance that he was a pupil at the Dublin Lying-in Hospital when Dr. Shekelton was master. We can certainly say that his teachings reflect great credit upon his Alma Mater."—*London Lancet*, April 11, 1868.

"This may be said to belong to a class of books 'after the practitioner's own heart.' In them he finds a wider range of cases than comes under his observation in ordinary practice; in them he learns the application of the most recent improvements of his art; in them he finds the counterpart of cases which have caused him the deepest anxiety; in them, too, he may find consolation, for the regret—the offspring of limited experience, which has always cast a shadow on the remembrance of some of his fatal cases—will pass away as he reads of similar ones in which far greater resources of every kind failed to avert a fatal termination.

"There are not many books of this kind in our language: they can probably all be numbered on the fingers of a single hand. * * * Many circumstances concur, therefore, to influence us to extend to this work a cheerful welcome, and to commend it as fully as possible. We do thus welcome it; as the production of a gentleman of great experience, acknowledged ability, and high position—as an emanation from one of the leading schools of our country, and as an honorable addition to our national medical literature."—*American Journal of Medical Science*, April, 1868.

"As the book now stands, it is invaluable for the practitioner of obstetrics, for he will hardly ever in practice find himself in a tight place, the counterpart of which he will not find in Dr. Elliot's book."—*New York Medical Journal*, February, 1868.

"The book has the freshness of hospital practice throughout, in reference to diagnosis, pathology, therapeutical and operative proceedings. It will be found to possess a great amount of valuable information in the department of obstetrics, in an attractive and easy style, according to the most modern and improved views of the profession."—*Cincinnati Lancet and Observer*, April, 1868.

"As a whole, we know of no similar work which has issued from the American press, which can be compared with it. It ought to be in the hands of every practitioner of midwifery in the country."—*Boston Medical and Surgical Journal*.

"One of the most attractive as well as forcibly instructive works we have had the pleasure of reading. In conclusion, we recommend it as one having no equal in the English language, as regards clinical instruction in obstetrics."—*Am. Jour. of Obstetrics*, Aug., 1868.

"Many ripe, elderly practitioners might, but few young could, write a book so distinguished by candor, want of prejudice, kindly feeling, soundness of judgment, and extent of erudition. While we do not say the book is faultless, we say there is no book in American obstetrical literature that surpasses this one. * * * The work now under review is his first-born book or volume, and shows how fine opportunities he has had, chiefly at Bellevue Hospital, for acquiring experience, and how diligently he has availed himself of them. But his book shows much more. It is the work of a physician of high education, a qualification in which obstetric authors are often deficient—it shows qualities of mind and skill of hand rarely attained by so young a man."—*Edinburgh Medical Journal*, Feb., 1868.

D. APPLETON & CO.'S PUBLICATIONS.

THE PHYSIOLOGY OF MAN;

DESIGNED

TO REPRESENT THE EXISTING STATE OF PHYSIOLOGICAL SCIENCE, AS APPLIED TO THE FUNCTIONS OF THE HUMAN BODY.

By AUSTIN FLINT, Jr., M. D.

Alimentation; Digestion; Absorption; Lymph and Chyle.

1 volume, 8vo. Cloth. Price, $4.50.

RECENTLY PUBLISHED.

THE FIRST VOLUME OF THE SERIES

BY

AUSTIN FLINT, Jr., M. D.,

CONTAINING

Introduction; The Blood; The Circulation; Respiration.

Three Volumes now ready. Cloth. Price, $4.50 each.
To be completed in Four Volumes.

"Professor Flint is engaged in the preparation of an extended work on human physiology, in which he professes to consider all the subjects usually regarded as belonging to that department of physical science. The work will be divided into separate and distinct parts, but the several volumes in which it is to be published will form a connected series."—*Providence Journal.*

It is free from technicalities and purely professional terms, and instead of only being adapted to the use of the medical faculty, will be found of interest to the general reader who desires clear and concise information on the subject of man physical."—*Evening Post.*

"Digestion is too little understood, indigestion too extensively suffered, to render this a work of supererogation. Stomachs will have their revenge, sooner or later, if Nature's laws are infringed upon through ignorance or stubbornness, and it is well that all should understand how the penalty for 'high living' is assessed."—*Chicago Evening Journal.*

"A year has elapsed since Dr. Flint published the first part of his great work upon human physiology. It was an admirable treatise—distinct in itself—exhausting the special subjects upon which it treated."—*Philadelphia Inquirer.*

CATALOGUE OF MEDICAL WORKS.

ANSTIE.

Neuralgia, *and Diseases which resemble it.*

By FRANCIS E. ANSTIE, M. D., F. R. C. P.,

Senior Assistant Physician to Westminster Hospital; Lecturer on Materia Medica in Westminster Hospital School; and Physician to the Belgrave Hospital for Children; Editor of "The Practitioner" (London), etc.

1 vol., 12mo. Cloth, $2.50.

"It is a valuable contribution to scientific medicine."—*The Lancet (London).*

"His work upon Neuralgia is one of the most interesting, instructive, and practical, we have seen for a long time. We have given it careful reading and thoughtful study, and, for a treatise of its size, we are free to say that we have never met one that gives more practical information and is fuller of useful suggestions."—*Medical Record.*

BARKER.

On Sea-sickness.

By FORDYCE BARKER, M. D.,

Clinical Professor of Midwifery and the Diseases of Women in the Bellevue Hospital Medical College, etc.

1 vol., 16mo. 36 pp. Flexible Cloth, 75 cents.

Reprinted from the NEW YORK MEDICAL JOURNAL. By reason of the great demand for the number of that journal containing the paper, it is now presented in book form, with such prescriptions added as the author has found useful in relieving the suffering from sea-sickness.

BARNES.

Obstetric Operations, *including the Treatment of Hæmorrhage.*

By ROBERT BARNES, M. D., F. R. C. P., LONDON,

Obstetric Physician to and Lecturer on Midwifery and the Diseases of Women and Children at St. Thomas's Hospital; Examiner on Midwifery to the Royal College of Physicians and to the Royal College of Surgeons; formerly Obstetric Physician to the London Hospital, and late Physician to the Eastern Division of the Royal Maternity Charity.

WITH ADDITIONS, by BENJAMIN F. DAWSON, M. D.,

Late Lecturer on Uterine Pathology in the Medical Department of the University of New York; Assistant to the Clinical Professor of Diseases of Children in the College of Physicians and Surgeons, New York; Physician for the Diseases of Children to the New York Dispensary; Member of the New York Obstetrical Society, of the Medical Society of the County of New York, etc., etc.

Second American Edition. 1 vol., 8vo. 503 pp. Cloth, $4.50.

To the student and practitioner this work will prove of the greatest value, being, as it is, a most perfect text-book on "Obstetric Operations," by one who has fairly earned the right to assume the position of a teacher.

"Such a work as Dr. Barnes's was greatly needed. It is calculated to elevate the practice of the obstetric art in this country, and to be of great service to the practitioner."—*Lancet.*

D. Appleton & Co.'s Medical Publications.

Bellevue and Charity Hospital Reports.

The volume of Bellevue and Charity Hospital Reports for 1870, containing valuable contributions from

ISAAC E. TAYLOR, M. D.,   WILLIAM A. HAMMOND, M. D.,
AUSTIN FLINT, M. D.,   T. GAILLARD THOMAS, M. D.,
LEWIS A. SAYRE, M. D.,   FRANK H. HAMILTON, M. D.,

and others.

1 vol., 8vo. Cloth, $4.00.

"These institutions are the most important, as regards accommodations for patients and variety of cases treated, of any on this continent, and are surpassed by but few in the world. The gentlemen connected with them are acknowledged to be among the first in their profession, and the volume is an important addition to the professional literature of this country."—*Psychological Journal.*

BENNET

Winter and Spring on the Shores of

the Mediterranean; or, the Riviera, Mentone, Italy, Corsica, Sicily, Algeria, Spain, and Biarritz, as Winter Climates.

By J. HENRY BENNET, M. D.,

Member of the Royal College of Physicians, London; late Physician-Accoucher to the Royal Free Hospital; Doctor of Medicine of the University of Paris; formerly Resident Physician to the Paris Hospitals (ex-Interne des Hôpitaux de Paris), etc.

This work embodies the experience of ten winters and springs passed by Dr. Bennet on the shores of the Mediterranean, and contains much valuable information for physicians in relation to the health-restoring climate of the regions described.

1 vol., 12mo. 621 pp. Cloth, $3.50.

"Exceedingly readable, apart from its special purposes, and well illustrated."—*Evening Commercial.*

"It has a more substantial value for the physician, perhaps, than for any other class or profession. . . . We commend this book to our readers as a volume presenting two capital qualifications—it is at once entertaining and instructive."—*N. Y. Medical Journal.*

On the Treatment of Pulmonary Con-

sumption, by Hygiene, Climate, and Medicine, in its Connection with Modern Doctrines.

By JAMES HENRY BENNET, M. D.,

Member of the Royal College of Physicians, London; Doctor of Medicine of the University of Paris, etc., etc.

1 vol., thin 8vo. Cloth, $1.50.

An interesting and instructive work, written in the strong, clear, and lucid manner which appears in all the contributions of Dr. Bennet to medical or general literature.

"We cordially commend this book to the attention of all, for its practical common-sense views of the nature and treatment of the scourge of all temperate climates, pulmonary consumption."—*Detroit Review of Medicine.*

D. Appleton & Co.'s Medical Publications.

BILLROTH.
General Surgical Pathology and Therapeutics, *in Fifty Lectures. A Text-book for Students and Physicians.*

By Dr. THEODOR BILLROTH,
Professor of Surgery in Vienna.

Translated from the Fourth German Edition, with the special permission of the Author, by

CHARLES E. HACKLEY, A. M., M. D.,
Surgeon to the New York Eye and Ear Infirmary; Physician to the New York Hospital; Fellow of the New York Academy of Medicine, etc.

1 vol., 8vo. 676 pp., and 152 Woodcuts. Cloth, $5.00.

Professor Theodor Billroth, one of the most noted authorities on Surgical Pathology, gives in this volume a complete *résumé* of the existing state of knowledge in this branch of medical science. The fact of this publication going through four editions in Germany, and having been translated into French, Italian, Russian, and Hungarian, should be some guarantee for its standing.

SPECIMEN OF ILLUSTRATIONS.

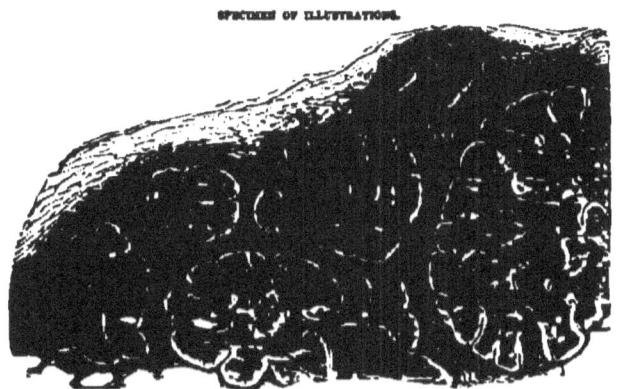

Mammary Cancer, acinous form, magnified 50 diameters.

"The want of a book in the English language, presenting in a concise form the views of the German pathologists, has long been felt; and we venture to say no book could more perfectly supply that want than the present volume. . . . . We would strongly recommend it to all who take any interest in the progress of thought and observation in surgical pathology and surgery."—*The Lancet.*

"A great addition to our literature."—*N. Y. Medical Journal.*

"We can assure our readers that they will consider neither money wasted in its purchase, nor time in its perusal."—*The Medical Investigator.*

D. Appleton & Co.'s Medical Publications.

COMBE.

The Management of Infancy, *Physiological and Moral. Intended chiefly for the Use of Parents.*

By ANDREW COMBE, M. D.

REVISED AND EDITED

By SIR JAMES CLARK, K. C. B., M. D., F. R. S.,

Physician-in-ordinary to the Queen.

First American from the Tenth London Edition. 1 vol., 12mo. 302 pp. Cloth, $1.50.

"In the following pages I have addressed myself chiefly to parents and to the younger members of the medical profession; but it is not to them alone that the subject ought to prove attractive. The study of infancy, considered even as an element in the history and philosophy of man, abounds in interest, and is fertile in truths of the highest practical value and importance."—*Extract from Author's Preface.*

"This excellent little book should be in the hand of every mother of a family; and if some of our lady friends would master its contents, and either bring up their children by the light of its teachings, or communicate the truths it contains to the poor by whom they are surrounded, we are convinced that they would effect infinitely more good than by the distribution of any number of tracts whatever.... We consider this work to be one of the few popular medical treatises that any practitioner may recommend to his patients; and, though, if its precepts are followed, he will probably lose a few guineas, he will not begrudge them if he sees his friends' children grow up healthy, active, strong, and both mentally and physically capable."—*The Lancet.*

DAVIS.

Conservative Surgery, *as exhibited in remedying some of the Mechanical Causes that operate injuriously both in Health and Disease. With Illustrations.*

By HENRY G. DAVIS, M. D.,

Member of the American Medical Association, etc., etc.

1 vol., 8vo. 315 pp. Cloth, $3.00.

The Author has enjoyed rare facilities for the study and treatment of certain classes of disease, and the records here presented to the profession are the gradual accumulation of over thirty years' investigation.

"Dr. Davis, bringing, as he does to his specialty, a great aptitude for the solution of mechanical problems, takes a high rank as an orthopedic surgeon, and his very practical contribution to the literature of the subject is both valuable and opportune. We deem it worthy of a place in every physician's library The style is unpretending, but trenchant, graphic, and, best of all, quite intelligible."—*Medical Record.*

D. Appleton & Co.'s Medical Publications.

FLINT.

The Physiology of Man. *Designed to represent the Existing State of Physiological Science as applied to the Functions of the Human Body.*

By AUSTIN FLINT, JR., M. D.,

Professor of Physiology and Microscopy in the Bellevue Hospital Medical College, and in the Long Island College Hospital; Fellow of the New York Academy of Medicine; Microscopist to Bellevue Hospital.

In Five Volumes. 8vo. Tinted Paper.

Volume I.—*The Blood; Circulation; Respiration.*

8vo. 502 pp. Cloth, $4.50.

SPECIMEN OF ILLUSTRATIONS.

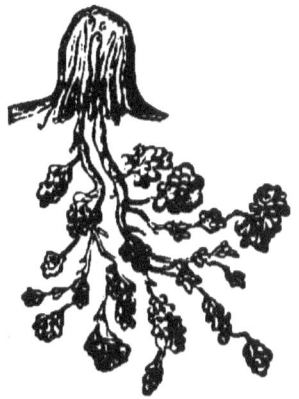

Ducts and Acini of the Mammary Organs.

"If the remaining portions of this work are compiled with the same care and accuracy, the whole may vie with any of those that have of late years been produced in our own or in foreign languages."—*British and Foreign Medico-Chirurgical Review.*

"As a book of general information it will be found useful to the practitioner, and, as a book of reference, invaluable in the hands of the anatomist and physiologist."—*Dublin Quarterly Journal of Medical Science.*

"The complete work will prove a valuable addition to our systematic treatises on human physiology."—*The Lancet.*

"To those who desire to get in one volume a concise and clear, and at the same time sufficiently full *résumé* of 'the existing state of physiological science,' we can heartily recommend Dr. Flint's work. Moreover, as a work of typographical art it deserves a prominent place upon our library-shelves. Messrs. Appleton & Co. deserve the thanks of the profession for the very handsome style in which they issue medical works. They give us hope of a time when it will be very generally believed by publishers that physicians' eyes are worth saving."—*Medical Gazette.*

D. Appleton & Co.'s Medical Publications.

Flint's Physiology. Volume II.—*Alimentation; Digestion; Absorption; Lymph and Chyle.*

8vo. 556 pp. Cloth, $4.50.

"The second instalment of this work fulfils all the expectations raised by the perusal of the first. . . . The author's explanations and deductions bear evidence of much careful reflection and study. . . . The entire work is one of rare interest. The author's style is as clear and concise as his method is studious, careful, and elaborate."—*Philadelphia Inquirer.*

"We regard the two treatises already issued as the very best on human physiology which the English or any other language affords, and we recommend them with thorough confidence to students, practitioners, and laymen, as models of literary and scientific ability."—*N. Y. Medical Journal.*

"We have found the style easy, lucid, and at the same time terse. The practical and positive results of physiological investigation are succinctly stated, without, it would seem, extended discussion of disputed points."—*Boston Medical and Surgical Journal.*

"It is a volume which will be welcome to the advanced student, and as a work of reference."—*The Lancet.*

"The leading subjects treated of are presented in distinct parts, each of which is designed to be an exhaustive essay on that to which it refers."—*Western Journal of Medicine.*

Volume III.—*Secretion; Excretion; Ductless Glands; Nutrition; Animal Heat; Movements; Voice and Speech.*

8vo. 526 pp. Cloth, $4.50.

"Dr. Flint's reputation is sufficient to give a character to the book among the profession, where it will chiefly circulate, and many of the facts given have been verified by the author in his laboratory and in public demonstrations."—*Chicago Courier.*

"The author bestows judicious care and labor. Facts are selected with discrimination, theories critically examined, and conclusions enunciated with commendable clearness and precision."—*American Journal of the Medical Sciences.*

"The work is calculated to attract other than professional readers, and is written with sufficient clearness and freedom from technical pedantry to be perfectly intelligible to any well-informed man."—*London Saturday Review.*

"From the extent of the author's investigations into the best theory and practice of the present day, the world over, and the candor and good judgment which he brings to bear upon the discussion of each subject, we are justified in regarding his treatises as standard and authoritative, so far as in this disputed subject authority is admissible.—*New York Times.*

Volume IV.—*The Nervous System.*

This volume is now ready. It is a work of great interest, and, in conjunction with the "Treatise on Diseases of the Nervous System," by Dr. Wm. A. Hammond, constitutes a complete work on "The Physiology and Pathology of the Nervous System."

Volume V.—*Generation.* (*In press.*)

FLINT.
Manual of Chemical Examination of
the Urine in Disease. With Brief Directions for the Examination of the most Common Varieties of Urinary Calculi.

By AUSTIN FLINT, JR., M. D.,

Professor of Physiology and Microscopy in the Bellevue Hospital Medical College; Fellow of the New York Academy of Medicine; Member of the Medical Society of the County of New York; Resident Member of the Lyceum of Natural History in the City of New York, etc.

Third Edition, revised and corrected. 1 vol., 12mo. 77 pp. Cloth, $1.00.

The chief aim of this little work is to enable the busy practitioner to make for himself, rapidly and easily, all ordinary examinations of Urine; to give him the benefit of the author's experience in eliminating little difficulties in the manipulations, and in reducing processes of analysis to the utmost simplicity that is consistent with accuracy.

"We do not know of any work in English so complete and handy as the Manual now offered to the profession by Dr. Flint, and the high scientific reputation of the author is a sufficient guarantee of the accuracy of all the directions given."—*Journal of Applied Chemistry.*

"We can unhesitatingly recommend this Manual."—*Psychological Journal.*

"Eminently practical."—*Detroit Review of Medicine.*

On the Physiological Effects of Severe
and Protracted Muscular Exercise. With Special Reference to its Influence upon the Excretion of Nitrogen.

By AUSTIN FLINT, JR., M. D.,

Professor of Physiology in the Bellevue Hospital Medical College, New York, etc., etc.

1 vol., 8vo. 91 pp. Cloth, $2.00.

This monograph on the relations of Urea to Exercise is the result of a thorough and careful investigation made in the case of Mr. Edward Payson Weston, the celebrated pedestrian. The chemical analyses were made under the direction of R. O. Doremus, M. D., Professor of Chemistry and Toxicology in the Bellevue Hospital Medical College, by Mr. Oscar Loew, his assistant. The observations were made with the coöperation of J. C. Dalton, M. D., Professor of Physiology in the College of Physicians and Surgeons; Alexander B. Mott, M. D., Professor of Surgical Anatomy; W. H. Van Buren, M. D., Professor of Principles of Surgery; Austin Flint, M. D., Professor of the Principles and Practice of Medicine; W. A. Hammond, M. D., Professor of Diseases of the Mind and Nervous System—all of the Bellevue Hospital Medical College.

"This work will be found interesting to every physician. A number of important results were obtained valuable to the physiologist."—*Cin. Med. Repertory.*

D. Appleton & Co.'s Medical Publications.

HAMMOND.

A Treatise on Diseases of the Nervous System.

By WILLIAM A. HAMMOND, M. D.,

Professor of Diseases of the Mind and Nervous System, and of Clinical Medicine, in the Bellevue Hospital Medical College; Physician-in-Chief to the New York State Hospital for Diseases of the Nervous System, etc., etc.

SECOND EDITION, REVISED AND CORRECTED.

With Forty-five Illustrations. 1 vol., 8vo. 750 pp. Cloth, $5.00.

The treatise embraces an introductory chapter, which relates to the instruments and apparatus employed in the diagnosis and treatment of diseases of the nervous system, and five sections. Of these, the first treats of diseases of the brain; the second, diseases of the spinal cord; the third, cerebro-spinal diseases; the fourth, diseases of nerve-cells; and the fifth, diseases of the peripheral nerves. One feature which may be claimed for the work is, that it rests, to a great extent, upon the personal observation and experience of the author, and is therefore no mere compilation.

"The author's clear and terse style of diction renders the book exceedingly readable, and the cases reported and cited add much to the interest of the text. ... There is so much that is entertaining in the mental and other manifestations of nervous disorder, especially when presented as they are here, that a work of this kind will find many readers outside the profession; and, it may be hoped, will serve not only to interest and amuse, but to induce a closer observance of those hygienic laws upon whose violation many of the ailments here treated of depend."—*New York Medical Journal.*

"The work is replete with useful knowledge, and every physician who expects to be called on, as an expert, to testify in cases of supposed insanity, after the commission of crimes, should give the book a thorough perusal."—*Leavenworth Medical Herald.*

"That a treatise by Prof. Hammond would be one of a high order was what we anticipated, and it affords us pleasure to state that our anticipations have been realized."—*Cincinnati Medical Repertory.*

"It affords a vast amount of information, is captivating, and worth reading"—*Cincinnati Lancet and Observer.*

"This is unquestionably the most complete treatise on the diseases to which it is devoted that has yet appeared in the English language; and its value is much increased by the fact that Dr. Hammond has mainly based it on his own experience and practice, which, we need hardly remind our readers, have been very extensive."—*London Medical Times and Gazette.*

"Free from useless verbiage and obscurity, it is evidently the work of a man who knows what he is writing about, and knows how to write about it."—*Chicago Medical Journal.*

D. Appleton & Co.'s Medical Publications.

HOLLAND.

Recollections of Past Life,

By SIR HENRY HOLLAND, Bart., M. D., F. R. S., K. C. B., etc.,

President of the Royal Institution of Great Britain, Physician-in-Ordinary to the Queen, etc., etc.

1 vol., 12mo, 351 pp. Price, Cloth, $2.00.

A very entertaining and instructive narrative, partaking somewhat of the nature of autobiography and yet distinct from it, in this, that its chief object, as alleged by the writer, is not so much to recount the events of his own life, as to perform the office of chronicler for others with whom he came in contact and was long associated.

The "Life of Sir Henry Holland" is one to be recollected, and he has not erred in giving an outline of it to the public."—*The Lancet.*

"His memory was—is, we may say, for he is still alive and in possession of all his faculties—stored with recollections of the most eminent men and women of this century. . . . A life extending over a period of eighty-four years, and passed in the most active manner, in the midst of the best society, which the world has to offer, must necessarily be full of singular interest; and Sir Henry Holland has fortunately not waited until his memory lost its freshness before recalling some of the incidents in it."—*The New York Times.*

HOWE.

Emergencies, and How to Treat Them.

The Etiology, Pathology, and Treatment of Accidents, Diseases, and Cases of Poisoning, which demand Prompt Attention. Designed for Students and Practitioners of Medicine.

By JOSEPH W. HOWE, M. D.,

Visiting Surgeon to Charity Hospital; Lecturer on Surgery in the Medical Department of the University of New York, etc.

1 vol., 8vo. 265 pp. Cloth, $3.00.

This volume is designed as a guide in the treatment of cases of emergency occurring in medical, surgical, or obstetrical practice. It combines all the important subjects, giving special prominence to points of practical interest in preference to theoretical considerations, and uniting, with the results of personal observation, the latest views of European and American authorities.

"The style is concise, perspicuous, and definite. Each article is written as though that particular emergency were present; there is no waste of words, nor temporizing with remedies of doubtful efficacy. The articles on œdema glottidis, asphyxia, and strangulated hernia, are particularly clear and practical, and furnish all the information required in the management of those urgent cases.

"It will be found invaluable to students and young practitioners, in supplying them with an epitome of useful knowledge obtainable from no other single work; while to the older members of the profession it will serve as a reliable and 'ready remembrancer.'"—*The Medical Record.*

D. Appleton & Co.'s Medical Publications.

HUXLEY AND YOUMANS.
The Elements of Physiology and Hygiene. With Numerous Illustrations.

By THOMAS H. HUXLEY, LL. D., F. R. S., and
WILLIAM JAY YOUMANS, M. D.

1 vol., 12mo. 420 pp. $1.75.

A text-book for educational institutions, and a valuable elementary work for students of medicine. The greater portion is from the pen of Professor Huxley, adapted by Dr. Youmans to the circumstances and requirements of American education.

"A valuable contribution to anatomical and physiological science."—*Religious Telescope.*

"A clear and well-arranged work, embracing the latest discoveries and accepted theories."—*Buffalo Commercial.*

"Teeming with information concerning the human physical economy."—*Evening Journal.*

HUXLEY.
The Anatomy of Vertebrated Animals,

By THOMAS HENRY HUXLEY, LL. D., F. R. S.,
Author of "Man's Place in Nature," "On the Origin of Species," "Lay Sermons and Addresses," etc.

1 vol., 12mo. Cloth, $2.00.

The former works of Prof. Huxley leave no room for doubt as to the importance and value of his new volume. It is one which will be very acceptable to all who are interested in the subject of which it treats.

SPECIMEN OF ILLUSTRATIONS.

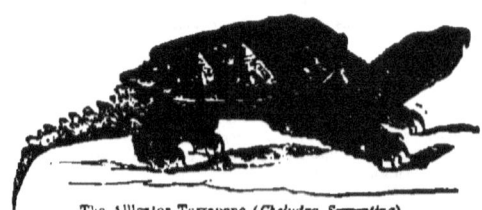

The Alligator Terrapene (*Chelydra Serpentina*).

"This long-expected work will be cordially welcomed by all students and teachers of Comparative Anatomy as a compendious, reliable, and, notwithstanding its small dimensions, most comprehensive guide on the subject of which it treats. To praise or to criticise the work of so accomplished a master of his favorite science would be equally out of place. It is enough to say that it realizes, in a remarkable degree, the anticipations which have been formed of it; and that it presents an extraordinary combination of wide, general views, with the clear, accurate, and succinct statement of a prodigious number of individual facts."—*Nature.*

D. Appleton & Co.'s Medical Publications.

JOHNSON.
The Chemistry of Common Life.
Illustrated with numerous Wood Engravings.

By JAMES F. JOHNSON, M. A., F. R. S., F. G. S., ETC., ETC.,

Author of "Lectures on Agricultural Chemistry and Geology," "A Catechism of Agricultural Chemistry and Geology," etc.

2 vols., 12mo. Cloth, $3.00.

It has been the object of the author in this work to exhibit the present condition of chemical knowledge, and of matured scientific opinion, upon the subjects to which it is devoted. The reader will not be surprised, therefore, should he find in it some things which differ from what is to be found in other popular works already in his hands or on the shelves of his library.

LETTERMAN.
Medical Recollections of the Army of the Potomac.

By JONATHAN LETTERMAN, M. D.,

Late Surgeon U. S. A., and Medical Director of the Army of the Potomac.

1 vol., 8vo. 194 pp. Cloth, $1.00.

"This account of the medical department of the Army of the Potomac has been prepared, amid pressing engagements, in the hope that the labors of the medical officers of that army may be known to an intelligent people, with whom to know is to appreciate; and as an affectionate tribute to many, long my zealous and efficient colleagues, who, in days of trial and danger, which have passed, let us hope never to return, evinced their devotion to their country and to the cause of humanity, without hope of promotion or expectation of reward."—*Preface.*

"We venture to assert that but few who open this volume of medical annals, pregnant as they are with instruction, will care to do otherwise than finish them at a sitting."—*Medical Record.*

"A graceful and affectionate tribute."—*N. Y. Medical Journal.*

LEWES.
The Physiology of Common Life.

By GEORGE HENRY LEWES,

Author of "Seaside Studies," "Life of Goethe," etc.

2 vols., 12mo. Cloth, $3.00.

The object of this work differs from that of all others on popular science in its attempt to meet the wants of the student, while meeting those of the general reader, who is supposed to be wholly unacquainted with anatomy and physiology.

D. Appleton & Co.'s Medical Publications.

MAUDSLEY.
The Physiology and Pathology of the Mind.

By HENRY MAUDSLEY, M. D., LONDON,

Physician to the West London Hospital; Honorary Member of the Medico-Psychological Society of Paris; formerly Resident Physician of the Manchester Royal Lunatic Hospital, etc.

1 vol., 8vo. 442 pp. Cloth, $3.50.

This work aims, in the first place, to treat of mental phenomena from a physiological rather than from a metaphysical point of view; and, secondly, to bring the manifold instructive instances presented by the unsound mind to bear upon the interpretation of the obscure problems of mental science.

"Dr. Maudsley has had the courage to undertake, and the skill to execute, what is, at least in English, an original enterprise."—*London Saturday Review.*

"It is so full of sensible reflections and sound truths that their wide dissemination could not but be of benefit to all thinking persons."—*Psychological Journal.*

"Unquestionably one of the ablest and most important works on the subject of which it treats that has ever appeared, and does credit to his philosophical acumen and accurate observation."—*Medical Record.*

"We lay down the book with admiration, and we commend it most earnestly to our readers as a work of extraordinary merit and originality—one of those productions that are evolved only occasionally in the lapse of years, and that serve to mark actual and very decided advances in knowledge and science."—*N. Y. Medical Journal.*

Body and Mind: *An Inquiry into their Connection and Mutual Influence, specially in reference to Mental Disorders; being the Gulstonian Lectures for 1870, delivered before the Royal College of Physicians. With Appendix.*

By HENRY MAUDSLEY, M. D., LONDON,

Fellow of the Royal College of Physicians; Professor of Medical Jurisprudence in University College, London; President-elect of the Medico-Psychological Association; Honorary Member of the Medico-Psychological Society of Paris, of the Imperial Society of Physicians of Vienna, and of the Society for the Promotion of Psychiatry and Forensic Psychology of Vienna; formerly Resident Physician of the Manchester Royal Lunatic Asylum, etc., etc.

1 vol., 12mo. 165 pp. Cloth, $1.00.

The general plan of this work may be described as being to bring man, both in his physical and mental relations, as much as possible within the scope of scientific inquiry.

"A representative work, which every one must study who desires to know what is doing in the way of real progress, and not mere chatter, about mental physiology and pathology."—*The Lancet.*

"It distinctly marks a step in the progress of scientific psychology."—*The Practitioner.*

D. Appleton & Co.'s Medical Publications.

MARKOE.
A Treatise on Diseases of the Bones.

By THOMAS M. MARKOE, M. D.,

Professor of Surgery in the College of Physicians and Surgeons, New York, etc.

WITH NUMEROUS ILLUSTRATIONS.

1 vol. 8vo. Cloth, $4.50.

SPECIMEN OF ILLUSTRATIONS.

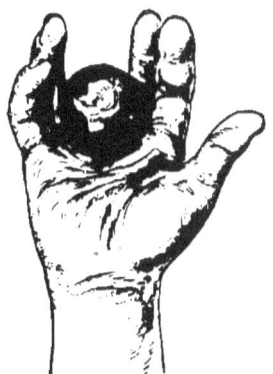

This valuable work is a treatise on Diseases of the Bones, embracing their structural changes as affected by disease, their clinical history and treatment, including also an account of the various tumors which grow in or upon them. None of the *injuries* of bone are included in its scope, and no *joint* diseases, excepting where the condition of the bone is a prime factor in the problem of disease. As the work of an eminent surgeon of large and varied experience, it may be regarded as the best on the subject, and a valuable contribution to medical literature.

"The book which I now offer to my professional brethren contains the substance of the lectures which I have delivered during the past twelve years at the college. . . . I have followed the leadings of my own studies and observations, dwelling more on those branches where I had seen and studied most, and perhaps too much neglecting others where my own experience was more barren, and therefore to me less interesting. I have endeavored, however, to make up the deficiencies of my own knowledge by the free use of the materials scattered so richly through our periodical literature, which scattered leaves it is the right and the duty of the systematic writer to collect and to embody in any account he may offer of the state of a science at any given period."—*Extract from Author's Preface.*

D. Appleton & Co.'s Medical Publications.

MEYER.
Electricity in its Relations to Practical Medicine.

By DR. MORITZ MEYER,
Royal Counsellor of Health, etc.

**Translated from the Third German Edition, with Notes and Additions.
A New and Revised Edition.**

By WILLIAM A. HAMMOND, M. D.,

Professor of Diseases of the Mind and Nervous System, and of Clinical Medicine, in the Bellevue Hospital Medical College; Vice-President of the Academy of Mental Sciences, National Institute of Letters, Arts, and Sciences; late Surgeon-General U. S. A., etc.

1 vol., 8vo. 497 pp. Cloth, $4.50.

"It is the duty of every physician to study the action of electricity, to become acquainted with its value in therapeutics, and to follow the improvements that are being made in the apparatus for its application in medicine, that he may be able to choose the one best adapted to the treatment of individual cases, and to test a remedy fairly and without prejudice, which already, especially in nervous diseases, has been used with the best results, and which promises to yield an abundant harvest in a still broader domain."—*From Author's Preface.*

SPECIMEN OF ILLUSTRATIONS.

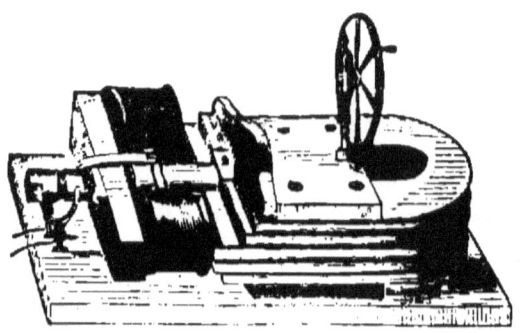

Saxton-Ettinghausen Apparatus.

"Those who do not read German are under great obligations to William A. Hammond, who has given them not only an excellent translation of a most excellent work, but has given us much valuable information and many suggestions from his own personal experience."—*Medical Record.*

"Dr. Moritz Meyer, of Berlin, has been for more than twenty years a laborious and conscientious student of the application of electricity to practical medicine, and the results of his labors are given in this volume. Dr. Hammond, in making a translation of the third German edition, has done a real service to the profession of this country and of Great Britain. Plainly and concisely written, and simply and clearly arranged, it contains just what the physician wants to know on the subject."—*N. Y. Medical Journal.*

"It is destined to fill a want long felt by physicians in this country."—*Journal of Obstetrics.*

D. Appleton & Co.'s Medical Publications.

NIEMEYER.
A Text-Book of Practical Medicine.
With Particular Reference to Physiology and Pathological Anatomy.

By the late Dr. FELIX VON NIEMEYER,

Professor of Pathology and Therapeutics; Director of the Medical Clinic of the University of Tübingen.

Translated from the Eighth German Edition, by special permission of the Author,

By GEORGE H. HUMPHREYS, M. D.,

Late one of the Physicians to the Bureau of Medical and Surgical Relief at Bellevue Hospital for the Out-door Poor; Fellow of the New York Academy of Medicine, etc.,

and

CHARLES E. HACKLEY, M. D.,

One of the Physicians to the New York Hospital; one of the Surgeons to the New York Eye and Ear Infirmary; Fellow of the New York Academy of Medicine, etc.

Revised Edition. 2 vols., 8vo. 1,528 pp. Cloth, $9.00; Sheep, $11.00.

The author undertakes, first, to give a picture of disease which shall be as lifelike and faithful to nature as possible, instead of being a mere theoretical scheme; secondly, so to utilize the more recent advances of pathological anatomy, physiology, and physiological chemistry, as to furnish a clearer insight into the various processes of disease.

The work has met with the most flattering reception and deserved success; has been adopted as a text-book in many of the medical colleges both in this country and in Europe; and has received the very highest encomiums from the medical and secular press.

"It is comprehensive and concise, and is characterized by clearness and originality."—*Dublin Quarterly Journal of Medicine.*

"Its author is learned in medical literature; he has arranged his materials with care and judgment, and has thought over them."—*The Lancet.*

"As a full, systematic, and thoroughly practical guide for the student and physician, it is not excelled by any similar treatise in any language."—*Appletons' Journal.*

"The author is an accomplished pathologist and practical physician; he is not only capable of appreciating the new discoveries, which during the last ten years have been unusually numerous and important in scientific and practical medicine, but, by his clinical experience, he can put these new views to a practical test, and give judgment regarding them."—*Edinburgh Medical Journal.*

"From its general excellence, we are disposed to think that it will soon take its place among the recognized text-books."—*American Quarterly Journal of Medical Sciences.*

"The first inquiry in this country regarding a German book generally is, 'Is it a work of practical value?' Without stopping to consider the justness of the American idea of the 'practical,' we can unhesitatingly answer, 'It is!'"—*New York Medical Journal.*

"The author has the power of sifting the tares from the wheat—a matter of the greatest importance in a text-book for students."—*British Medical Journal.*

"Whatever exalted opinion our countrymen may have of the author's talents of observation and his practical good sense, his text-book will not disappoint them, while those who are so unfortunate as to know him only by name, have in store a rich treat."—*New York Medical Record.*

D. Appleton & Co.'s Medical Publications.

NEUMANN.
Hand-Book of Skin Diseases.

By Dr. ISIDOR NEUMANN,
Lecturer on Skin Diseases in the Royal University of Vienna.

Translated from advanced sheets of the second edition, furnished by the Author; with Notes,

By LUCIUS D. BULKLEY, A. M., M. D.,
Surgeon to the New York Dispensary, Department of Venereal and Skin Diseases; Assistant to the Skin Clinic of the College of Physicians and Surgeons, New York; Member of the New York Dermatological Society, etc., etc.

1 vol., 8vo. About 450 pages and 66 Woodcuts. Cloth, $4.00.

SPECIMEN OF ILLUSTRATIONS.

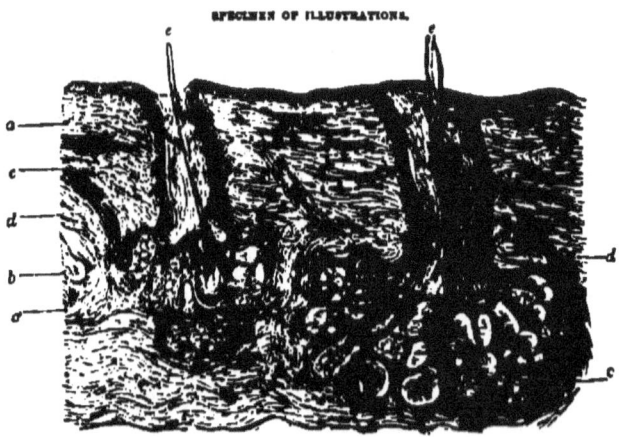

Section of skin from a bald head.

Prof. Neumann ranks second only to Hebra, whose assistant he was for many years, and his work may be considered as a fair exponent of the German practice of Dermatology. The book is abundantly illustrated with plates of the histology and pathology of the skin. The translator has endeavored, by means of notes from French, English, and American sources, to make the work valuable to the student as well as to the practitioner.

"It is a work which I shall heartily recommend to my class of students at the University of Pennsylvania, and one which I feel sure will do much toward enlightening the profession on this subject."—*Louis A. Duhring.*

"I know it to be a good book, and I am sure that it is well translated; and it is interesting to find it illustrated by references to the views of co-laborers in the same field."—*Erasmus Wilson.*

"So complete as to render it a most useful book of reference."—*T. McCall Anderson.*

"There certainly is no work extant which deals so thoroughly with the Pathological Anatomy of the Skin as does this hand-book."—*N. Y. Medical Record.*

"The original notes by Dr. Bulkley are very practical, and are an important adjunct to the text. . . . I anticipate for it a wide circulation."—*Silas Durkee, Boston.*

"I have already twice expressed my favorable opinion of the book in print, and am glad that it is given to the public at last."—*James C. White, Boston.*

"More than two years ago we noticed Dr. Neumann's admirable work in its original shape; and we are therefore absolved from the necessity of saying more than to repeat our strong recommendation of it to English readers."—*Practitioner.*

D. Appleton & Co.'s Medical Publications.

NEFTEL.

Galvano-Therapeutics. *The Physiological and Therapeutical Action of the Galvanic Current upon the Acoustic, Optic, Sympathetic, and Pneumogastric Nerves.*

By WILLIAM B. NEFTEL.

1 vol., 12mo. 161 pp. Cloth, $1.50.

This book has been published at the request of several aural surgeons and other professional gentlemen, and is a valuable treatise on the subjects of which it treats. Its author, formerly visiting physician to the largest hospital of St. Petersburg, has had the very best facilities for investigation.

"This little work shows, as far as it goes, full knowledge of what has been done on the subjects treated of, and the author's practical acquaintance with them."—*New York Medical Journal.*

"Those who use electricity should get this work, and those who do not should peruse it to learn that there is one more therapeutical agent that they could and should possess."—*The Medical Investigator.*

NIGHTINGALE.

Notes on Nursing: *What it is, and what it is not.*

By FLORENCE NIGHTINGALE.

1 vol., 12mo, 140 pp. Cloth, 75 cents.

Every day sanitary knowledge, or the knowledge of nursing, or, in other words, of how to put the constitution in such a state as that it will have no disease or that it can recover from disease, takes a higher place. It is recognized as the knowledge which every one ought to have—distinct from medical knowledge, which only a profession can have.

D. Appleton & Co.'s Medical Publications.

PEASLEE.

A Treatise on Ovarian Tumors. *Their Pathology, Diagnosis, and Treatment, with reference especially to Ovariotomy.*

By EDMUND R. PEASLEE, M. D., LL. D.,

Professor of Diseases of Women, in Dartmouth College ; one of the Consulting Surgeons to the N. Y. State Woman's Hospital; formerly Professor of Obstetrics and Diseases of Women, in the N. Y. Medical College; Corresponding Member of the Obstetrical Society of Berlin, etc.

In one large vol., 8vo., with Illustrations.

SPECIMEN OF ILLUSTRATIONS.

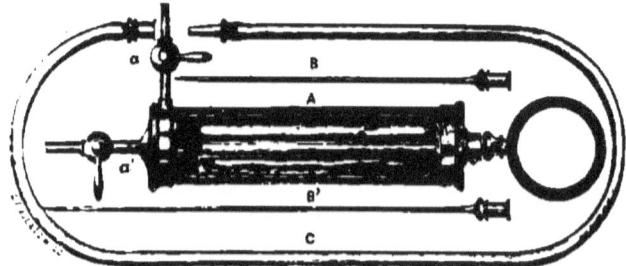

SYRINGE FOR EXPLORATION OF OVARIAN CYSTS.

A, instrument, 5¾ inches long ; *B*, gilded tube, 8 inches long, and 1/16 to 1/8 inch in diameter, with bevelled point ; *B'*, similar tube, 4¾ inches long ; *C*, rubber tube, to be attached to arm *a*, by which the fluid, drawn from the cyst through *a'*, is forced out. The stop-cocks at *a* and *a'* are both shown as closed.

This valuable work, embracing the results of many years of successful experience, in the department of which it treats, will prove most acceptable to the entire profession ; while the high standing of the author and his knowledge of the subject combine to make the book the best in the language. It is divided into two parts : the first, treating of Ovarian Tumors, their anatomy, pathology, diagnosis, and treatment, except by extirpation ; the second, of Ovariotomy, its history and statistics, and of the operation. Fully illustrated, and abounding with information the result of a prolonged study of the subject, the work should be in the hands of every physician in the country.

D. Appleton & Co.'s Medical Publications.

STROUD.
The Physical Cause of the Death of
Christ, and its Relations to the Principles and Practice of Christianity.

By WILLIAM STROUD, M. D.,

With a Letter on the Subject,

By Sir JAMES Y. SIMPSON, Bart., M. D.

1 vol., 12mo. 422 pp. Cloth, $2.00.

This important and remarkable book is, in its own place, a masterpiece, and will be considered as a standard work for many years to come.

"The principal point insisted upon is, that the death of Christ was caused by rupture or laceration of the heart. Sir James Y. Simpson, who had read the author's treatise and various comments on it, expressed himself very positively in favor of the views maintained by Dr. Stroud."—*Psychological Journal.*

SWETT.
A Treatise on the Diseases of the Chest.
Being a Course of Lectures delivered at the New York Hospital.

By JOHN A. SWETT, M. D.,

Professor of the Institutes and Practice of Medicine in the New York University; Physician to the New York Hospital; Member of the New York Pathological Society.

1 vol., 8vo. 587 pp. $3.50.

Embodied in this volume of lectures is the experience of ten years in hospital and private practice.

SAYRE.
A Practical Manual on the Treatment
of Club-Foot.

By LEWIS A. SAYRE, M. D.,

Professor of Orthopedic Surgery in Bellevue Hospital Medical College; Surgeon to Bellevue and Charity Hospitals, etc.

1 vol., 12mo. 91 pp. Cloth, $1.00.

"The object of this work is to convey, in as concise a manner as possible, all the practical information and instruction necessary to enable the general practitioner to apply that plan of treatment which has been so successful in my own hands."

"The book will very well satisfy the wants of the majority of general practitioners, for whose use, as stated, it is intended."—*New York Medical Journal.*

D. Appleton & Co.'s Medical Publications.

SIMPSON.

The Posthumous Works of Sir James Young Simpson, Bart., M. D. In Three Volumes.

Volume I.—*Selected Obstetrical and Gynæcological Works* of Sir James Y. Simpson, Bart., M. D., D. C. L., late Professor of Midwifery in the University of Edinburgh. Containing the substance of his Lectures on Midwifery. Edited by J. WATT BLACK, A. M., M. D., Member of the Royal College of Physicians, London; Physician-Accoucheur to Charing Cross Hospital, London; and Lecturer on Midwifery and Diseases of Women and Children in the Hospital School of Medicine.

1 vol., 8vo. 852 pp. Cloth, $3.00.

This volume contains all the more important of the contributions of Sir James Y. Simpson to the study of obstetrics and diseases of women, with the exception of his clinical lectures on the latter subject, which will shortly appear in a separate volume. This first volume contains many of the papers reprinted from his Obstetric Memoirs and Contributions, and also his Lecture Notes, now published for the first time, containing the substance of the practical part of his course of midwifery. It is a volume of great interest to the profession, and a fitting memorial of its renowned and talented author.

"To many of our readers, doubtless, the chief of the papers it contains are familiar. To others, although probably they may be aware that Sir James Simpson has written on the subjects, the papers themselves will be new and fresh. To the first class, we would recommend this edition of Sir James Simpson's works, as a valuable volume of reference; to the latter, as a collection of the works of a great master and improver of his art, the study of which cannot fail to make them better prepared to meet and overcome its difficulties."—*Medical Times and Gazette.*

Volume II.—*Anæsthesia, Hospitalism, etc.* Edited by Sir WALTER SIMPSON, Bart.

1 vol., 8vo. 560 pp. Cloth, $3.00.

"We say of this, as of the first volume, that it should find a place on the table of every practitioner; for, though it is patchwork, each piece may be picked out and studied with pleasure and profit."—*The Lancet (London).*

Volume III.—*The Diseases of Women.* Edited by ALEX. SIMPSON, M. D., Professor of Midwifery in the University of Edinburgh.

1 vol., 8vo., Cloth, $3.00.

One of the best works on the subject extant. Of inestimable value to every physician.

TILT.
A Hand-Book of Uterine Therapeutics and of Diseases of Women.

By EDWARD JOHN TILT, M. D.,

Member of the Royal College of Physicians; Consulting Physician to the Farringdon General Dispensary; Fellow of the Royal Medical and Chirurgical Society, and of several British and foreign societies.

1 vol., 8vo. 345 pp. Cloth, $3.50.

Second American edition, thoroughly revised and amended.

The main points developed in this work are:

1. The paramount importance of hygiene for the relief and cure of diseases of women.
2. The constitutional nature of many diseases of women, and the impossibility of curing them without constitutional remedies.
3. The manifest reaction of uterine diseases on the female system, and the impossibility of curing many uterine complaints, without surgical measures.
4. The great value of therapeutics to assuage and cure diseases of women, and the belief in the value of those remedial measures that are as old as medicine itself, such as venesection, emetics, and caustics.

"In giving the result of his labors to the profession the author has done a great work. Our readers will find its pages very interesting, and, at the end of their task, will feel grateful to the author for many very valuable suggestions as to the treatment of uterine diseases."—*The Lancet.*

"Dr. Tilt's 'Hand-book of Uterine Therapeutics' supplies a want which has often been felt. . . . It may, therefore, be read not only with pleasure and instruction, but will also be found very useful as a book of reference."—*The Medical Mirror.*

"Second to none on the therapeutics of uterine disease."—*Journal of Obstetrics.*

VAN BUREN.
Lectures upon Diseases of the Rectum.
Delivered at the Bellevue Hospital Medical College. Session of 1869-'70.

By W. H. VAN BUREN, M. D.,

Professor of the Principles of Surgery with Diseases of the Genito-Urinary Organs, etc., in the Bellevue Hospital Medical College; one of the Consulting Surgeons of the New York Hospital, of the Bellevue Hospital; Member of the New York Academy of Medicine, of the Pathological Society of New York, etc., etc.

1 vol., 12mo. 164 pp. Cloth $1.50.

Lecture I.—Pruritus Ani, Hæmorrhoids, etc. II.—Internal Hæmorrhoids. III.—Polypus. IV.—Fistula in Ano. V.—Fissure, or Irritable Ulcer. VI.—Stricture of the Rectum. VII.—Cancer. VIII.—Diagnosis, etc.

"It seems hardly necessary to more than mention the name of the author of this admirable little volume in order to insure the character of his book. No one in this country has enjoyed greater advantages, and had a more extensive field of observation in this specialty, than Dr. Van Buren, and no one has paid the same amount of attention to the subject. . . . Here is the experience of years summed up and given to the professional world in a plain and practical manner."—*Psychological Journal.*

D. Appleton & Co.'s Medical Publications.

VOGEL.

A Practical Treatise on the Diseases
of Children. Second American from the Fourth German Edition. Illustrated by Six Lithographic Plates.

By ALFRED VOGEL, M. D.,

Professor of Clinical Medicine in the University of Dorpat, Russia.

TRANSLATED AND EDITED BY

H. RAPHAEL, M. D.,

Late House Surgeon to Bellevue Hospital; Physician to the Eastern Dispensary for the Diseases of Children, etc., etc.

1 vol., 8vo. 611 pp. Cloth, $4.50.

The work is well up to the present state of pathological knowledge; complete without unnecessary prolixity; its symptomatology accurate, evidently the result of careful observation of a competent and experienced clinical practitioner. The diagnosis and differential relations of diseases to each other are accurately described, and the therapeutics judicious and discriminating. All polypharmacy is discarded, and only the remedies which appeared useful to the author commended.

This work of Vogel's contains much that must gain for it the merited praise of all impartial judges, and prove it to be an invaluable text-book for the student and practitioner, and a safe and useful guide in the difficult but all-important department of Pædiatrica.

"Rapidly passing to a fourth edition in Germany, and translated into three other languages, America now has the credit of presenting the first English version of a book which must take a prominent, if not the leading, position among works devoted to this class of disease."—*N. Y. Medical Journal.*

"The profession of this country are under many obligations to Dr. Raphael for bringing, as he has done, this truly valuable work to their notice."—*Medical Record.*

"The translator has been more than ordinarily successful, and his labors have resulted in what, in every sense, is a valuable contribution to medical science."—*Psychological Journal.*

"We do not know of a compact text-book on the diseases of children more complete, more comprehensive, more replete with practical remarks and scientific facts, more in keeping with the development of modern medicine, and more worthy of the attention of the profession, than that which has been the subject of our remarks."—*Journal of Obstetrics.*

NEW MEDICAL WORKS IN PRESS.

On Puerperal Diseases. *Clinical Lectures delivered at Bellevue Hospital.*

By FORDYCE BARKER, M. D.,

Clinical Professor of Midwifery and Diseases of Women in the Bellevue Hospital Medical College; Obstetric Physician to Bellevue Hospital; Consulting Physician to the N. Y. State Woman's Hospital, and to the N. Y. State Hospital for Diseases of the Nervous System; Honorary Member of the Edinburgh Obstetrical Society, etc., etc.

A course of lectures valuable alike to the student and the practitioner.

Hand-Book of the Histology and Histo-Chemistry of Man.

By Dr. HEINRICH FREY,
of Zurich.

Illustrated with 500 Woodcuts.

A Treatise on Obstetrics, *with an Introduction on the Pathology of Pregnancy and Childbirth.*

By Dr. KARL SCHROEDER,
of the University of Erlangen, Bavaria.

On Surgical Diseases of the Male Genito-Urinary Organs, including Syphilis.

By W. H. VAN BUREN, M. D., and EDW. L. KEYES, M. D.

A New Work on the Anatomy, Pathology, and Treatment of Diseases of the Ovaries.

By T. SPENCER WELLS, M. D.,

Surgeon-in-Ordinary to Her Majesty's Household; Surgeon to the Samaritan Hospital for Women; Member of the Royal Institutions, etc., etc.

Chemical Technology.

By RUDOLF WAGNER.

Translated by WM. CROOKES, F. R. S.

THE NEW YORK MEDICAL JOURNAL.

WM. T. LUSK, M.D.,
JAS. B. HUNTER, M.D., } *Editors.*

Published Monthly. Volumes begin in January and July.

"Among the numerous records of Medicine and the collateral sciences published in America, the above Journal occupies a high position, and deservedly so."—*The Lancet* (*London*).

Terms, $4.00 per Annum. Specimen Copies, 25 Cents.

THE JOURNAL OF PSYCHOLOGICAL MEDICINE:

A QUARTERLY REVIEW OF

DISEASES OF THE NERVOUS SYSTEM, MEDICAL JURIS-
PRUDENCE, AND ANTHROPOLOGY.

EDITED BY

WILLIAM A. HAMMOND, M.D.

"A Quarterly that does honor to the professions to which it is chiefly addressed."—*New York World.*

Terms, $5.00 per Annum. Specimen Copies, $1.00.

THE POPULAR SCIENCE MONTHLY,

Conducted by Prof. E. L. Youmans.

Published Monthly. Each Number contains 128 pages.

OPINIONS OF THE PRESS.

"Just the publication needed at the present day."—*Montreal Gazette.*
"It is, beyond comparison, the best attempt at journalism of the kind ever made in this country."—*Home Journal.*
"The initial number is admirably constituted."—*Evening Mail.*
"In our opinion, the right idea has been happily hit in the plan of this new monthly.'
—*Buffalo Courier.*
"A journal which promises to be of eminent value to the cause of popular education in this country."—*N. Y. Tribune.*

THE POPULAR SCIENCE MONTHLY *is published in a large octavo, handsomely printed on clear type. Terms, Five dollars per annum, or Fifty Cents per copy.*

New York Medical Journal and Psychological Journal................................$8 00
New York Medical Journal and Appletons' Weekly Journal of Literature, Science,
  and Art.. 7 00
Psychological Journal and Appletons' Weekly Journal.............................. 8 00
Psychological, Medical, and Weekly Journal.. 10 00
Psychological, Medical, Popular Science Monthly, and Weekly Journal............. 14 50

☞ *Payment, in all cases, must be in advance.*

Remittances should be made by postal money-order or check to the Publishers,

D. APPLETON & CO., 549 and 551 Broadway, N. Y.

www.ingramcontent.com/pod-product-compliance
Lightning Source LLC
Chambersburg PA
CBHW031943290426
44108CB00011B/659